Thoracic Imaging
Case Review Series

Thoracic Imaging
Case Review Series

THIRD EDITION

JUSTIN T. STOWELL, MD
Assistant Professor of Radiology
Consultant
Division of Cardiothoracic Imaging,
Department of Radiology,
Mayo Clinic
Jacksonville, Florida

JONATHAN H. CHUNG, MD
Professor of Radiology
Chief Quality Officer, Department of Radiology
Section Chief, Thoracic Radiology
The University of Chicago Medicine
Chicago, Illinois

JEFFREY P. KANNE, MD, FACR, FCCP
Professor of Radiology
Chief of Thoracic Imaging
University of Wisconsin School of Medicine and Public Health
Madison, Wisconsin

THERESA C. MCLOUD, MD
Professor of Radiology
Harvard Medical School
Senior Advisor for Faculty Affairs and Thoracic Radiologist
Massachusetts General Hospital
Boston, Massachusetts

GERALD F. ABBOTT, MD, FACR
Associate Professor
Harvard Medical School
Division of Thoracic Imaging and Intervention
Massachusetts General Hospital
Boston, Massachusetts

ELSEVIER

Elsevier
1600 John F. Kennedy Blvd.
Ste 1800
Philadelphia, PA 19103-2899

THORACIC IMAGING: CASE REVIEW SERIES, THIRD EDITION   ISBN: **978-0-323-42879-8**

Previous editions copyrighted 2011, 2001

Senior Content Development Manager: Somodatta Roy Choudhury
Senior Content Strategist: Melanie Tucker
Senior Content Development Specialist: Priyadarshini Pandey
Publishing Services Manager: Shereen Jameel
Project Manager: Vishnu T. Jiji
Senior Designer: Amy L. Buxton

Printed in India

Last digit is the print number: 9   8   7   6   5   4   3   2   1

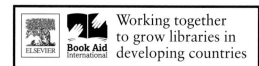

This book is dedicated to radiology residents and other trainees and practitioners in related fields with the hope that the provided cases and discussions will expose them to the rich variety of imaging findings in thoracic imaging and their relevant clinical features.

Justin T. Stowell, MD

Jonathan H. Chung, MD

Jeffrey P. Kanne, MD, FACR, FCCP

Theresa C. McLoud, MD

Gerald F. Abbott, MD, FACR

Foreword

What is more fundamental to radiology than thoracic imaging? Radiology imaging no doubt starts here for most residents, and yet the depth of investigation into cardiopulmonary pathology stretches into the final year of residency (or fellowship) training. The lungs and heart yield ever greater challenges to the reader, even as our imaging modalities get more and more sophisticated. So it is that *Thoracic Imaging: Case Review Series*, Third Edition, serves the needs of all resident levels, fellows, and practicing radiologists. This is a book for the ages. There are new COVID-like pearls and all kinds of new autoimmune and infectious agents that are explored in the latest edition.

Congratulations to Drs. Gerald F. Abbott, Jonathan H. Chung, Jeffrey P. Kanne, Theresa C. McLoud (goddess of thoracic radiology), and Justin T. Stowell for their latest contributions to the ever-vibrant Case Review Series. These books are perfect for the current generation of learners who want the short, pertinent hits that they can enjoy during breaks from clinical cases or video games or TikTok submissions. The series keeps your attention by stimulating you, like with ongoing longitudinal assessments, for a few images, quick questions, short blurb, and relevant reference. Boom. Move on to next case. Thank you to the authors for their hard work.

To our readers, I hope you enjoy *Thoracic Imaging: Case Review Series*, Third Edition, whether you are currently reading hard copy or Soft Copy … or both. Live, love, LEARN, and leave a legacy.

David M. Yousem, MD, MBA

Preface

The publication of the third edition of *Thoracic Imaging: The Requisites* in 2019 by our close friend and colleague, Jo-Anne O. Shepard, MD, was a major undertaking and involved the collaboration of numerous other experts in thoracic imaging. The many co-editors and contributors to that work all share close ties to the Massachusetts General Hospital (MGH) Department of Thoracic Imaging and Intervention (Boston, MA). We are pleased to present the long-awaited accompanying *Thoracic Imaging: Case Review Series*, Third Edition.

Similar to the third edition of *Thoracic Imaging: The Requisites*, this Case Review book has been extensively edited to include the latest updates in the expanding subspecialty of thoracic imaging. This edition has been completely rewritten and supplemented with hundreds of new images. Firstly, it maintains the two primary goals of the previous editions. These include a case format presentation to illustrate and review the imaging features of disorders that span the spectrum of thoracic diseases. Secondly, it is our goal to help the reader develop a sound framework with which to approach imaging interpretation in thoracic radiology.

The evolution of complex thoracic diseases and treatments, including lung cancer, interstitial lung disease, and heart and lung transplant, must be emphasized in both residency and fellowship curricula. Lung cancer screening continues to expand to more eligible patients with risk factors for lung cancer. The critical role of radiology has been emphasized, and the art and science of radiologic staging is illustrated in several cases. Pulmonary nodule management strategies and interstitial lung disease classifications have been updated by multidisciplinary societies and are included in this edition. This update is composed of a diverse group of more than 140 cases using multimodality imaging from radiography to magnetic resonance imaging. As is standard for the Case Review Series, the book is organized by the level of difficulty: Opening Round, Fair Game, and Challenge cases. Each case is accompanied by a series of multiple-choice questions with answers on the opposite page. Answers are followed by a brief discussion to highlight imaging features, differential diagnostic considerations, and key points from each case. Additional references are provided for those who desire more information about each topic, and cross-references to *Thoracic Imaging: The Requisites* are also provided.

We hope that this latest edition of *Thoracic Imaging* will continue to serve as a valuable tool for lifelong learning of thoracic imaging.

Justin T. Stowell, MD
Jonathan H. Chung, MD
Jeffrey P. Kanne, MD, FACR, FCCP
Theresa C. McLoud, MD
Gerald F. Abbott, MD, FACR

Contents

Supplemental figures can be accessed at
Elsevier eBooks+ (eBooks.Health.Elsevier.com)

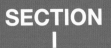
Case 1

History: Hemoptysis.

1. Which of the following should be included in the differential diagnosis? (Figs. 1.1, 1.2, 1.3 and 1.4) (Choose all that apply.)
   A. Lung carcinoma
   B. Infection
   C. Silicosis
   D. Pulmonary sequestration
2. What is the most common histologic type of lung carcinoma?
   A. Adenocarcinoma
   B. Squamous cell carcinoma
   C. Small cell carcinoma
   D. Carcinoid
3. What is the greatest risk factor for developing lung carcinoma?
   A. Coal
   B. Asbestos
   C. Smoking
   D. Obesity
4. Which factor best predicts 5-year survival for patients with lung carcinoma?
   A. Smoking history
   B. Histologic type
   C. Grade of neoplasm
   D. Stage at diagnosis

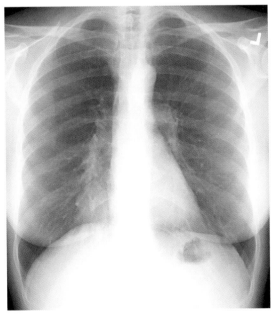

Fig. 1.1

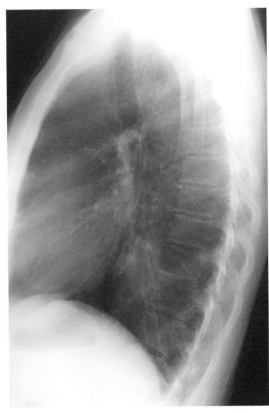

Fig. 1.2

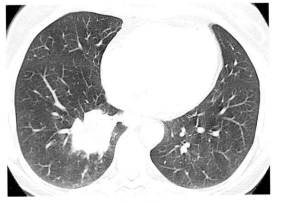

Fig. 1.3

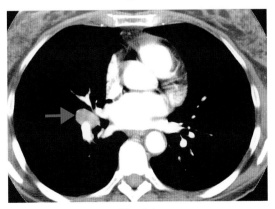

Fig. 1.4

Case 2

History: A 28-year old man has acute chest pain while playing basketball.

1. What is the most likely diagnosis (Figs. 2.1 and 2.2)?
   A. Traumatic pneumatocele
   B. Pneumomediastinum
   C. Spontaneous tension pneumothorax
   D. Swyer-James-McLeod syndrome
2. What is the likely mechanism involved in producing a traumatic pneumatocele?
   A. Penetrating trauma to the lung
   B. Compression-decompression trauma causing rupture of small airways
   C. Extension of pneumomediastinum into lung parenchyma
   D. Expansion of a preexisting bulla
3. What is the causative pathologic process in Swyer-James-McLeod syndrome?
   A. Blunt force trauma
   B. Postinfectious bronchiolitis
   C. Congenital bronchial atresia
   D. Incomplete interlobar fissures
4. Which radiographic finding occurs in tension pneumothorax? (Choose all that apply.)
   A. Contralateral shift of the mediastinum
   B. Downward displacement of the ipsilateral hemidiaphragm
   C. Ipsilateral widening of intercostal space (between ribs)
   D. All of the above

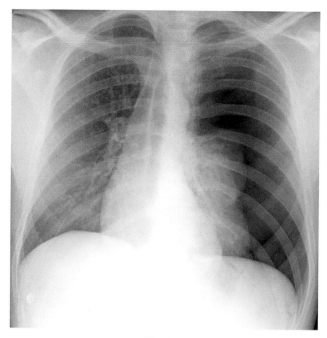

Fig. 2.2

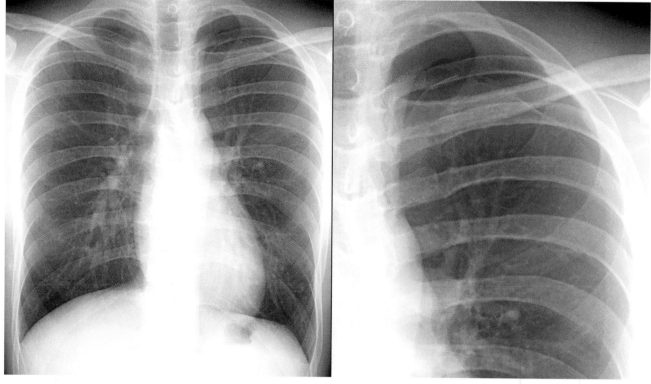

Fig. 2.1

Case 3

History: Asymptomatic 63-year-old man.

1. Based on the radiographic and computed tomography CT findings (Fig. 3.1), what is the most likely diagnosis?
   A. Fibrothorax
   B. Previous pleurodesis
   C. Asbestos-related pleural plaques
   D. Metastases
2. What percentage of patients diagnosed with the pleural malignancy caused by mesothelioma will have concomitant pleural plaques?
   A. 0%
   B. 5%
   C. 25%
   D. 100%

3. What is the characteristic latency period between a person's occupational exposure to asbestos and the development of mesothelioma?
   A. 1–2 years
   B. 5–10 years
   C. 10–15 years
   D. 30–40 years
4. Which of the following occupations has been associated with asbestos exposure in past decades? (Choose all that apply.)
   A. Construction worker
   B. Firefighter
   C. Shipyard worker
   D. Textile mill worker
   E. All of the above

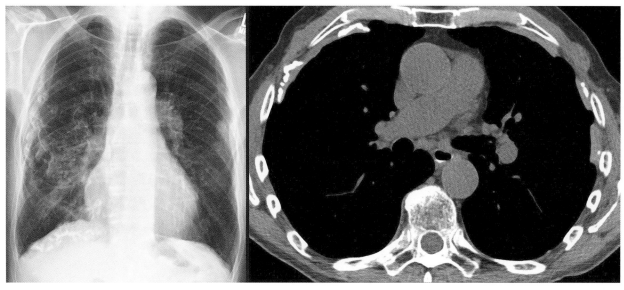

Fig. 3.1

Case 4

History: 60-year-old man with dyspnea.

1. Which of the following conditions is associated with hyperinflated lungs? (Choose all that apply.)
   A. Centrilobular emphysema
   B. Fibrotic hypersensitivity pneumonitis
   C. Lymphangioleiomyomatosis
   D. Asthma
2. What is the characteristic etiology of Swyer-James-McLeod syndrome?
   A. Follicular bronchiolitis
   B. Postinfectious bronchiolitis
   C. Broncholithiasis with air trapping
   D. Bronchial atresia
3. Which of the following is not always a smoking-related disease?
   A. Centrilobular emphysema
   B. Paraseptal emphysema
   C. Panlobular emphysema
   D. Desquamative interstitial pneumonia (DIP)
4. Which of the following are characteristic radiographic findings of advanced centrilobular emphysema in a patient who smokes (Fig. 4.1)? (Choose all that apply.)
   A. Hyperinflation
   B. Hyperlucency of upper lung zones
   C. Rapid tapering and attenuation of pulmonary vessels in affected lung
   D. Flattened hemidiaphragms

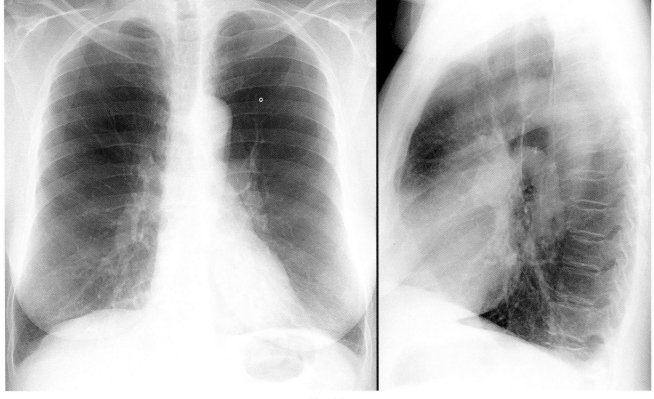

Fig. 4.1

Case 5

History: Asymptomatic 29-year-old woman.

1. Based on the clinical setting and imaging findings (Fig. 5.1), what is the most likely diagnosis?
   A. Castleman disease
   B. Lymphoma
   C. Sarcoidosis
   D. Silicosis
2. Which of the following malignancies may manifest with metastatic mediastinal and hilar lymphadenopathy? (Choose all that apply.)
   A. Head and neck malignancies
   B. Melanoma
   C. Breast cancer
   D. Genitourinary malignancies
   E. All of the above
3. Which of the following endemic fungal infections is most associated with lymphadenopathy?
   A. Blastomycosis
   B. Coccidioidomycosis
   C. Histoplasmosis
4. Which of the following may manifest with asymmetric bilateral hilar lymphadenopathy? (Choose all that apply.)
   A. Lymphoma
   B. Sarcoidosis
   C. Metastatic disease
   D. All of the above

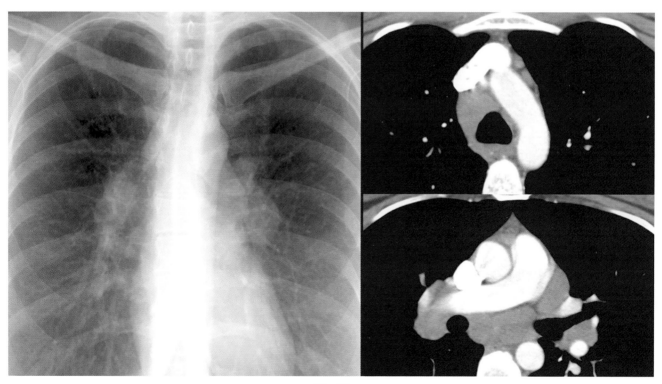

Fig. 5.1

Case 6

History: 66-year-old man with weight loss.

1. Which of the following imaging features are characteristic of pleural malignancy (Figs. 6.1A and 6.1B)? (Choose all that apply.)
   A. >1 cm in thickness
   B. Nodularity
   C. Circumferential growth pattern within the involved hemithorax
   D. Involvement of the mediastinal pleural
2. Which of the following is most common?
   A. Mesothelioma
   B. Pleural lymphoma
   C. Pleural metastasis
   D. Solitary fibrous tumor of the pleura
3. What percentage of patients with pleural mesothelioma also have pleural plaques as a manifestation of prior asbestos exposure?
   A. 10%
   B. 25%
   C. 50%
   D. 100%
4. Which of the following is the most common histologic sub-type of mesothelioma?
   A. Epithelioid
   B. Sarcomatoid
   C. Adenomatoid
   D. Mixed (biphasic)

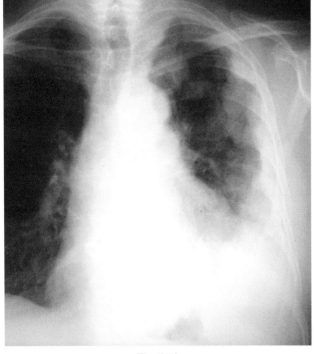

Fig. 6.1A

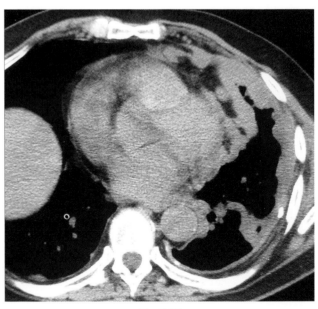

Fig. 6.1B

Case 7

History: 28-year-old man with cough.

1. Based on the structures indicated (arrow and arrowhead Fig. 7.1), what is the most likely diagnosis?
   A. Pneumomediastinum
   B. Pneumothorax
   C. Esophageal dilatation
   D. Normal study
2. Which of the following etiologies are associated with pneumomediastinum? (Choose all that apply.)
   A. Inhalational drug use
   B. Weightlifting
   C. Obstructive lung disease
   D. Pulmonary fibrosis
3. In Dr. Benjamin Felson's original system for evaluating mediastinal abnormalities on lateral chest radiography, which of the following courses of a boundary line separates the anterior mediastinum from the middle mediastinum?
   A. Anterior to the trachea and anterior to the heart
   B. Anterior to the trachea and posterior to the heart
   C. Posterior to the trachea and anterior to the heart
   D. Posterior to the trachea and posterior to the heart
4. Which of the following radiographic findings typically occur in total atelectasis of the right or left lung?
   A. Contralateral displacement of the anterior junction line
   B. Ipsilateral displacement of the anterior junction line
   C. Downward displacement of the ipsilateral hemidiaphragm
   D. Downward displacement of the contralateral hemidiaphragm

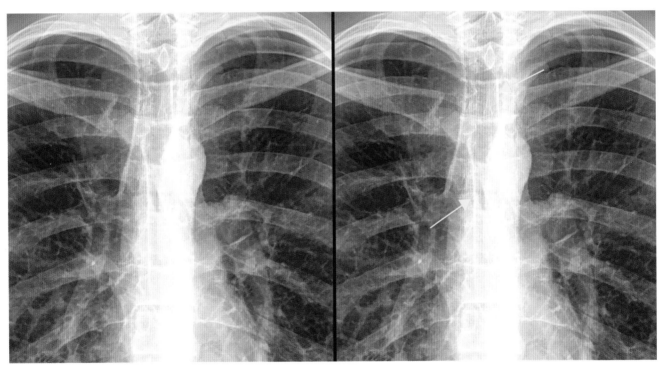

Fig. 7.1

Case 8

History: 70-year-old man with 30-pack year history of cigarette smoking. Finding detected on initial lung cancer screening computed tomography (CT) study (Fig. 8.1).

1. What is the most likely diagnosis?
   A. Lepidic adenocarcinoma
   B. Carcinoid tumor
   C. Hamartoma
   D. Lipoid pneumonia
2. Which of the following may show fluorodeoxyglucose (FDG)-avidity on positron emission tomography (PET) imaging? (Choose all that apply.)
   A. Lepidic adenocarcinoma
   B. Carcinoid tumor
   C. Lipoid pneumonia

   D. Hamartoma
   E. All of the above
3. What is the range of fat attenuation on the Hounsfield scale of CT numbers?
   A. -300 to -200
   B. -200 to -100
   C. -100 to -50
   D. -40 to 0
4. What is the percentage of hamartomas detected by thin-section CT exhibit fat attenuation?
   A. 9%
   B. 29%
   C. 59%
   D. 79%

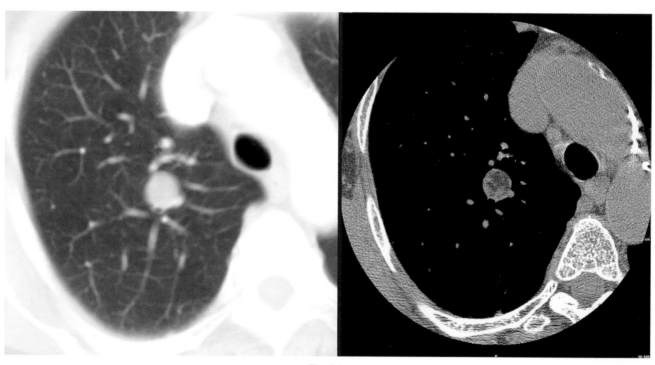

Fig. 8.1

Case 9

History: 22-year-old man with chronic cough.

1. Based on the radiographic findings (Fig. 9.1), what is the most likely diagnosis?
   A. Lymphangioleiomyomatosis
   B. Cystic fibrosis
   C. Centrilobular emphysema
   D. Pulmonary Langerhans cell histiocytosis
2. Which of the following computed tomography (CT) techniques is most helpful in the detection of bronchiectasis?
   A. Maximum-intensity projection images (MIPs)
   B. Minimum-intensity projection images (MinIPs)
   C. Multiplanar reformations
   D. Expiratory images
3. Which of the following conditions are associated with bronchial artery dilatation? (Choose all that apply.)
   A. Bronchiectasis
   B. Cavitary infection
   C. Cavitary sarcoidosis
   D. Lung cancer
   E. All of the above
4. Which of the following abnormalities are associated with cystic fibrosis? (Choose all that apply.)
   A. Mediastinal/hilar lymphadenopathy
   B. Pansinusitis
   C. Biliary cirrhosis
   D. Infertility
   E. All of the above

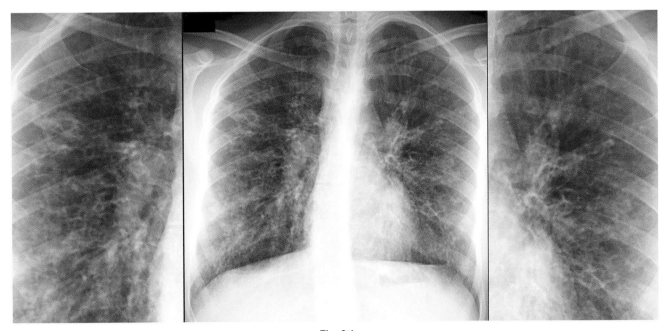

Fig. 9.1

Case 10

History: 66-year-old man with substernal chest pain.

1. Dr. Benjamin Felson introduced the concept of mediastinal compartments by using normal anatomic landmarks on the lateral chest radiograph. What is the course of the line Felson used to separate the anterior mediastinum from the middle mediastinum?
   A. Anterior to the trachea and anterior to the heart
   B. Anterior to the trachea and posterior to the heart
   C. Posterior to the trachea and anterior to the heart
   D. Posterior to the trachea and posterior to the heart

2. Which of the following diagnoses is most consistent with the radiographic finding of diffuse mediastinal widening (Fig. 10.1)?
   A. Thymoma
   B. Bronchogenic cyst
   C. Metastatic lymphadenopathy
   D. Esophageal varices

3. What percentage of mediastinal abnormalities are vascular lesions?
   A. 10%
   B. 20%
   C. 30%
   D. 40%

4. Which of the following are most characteristic of patient age encountered in cases of thymoma and teratoma?
   A. Over and under the age of 20 years, respectively
   B. Under and over the age of 40 years, respectively
   C. Over and under the age of 40 years, respectively
   D. Under and over the age of 20 years, respectively

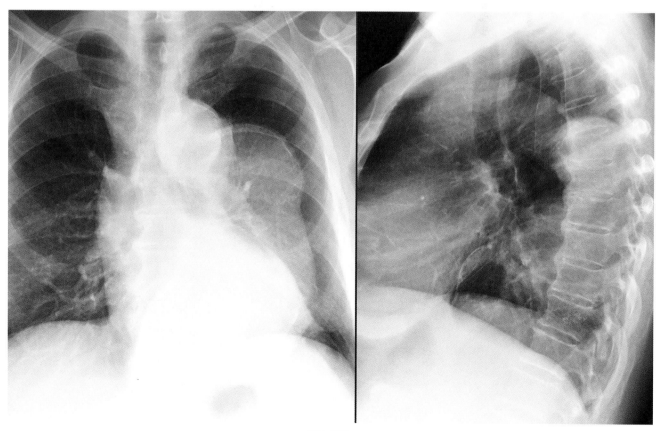

Fig. 10.1

Case 11

History: 46-year-old man was struck by a motorcycle.

1. What is the most likely cause of the ground-glass opacity and consolidation in the left lung (Figs. 11.1A and 11.1B)?
   A. Aspiration
   B. Atelectasis
   C. Pulmonary contusion
   D. Lung cancer
2. What is the most likely cause of the focal lucency within the parenchymal consolidation?
   A. Bronchiectasis
   B. Bullous emphysema
   C. Post-traumatic pneumatocele
   D. Cystic neoplasm
3. Pulmonary contusion should begin to resolve within how much time from injury?
   A. 4 hours
   B. 12 hours
   C. 24 hours
   D. 48 hours
4. Which of the following may manifest as cysts on computed tomography (CT)?
   A. Desquamative interstitial pneumonia (DIP)
   B. Lymphocytic interstitial pneumonia (LIP)
   C. Pulmonary Langerhans cell histiocytosis (PLCH)
   D. All of the above

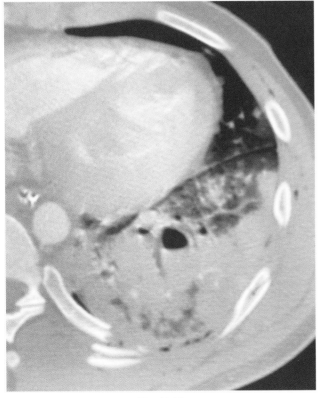

Fig. 11.1A

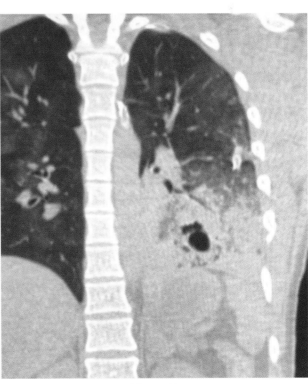

Fig. 11.1B

Case 12

History: Recent central line placement.

1. Where does the central line terminate (Figs. 12.1 and 12.2)?
   A. Superior vena cava (SVC)
   B. Azygos vein
   C. Great cardiac vein
   D. Brachiocephalic vein
2. What is the ideal location for the termination of a central venous line in most cases?
   A. Subclavian vein
   B. Azygos vein
   C. Brachiocephalic vein
   D. Cavoatrial junction
3. What is the most likely complication of a central venous line placed in the right atrium?
   A. Cardiac arrhythmia
   B. Cardiac thrombus
   C. Cardiac rupture
   D. Cardiac tamponade
4. A subclavian central catheter is placed for administration of chemotherapy for lung cancer. Pulsatile, bright, red blood is noted from the catheter immediately after placement. Of the listed choices, what is the next best step in management?
   A. Use the catheter for drug administration
   B. Remove the line immediately
   C. Contact vascular surgery
   D. Vigorously flush the catheter

See Supplemental Figures section for additional figures for this case. **[E-book/Inkling: Link to supplemental figures, Case 12]**

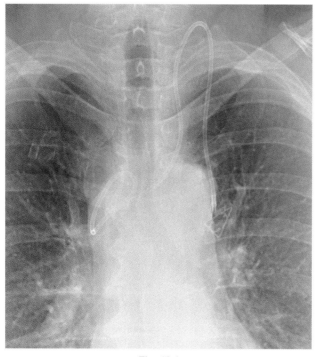

Fig. 12.1

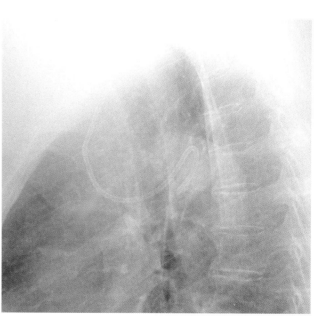

Fig. 12.2

Case 13

History: History withheld.

1. Which of the following could cause this imaging finding (Figs. 13.1, 13.2 and 13.3)?
   A. Achalasia
   B. Spinal fracture
   C. Metastatic disease
   D. Aortic aneurysm

2. What classic sign of posterior mediastinal lesions is present in this case?
   A. Cervicothoracic sign
   B. Thoracoabdominal sign
   C. Cervicoabdominal sign
   D. Cervicothoracoabdominal sign

3. What is the most sensitive modality to detect acute spinal fractures?
   A. Radiography
   B. Fluoroscopy
   C. Computed tomography (CT)
   D. Magnetic resonance imaging (MRI)

4. An increase in tube potential does what to radiation dose?
   A. Increase on radiography and CT
   B. Decrease on radiography and CT
   C. Increase on radiography but decrease on CT
   D. Decrease on radiography but increase on CT

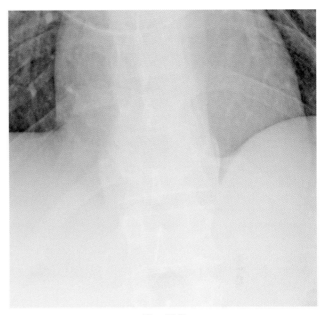

Fig. 13.2

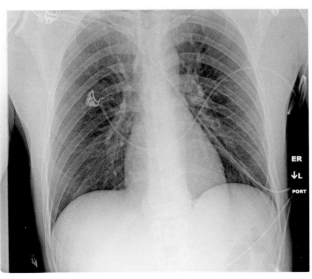

Fig. 13.1

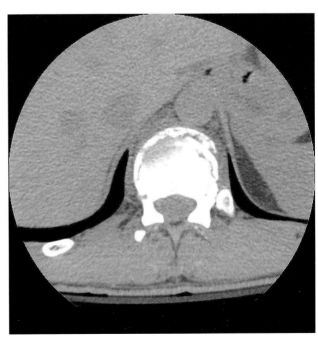

Fig. 13.3

13

Case 14

History: 53-year-old man with cough and shortness of breath.

1. Which of the following should be included in the differential diagnosis for this patient (Figs. 14.1 and 14.2)? (Choose all that apply.)
   A. Emphysema
   B. Pulmonary edema
   C. Tuberculosis
   D. Metastases
2. The computed tomography (CT) chest pattern is best described as:
   A. Tree-in-bud
   B. Random
   C. Perilymphatic
   D. Centrilobular
3. A tree-in-bud pattern on CT is most suggestive of which of the below conditions?
   A. Aspiration
   B. Edema
   C. Metastases
   D. Hemorrhage
4. What does a random pattern of diffuse nodular lung disease imply?
   A. Lymphatic spread
   B. Hematogenous spread
   C. Aerogenous spread
   D. Mixed spread

See Figure S14.1. See Supplemental Figures section for additional figures for this case. [**E-book/Inkling – Link to supplemental figures Case 14**]

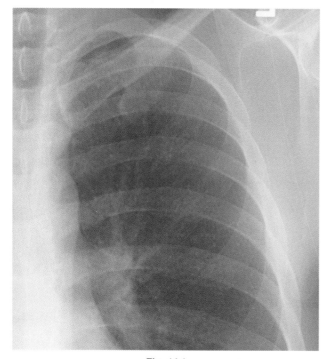

Fig. 14.1

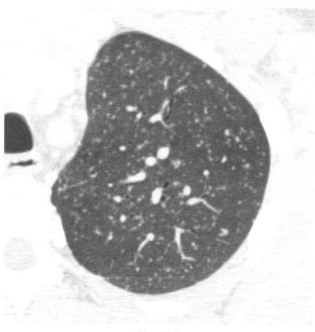

Fig. 14.2

Case 15

History: History withheld.

1. Which of the following should be included in the differential diagnosis for this patient (Figs. 15.1A and 15.1B)? (Choose all that apply.)
   A. Pulmonary metastases
   B. Neurofibromatosis
   C. Pleural metastases
   D. Pulmonary histoplasmosis

2. What imaging sign is exemplified in this case example?
   A. Incomplete border
   B. Hilar overlay
   C. Cervicothoracic
   D. Monod

3. Which of the following is least common in neurofibromatosis 1?
   A. Café-au-lait spots
   B. Scoliosis
   C. Acoustic neuromas
   D. Optic gliomas

4. Two symmetrically located nodules are noted overlying the lower thorax; both are well-defined laterally but poorly defined medially. What is the next step in management?
   A. In-and-out of phase magnetic resonance imaging (MRI)
   B. Chest computed tomography (CT) with contrast
   C. Chest radiograph with BB markers
   D. Positron emission tomography (PET)/CT

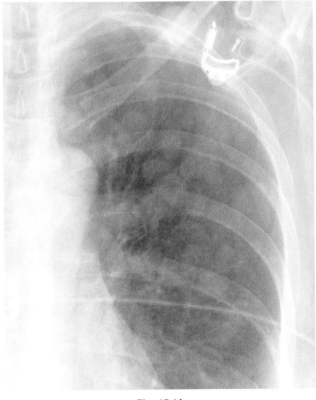

Fig. 15.1A

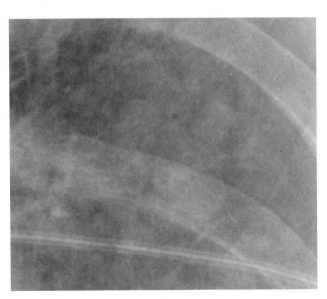

Fig. 15.1B

Case 16

History: Outpatient radiograph in a 55-year-old man with subacute cough.

1. Based on the radiograph (Fig. 16.1), which of the following should be included in the differential diagnosis?
   A. Pneumonia
   B. Atelectasis
   C. Pleural effusion
   D. Chest wall mass
2. What is the most likely cause of this condition in this man (Fig. 16.2)?
   A. Aspiration
   B. Hypoventilation
   C. Lung cancer
   D. Carcinoid tumor

3. What would be the most likely cause of this condition in a child?
   A. Aspiration
   B. Hypoventilation
   C. Lung Cancer
   D. Carcinoid tumor
4. Which of the following signs is associated with this condition?
   A. Cervicothoracic sign
   B. S sign of Golden
   C. Luftsichel sign
   D. Flat waist sign

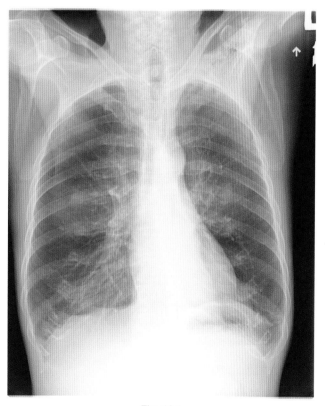

Fig. 16.1

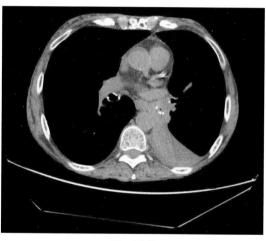

Fig. 16.2

Case 17

History: Chronic dyspnea.

1. What is the diagnosis (Fig. 17.1)?
   A. Pulmonary hypertension
   B. Aortic dissection
   C. Pulmonary stenosis
   D. Sarcoidosis
2. Which of the following is *not* a cause for this condition?
   A. Left-to-right shunt
   B. Mitral stenosis
   C. Calcium channel blockers
   D. Sleep apnea
3. What is the upper limit of normal for main pulmonary artery size on computed tomography (CT)?
   A. 2 cm
   B. 2.5 cm
   C. 3 cm
   D. 3.5 cm
4. Which of the following is a secondary cause of pulmonary hypertension?
   A. Portopulmonary hypertension
   B. Renopulmonary hypertension
   C. Adrenopulmonary hypertension
   D. Splenopulmonary hypertension

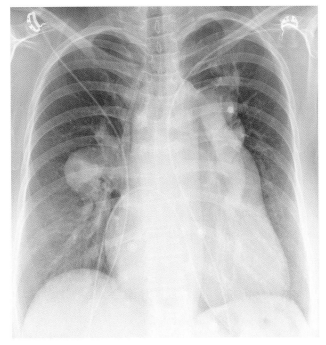

Fig. 17.1

Case 18

History: Middle-aged man with fever and cough.

1. What is the differential diagnosis for cavitary nodule(s) (Fig. 18.1)?
   A. Vasculitis
   B. Necrobiotic nodules
   C. Metastatic disease
   D. Abscess
2. Which primary tumor is *least* likely to cause cavitary lung metastases?
   A. Sarcoma
   B. Transitional cell carcinoma
   C. Melanoma
   D. Squamous cell carcinoma

3. What is the most common predisposing cause or factor in formation of a lung abscess (Fig. 18.2)?
   A. Trauma
   B. Pulmonary embolism
   C. Aspiration
   D. Air-trapping
4. In which lung segment is a lung abscess *least* likely to develop?
   A. Anterior segment, right upper lobe
   B. Superior segment, right lower lobe
   C. Posterior segment, right upper lobe
   D. Lateral basilar segment, right lower lobe

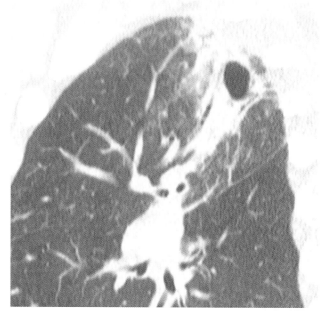

Fig. 18.1

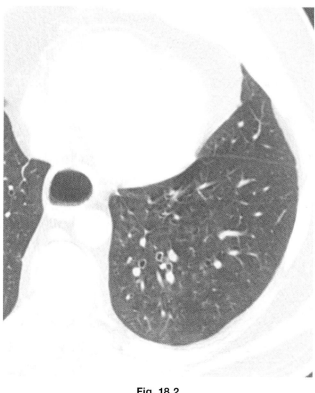

Fig. 18.2

Case 19

History: Patient with long history of asthma with new-onset chest pain.

1. Which of the following could be a cause this imaging finding (Figs. 19.1 and 19.2)?
   A. Asthma
   B. Esophageal rupture
   C. Ruptured bleb
   D. Tracheal rupture
2. Which of the following ectopic gas collections will *not* shift with patient position?
   A. Pneumomediastinum
   B. Pneumoperitoneum
   C. Pneumothorax
   D. Pneumopericardium
3. Which anatomic landmark represents the upper limit of visualized gas in a pneumopericardium?
   A. Tracheal carina
   B. Left atrial appendage
   C. Aortic arch
   D. Coronary sinus
4. Which of the following signs can be seen in either pneumomediastinum or pneumopericardium?
   A. Naclerio V sign
   B. Continuous diaphragm sign
   C. Deep sulcus sign
   D. Ring around the artery sign

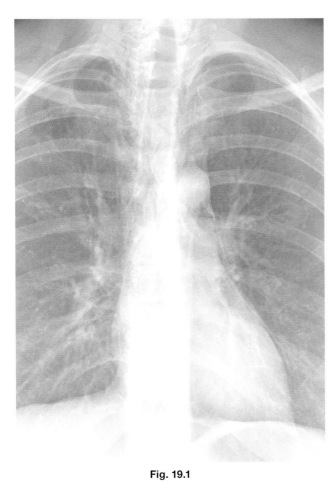

Fig. 19.1

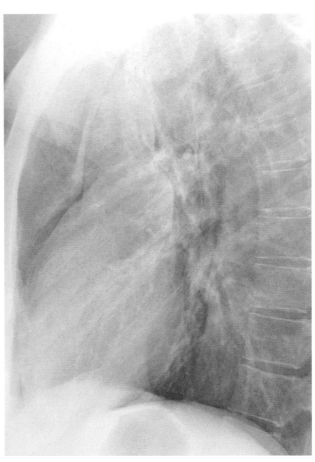

Fig. 19.2

Case 20

History: Acute onset shortness of breath.

1. Which of the following is the most likely cause this imaging finding (Fig. 20.1)?
   A. Liver mass
   B. Pleural effusion
   C. Diaphragmatic paralysis
   D. Diaphragmatic eventration
2. What is the most sensitive radiographic technique to detect pleural effusion?
   A. Oblique
   B. Posteroanterior (PA)
   C. Anteroposterior (AP)
   D. Lateral decubitus
3. What is the most common cause of transudative pleural effusion?
   A. Congestive heart failure
   B. Nephrotic syndrome
   C. Hepatic hydrothorax
   D. Hypoalbuminemia
4. What is the most common cause of exudative pleural effusion?
   A. Pneumonia
   B. Lung cancer
   C. Pulmonary infarct
   D. Collagen vascular disease

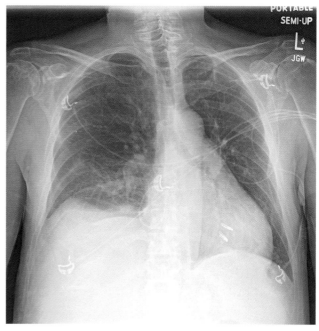

Fig. 20.1

Case 21

History: Decreased left-sided breath sounds on auscultation.

1. Which of the following could cause this imaging finding (Figs. 21.1 and 21.2)?
   A. Pneumothorax
   B. Pleural effusion
   C. Pneumoperitoneum
   D. Basilar emphysema
2. What is the most sensitive radiographic technique to detect pneumothorax?
   A. Oblique
   B. Posteroanterior (PA)
   C. Expiration PA
   D. Lateral decubitus

3. In a young patient, what is the most common cause of pneumothorax?
   A. Primary spontaneous
   B. Secondary spontaneous
   C. Traumatic
   D. Iatrogenic
4. Which sign is diagnostic of a pneumothorax on supine radiographs?
   A. Ring around the artery sign
   B. Deep sulcus sign
   C. Westermark sign
   D. Air crescent sign

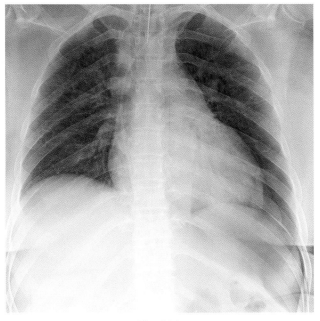

Fig. 21.1

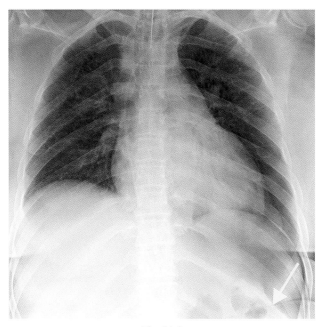

Fig. 21.2

Case 22

History: History of pulmonary hypertension.

1. What is the location of the abnormality on the right (Figs. 22.1, 22.2 and 22.3)?
   A. Right upper lobe
   B. Right middle lobe
   C. Right lower lobe
   D. None of the above
2. Which of the following is the most likely diagnosis?
   A. Lung cancer
   B. Pulmonary hamartoma
   C. Pseudotumor
   D. Metastatic disease
3. What is the most common malignancy to involve the pleura?
   A. Mesothelioma
   B. Solitary fibrous tumor
   C. Metastatic disease
   D. Sarcoma
4. What is the most common type of accessory pulmonary fissure?
   A. Azygos fissure
   B. Superior accessory fissure
   C. Inferior accessory fissure
   D. Left minor fissure

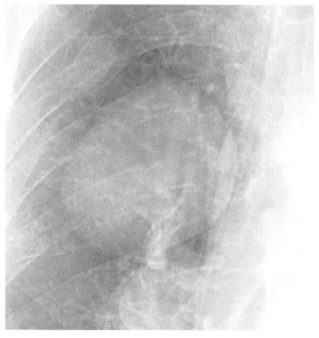

Fig. 22.2

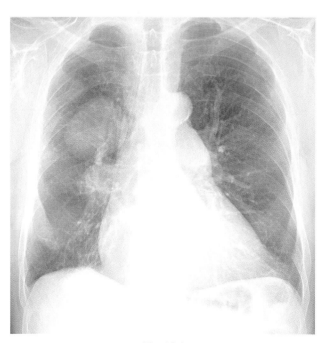

Fig. 22.1

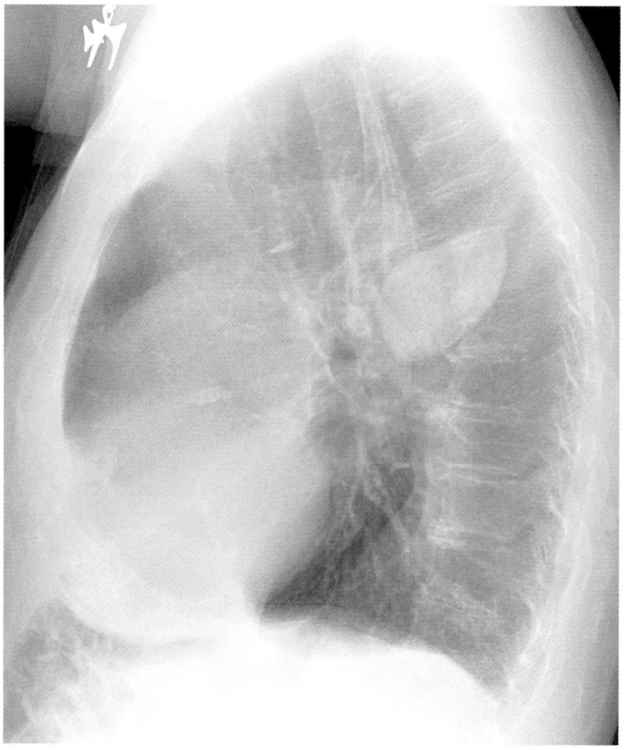

Fig. 22.3

Case 23

History: History of dysphagia and gastroesophageal reflux.

1. What diagnoses should be included in the differential diagnosis based on the scout image (Figs. 23.1 and 23.2)?
   A. Esophageal cancer
   B. Lung cancer
   C. Bronchogenic cyst
   D. Thymoma
2. Which of the following is true regarding fluorodeoxyglucose (FDG)-positron emission tomography (PET) FDG-PET imaging in the setting of esophageal cancer?
   A. High accuracy for T staging
   B. High accuracy for N staging
   C. High accuracy for M staging
   D. Not useful for TNM staging
3. What is the most common process causing abnormal convexity along the inferior aspect of the azygoesophageal recess?
   A. Hiatal hernia
   B. Left atrial dilation
   C. Esophageal cancer
   D. Lymphadenopathy
4. Regarding the differences between squamous cell carcinoma (SCC) and adenocarcinoma (AC) of the esophagus, which of the following is true?
   A. SCC is more common in the lower third of the esophagus than AC.
   B. AC is more common than SCC world-wide.
   C. The most common risk factor for AC is gastroesophageal reflux.
   D. SCC has a better prognosis than AC.

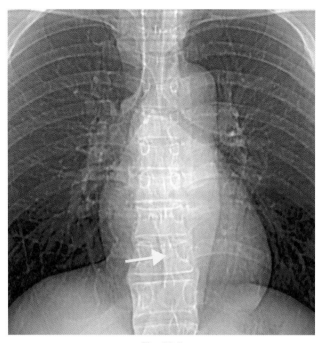

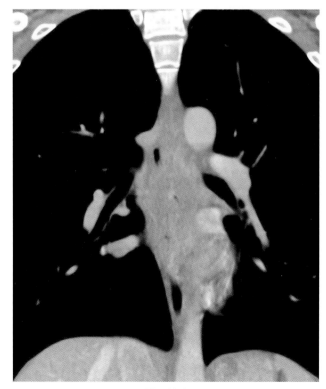

Fig. 23.2

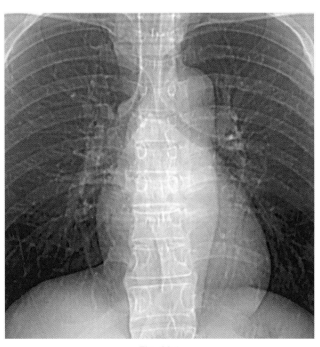

Fig. 23.1

Fig. 23.3

Case 24

History: Preoperative evaluation.

1. Which of the following should be included in the differential diagnosis for this patient (Fig. 24.1)? (Choose all that apply.)
    A. Hamartoma
    B. Adenocarcinoma
    C. Calcified granuloma
    D. Calcified pleural plaque
2. Which of the following is *not* a benign pattern of calcification in smoothly marginated lung nodules?
    A. Diffuse
    B. Central
    C. Stippled
    D. Laminar
3. Which of the following features on computed tomography (CT) is the *most* suggestive that a solitary lung nodule is benign?
    A. Eccentric calcification
    B. Smooth margins
    C. Mixed solid and ground-glass attenuation
    D. Fat attenuation
4. Which of the following characteristics is associated with the *highest* likelihood ratio that a solitary lung nodule is malignant?
    A. Size >3 cm
    B. Spiculated margins
    C. Doubling time less than 30 days
    D. Upper lobe location

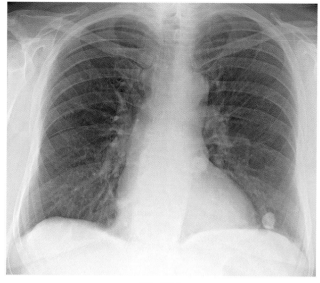

Fig. 24.1

Case 25

History: Lung cancer.

1. Which of the following should be included in the differential diagnosis for this patient (Figs. 25.1 and 25.2)? (Choose all that apply.)
   A. Sarcoidosis
   B. Idiopathic pulmonary fibrosis
   C. Radiation pneumonitis
   D. Infectious pneumonia
2. At what time point following completion of radiation therapy is radiation pneumonitis usually detectable by chest radiography?
   A. >1 week
   B. 2–4 weeks
   C. 6–8 weeks
   D. >8 weeks

3. Which of the following factors plays the *least* direct role in contributing to risk for developing radiation pneumonitis?
   A. Tumor histology
   B. Concomitant chemotherapy
   C. Radiation dose
   D. Size of tumor
4. Which of the following statements regarding radiation-induced lung disease is *true*?
   A. Radiation pneumonitis is a prerequisite for developing radiation fibrosis.
   B. A normal chest radiograph excludes the diagnosis of radiation pneumonitis.
   C. Radiation fibrosis is a progressive condition that often results in respiratory failure.
   D. Radiation fibrosis usually develops 6 to 12 months after the completion of therapy.

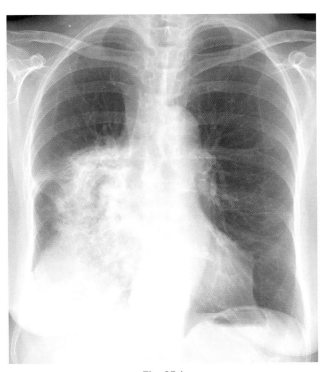

Fig. 25.1

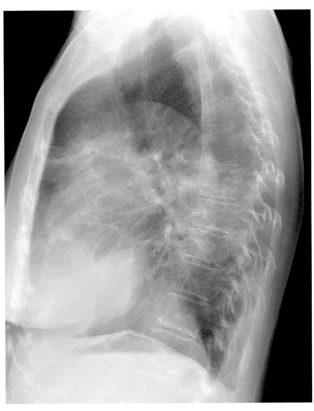

Fig. 25.2

Case 26

History: Hypoxia and failure to wean from ventilator.

1. Which of the following should be included in the differential diagnosis for this patient (Fig. 26.1)? (Choose all that apply.)
   A. Acute respiratory distress syndrome (ARDS)
   B. Aspiration
   C. Sarcoidosis
   D. Bacterial pneumonia

2. Aside from diffuse lung opacities, what other abnormality is present on this patient's chest radiograph? (Choose all that apply.)
   A. Pneumomediastinum
   B. Pneumopericardium
   C. Pneumoperitoneum
   D. Pneumothorax

3. What is the most likely cause of pneumothorax in this patient?
   A. Central venous catheter placement
   B. Barotrauma
   C. Bronchial rupture
   D. Pulmonary laceration

4. Which of the following is *not* a criterion for the diagnosis of ARDS?
   A. $Pao_2/Fio_2 \leq 300$ mmHg
   B. Bilateral lung opacity on chest radiography
   C. Hypoxemic respiratory failure within one week of insult
   D. Pleural effusion

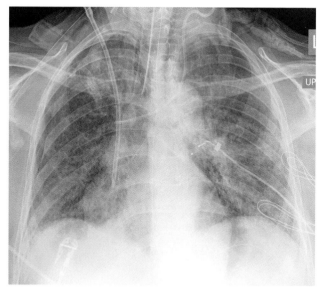

Fig. 26.1

Case 27

History: 55-year-old man with worsening cough and weight loss. Query lung carcinoma.

1. Which of the following should be included in the differential diagnosis of this patient (Figs. 27.1 and 27.2)? (Choose all that apply.)
   A. Lung cancer
   B. Granulomatosis with polyangiitis
   C. Sarcoidosis
   D. Tuberculosis
2. Which cell type of lung cancer is *most* closely associated with the presence of cavitation?
   A. Adenocarcinoma
   B. Small cell carcinoma
   C. Squamous cell carcinoma
   D. Large cell carcinoma
3. Which one of the following is *most* suggestive of a malignant cavitary lesion?
   A. Thick (>4 mm) wall
   B. Intracavitary fluid level
   C. Development in a preexisting area of consolidation
   D. Lower lobe location
4. Which of the following is the next best step in the management of this patient?
   A. Bronchoscopy with bronchoalveolar lavage
   B. Transthoracic fine needle aspiration
   C. Respiratory isolation
   D. Fluorodeoxyglucose (FDG)-positron emission tomography (PET)/computed tomography (CT)

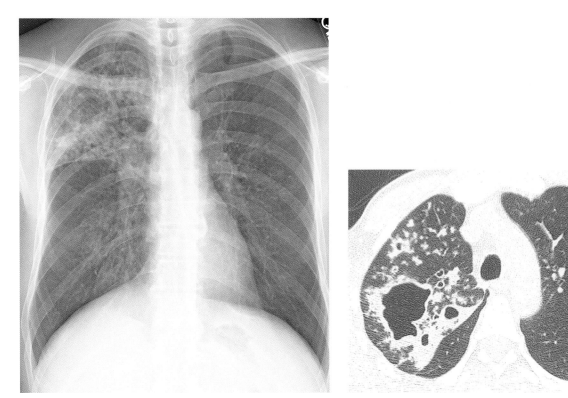

Fig. 27.1   Fig. 27.2

Case 28

History: Hemoptysis.

1. Which of the following should be included in the differential diagnosis for this patient (Figs. 28.1, 28.2 and 28.3)? (Choose all that apply.)
   A. Lung carcinoma
   B. Progressive massive fibrosis
   C. Mycetoma
   D. Pulmonary Langerhans cell histiocytosis
2. Which organism is most commonly associated with mycetoma?
   A. *Aspergillus*
   B. *Blastomyces*
   C. *Candida*
   D. *Coccidioides*
3. What one of the following is the most common complication of a mycetoma?
   A. Spread of infection to others
   B. Hemoptysis
   C. Dissemination of infection
   D. Lung carcinoma
4. Which of the following is preferred first-line therapy for patients with mycetoma and acute severe hemoptysis?
   A. Antifungal therapy
   B. Pneumonectomy
   C. Bronchial artery embolization
   D. Radiation therapy

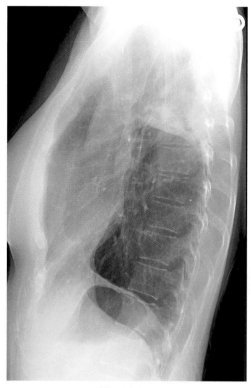

Fig. 28.2

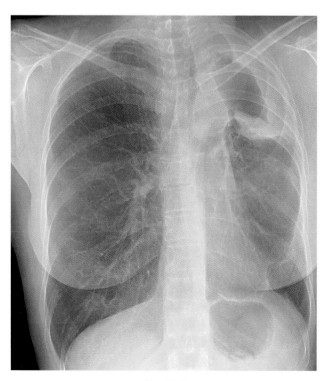

Fig. 28.1

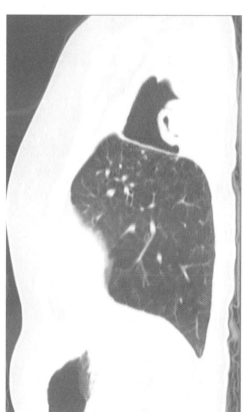

Fig. 28.3

Case 29

History: 33-year-old man presenting for employment physical examination.

1. Based on the chest radiograph (Fig. 29.1), which of the following should be included in the differential diagnosis for this patient? (Choose all that apply.)
   A. Pericardial cyst
   B. Lymphoma
   C. Paraganglioma
   D. Morgagni hernia
2. Based on the computed tomography (CT) scan image, what one of the following is the *best* diagnosis for this patient (Fig. 29.2)?
   A. Pericardial cyst
   B. Lymphoma
   C. Paraganglioma
   D. Morgagni hernia
3. Which of the following is *true* regarding pericardial cysts?
   A. Pericardial cysts occur more commonly in the left pericardiophrenic space.
   B. Most pericardial cysts communicate with the pericardium.
   C. Most pericardial cysts attach to the parietal pericardium.
   D. Most pericardial cysts cause symptoms.
4. Which of the following MR = magnetic resonance findings of pericardial cysts is correct?
   A. Most pericardial cysts have high signal intensity on T1-weighted imaging.
   B. T2-signal intensity is heterogeneous.
   C. T1 postcontrast images show thin capsular enhancement.
   D. T1 postcontrast images show no internal enhancement.

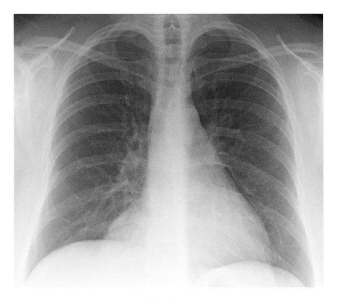

Fig. 29.1

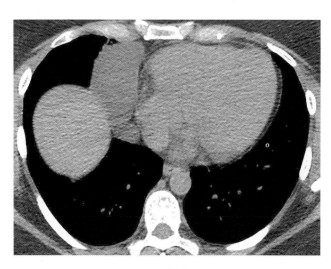

Fig. 29.2

Case 30

History: 20-year-old female with fever and cough.

1. Which of the following should be included in the differential diagnosis for this patient? (Choose all that apply.)
   A. Acute histoplasmosis
   B. Community-acquired pneumonia
   C. Pleural effusion
   D. Septic emboli
2. What is the term used to describe the air-filled, tubular, branching structures that are visible within the right lower lobe (Figs. 30.1 and 30.2)?
   A. Air bronchogram
   B. Pseudocavitation
   C. Pulmonary interstitial emphysema
   D. Black bronchus sign
3. Which organism is most often associated with lobar pneumonia in the normal (immunocompetent) host?
   A. *Aspergillus fumigatus*
   B. *Legionella pneumophila*
   C. *Staphylococcus aureus*
   D. *Streptococcus pneumoniae*
4. What sign is used to describe obscuration of the right hemidiaphragm on the posteroanterior (PA) view?
   A. Sail sign
   B. Spine sign
   C. Silhouette sign
   D. Continuous hemidiaphragm sign

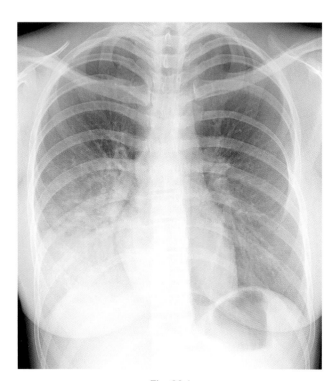

Fig. 30.1

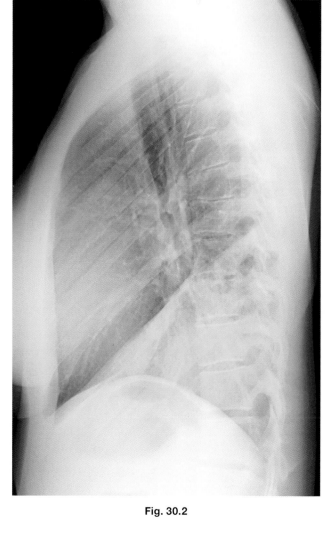

Fig. 30.2

Case 31

History: Leukocytosis and cough.

1. Which of the following should be included in the differential diagnosis for this patient (Fig. 31.1)? (Choose all that apply.)
   A. Chylothorax
   B. Empyema
   C. Malignant effusion
   D. Hemothorax
2. Which of the following best suggests empyema on computed tomography (CT)?
   A. Gravitational layering of fluid
   B. Lenticular shape of pleural collection
   C. Gas within the pleural collection
   D. Compressive atelectasis of adjacent lung
3. What is the most likely cause of an air fluid level within a pleural fluid collection?
   A. Gas-forming organisms
   B. Pulmonary gangrene
   C. Pleurocutaneous fistula
   D. Bronchopleural fistula
4. What is the most likely type of organism causing this abnormality?
   A. Bacterial
   B. Fungal
   C. Parasitic
   D. Viral

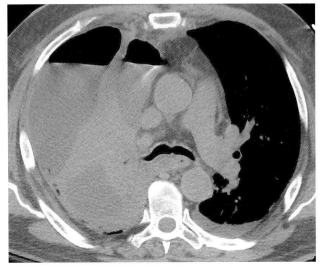

Fig. 31.1

Case 32

History: Chest pain.

1. Which of the following should be included in the differential diagnosis for this patient (Figs. 32.1, 32.2 and 32.3)? (Choose all that apply.)
   A. Schwannoma
   B. Thymoma
   C. Ganglioneuroma
   D. Germ cell tumor
2. In which mediastinal compartment is the mass?
   A. Anterior mediastinum
   B. Middle mediastinum
   C. Posterior mediastinum
   D. Inferior mediastinum
3. Which of the following is the next best step in management of this patient?
   A. Chest computed tomography (CT)
   B. Thoracic spine magnetic resonance imaging (MRI)
   C. Fluorodeoxyglucose-positron emission tomography (FDG-PET)/CT
   D. Biopsy
4. Which of the following regarding neurogenic tumors is true?
   A. Most neurogenic tumors are malignant.
   B. Rib spreading and erosions imply malignancy.
   C. Tumors of the sympathetic chain often widen the neural foramen.
   D. Calcification is more common in sympathetic chain tumors than peripheral nerve tumors.

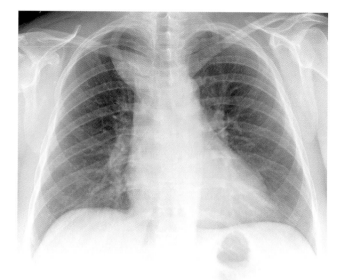

Fig. 32.1

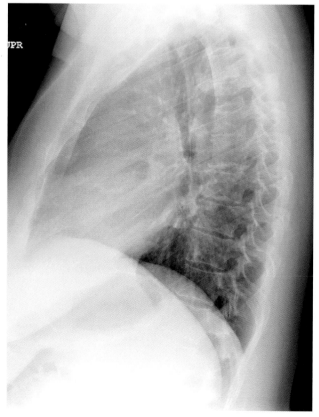

Fig. 32.2

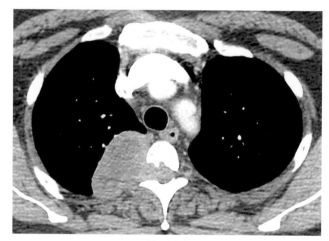

Fig. 32.3

Case 33

History: 50-year-old male with dyspnea and cough with increasing chest pain three days after slipping on ice.

1. Which of the following should be included in the differential diagnosis for this patient (Fig. 33.1)? (Choose all that apply.)
   A. Hemothorax
   B. Empyema
   C. Chylothorax
   D. Solitary fibrous tumor
2. Which of the following most likely suggests hemothorax?
   A. Rapidly enlarging pleural collection following heart surgery
   B. Slowly enlarging pleural collection over several weeks
   C. Pleural collection loculated in the major fissure
   D. Homogeneous, low-attenuation pleural collection on computed tomography (CT)
3. What sign describes layers of different attenuation in a hemothorax?
   A. Split pleura sign
   B. Dependent viscera sign
   C. Collar sign
   D. Hematocrit sign
4. What is the next best management for this hemodynamically stable patient?
   A. Thoracotomy
   B. Tube thoracostomy
   C. Transcatheter embolization
   D. Talc pleurodesis

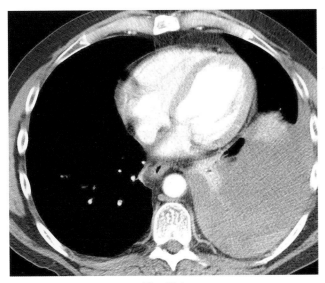

Fig. 33.1

Case 34

History: Multiple skin lesions.

1. Which of the following should be included in the differential diagnosis for this patient (Fig. 34.1)? (Choose all that apply.)
   A. Tuberous sclerosis complex
   B. Metastases
   C. Neurofibromatosis type 1 (NF-1)
   D. Takayasu arteritis
2. Which of the following is *not* an osseous manifestation of NF-1?
   A. Widened neural foramen
   B. Rib erosion
   C. Vertebra plana
   D. Scoliosis
3. What is the most common cause of destruction of a rib in an adult?
   A. Primary bone sarcoma
   B. Metastases
   C. Multiple myeloma
   D. Metabolic bone disease
4. What congenital aortic anomaly is associated with rib notching?
   A. Right aortic arch
   B. Cervical aortic arch
   C. Aberrant subclavian artery
   D. Aortic coarctation

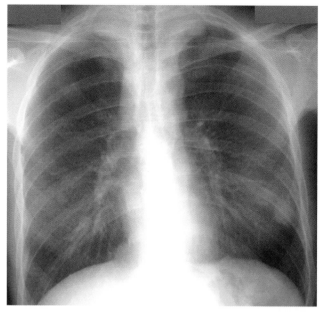

Fig. 34.1

Case 35

History: 60-year-old man with cough.

1. Which radiographic sign is demonstrated (Fig. 35.1)?
   A. S-sign of Golden
   B. Rock of Gibraltar
   C. Luftsichel sign
   D. Flat waist sign
2. In an adult *outpatient*, which is the most likely cause for lobar atelectasis?
   A. Aspirated foreign body
   B. Endobronchial mucus plug
   C. Lung cancer
   D. Bronchomalacia
3. In an adult *inpatient*, which is the most likely cause for lobar atelectasis?
   A. Aspirated foreign body
   B. Endobronchial mucus plug
   C. Lung cancer
   D. Bronchomalacia
4. The revised 8th edition *TNM Staging Classification for Lung Cancer* considers any degree of post-obstructive atelectasis or pneumonitis extending to the hilum to represent *at least* what T (tumor) stage?
   A. T1
   B. T2
   C. T3
   D. T4

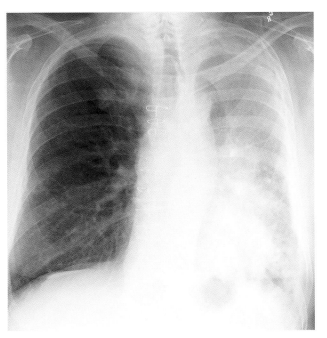

Fig. 35.1

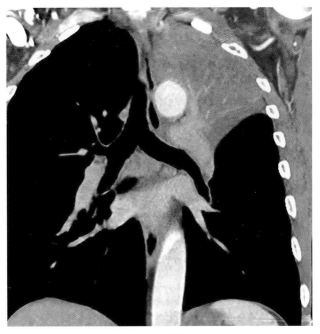

Fig. 35.2

Case 36

History: Shortness of breath in 48-year-old man.

1. Based on the radiographic appearance, what is the most likely diagnosis (Fig. 36.1)?
   A. Cardiogenic pulmonary edema
   B. Noncardiogenic pulmonary edema
   C. Lymphangitic carcinomatosis
   D. Community acquired pneumonia
2. What of the following is *not* a typical radiologic feature of this entity?
   A. Architectural distortion
   B. Perihilar haze
   C. Septal thickening
   D. Cardiomegaly
3. What is the most common cause for this radiographic appearance?
   A. Drug toxicity
   B. Left heart disease
   C. Neurologic disease
   D. Inhalational injury
4. Which of the following is true regarding the imaging features of this entity? (Choose all that apply.)
   A. Associated with increased hydrostatic pressure in pulmonary capillaries
   B. Affects the axial, peripheral, and parenchymal interstitium
   C. Widening of the vascular pedicle to greater than 58 mm is a marker for increased central vascular pressure
   D. Radiographic improvement may lag behind clinical parameters
   E. All of the above

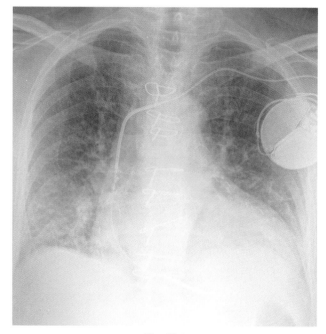

Fig. 36.1

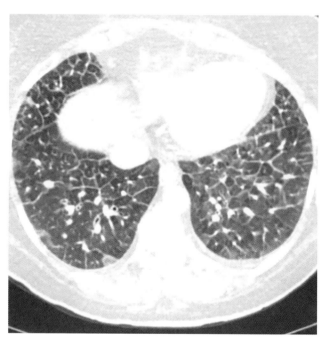

Fig. 36.2

Case 37

History: Elderly woman with incidental finding on chest radiography.

1. What radiographic sign is demonstrated (Fig. 37.1)?
   A. Thoracoabdominal sign
   B. Hilum convergence sign
   C. Hilum overlay sign
   D. Cervicothoracic sign
2. In which radiographic space is the abnormality located on the lateral radiograph (Fig. 37.2)?
   A. Retrotracheal space
   B. Retrosternal space
   C. Infrahilar window
   D. Paravertebral space
3. In which anatomic compartment is the abnormality located?
   A. Prevascular mediastinum
   B. Visceral mediastinum
   C. Paravertebral mediastinum
   D. Pleural space

4. Which of the following imaging features of this entity might prospectively predict the need for sternotomy in the surgical management of this lesion?
   A. Tracheal deviation
   B. Visceral mediastinal extension
   C. Paravertebral mediastinal extension
   D. Subcarinal extension
   E. Intrathoracic component larger than thoracic inlet
   F. Dumbbell or "conical" shape
   G. B, C, D, E, and F
   H. All of the above

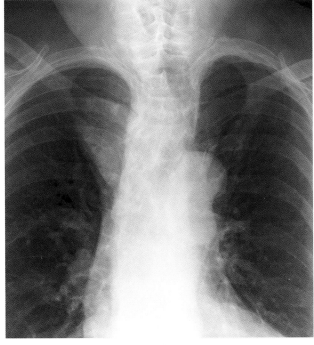

Fig. 37.1

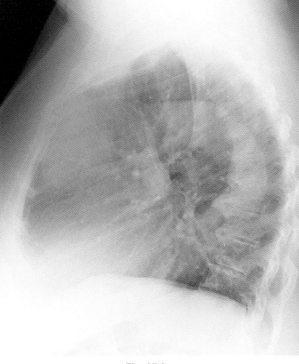
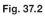

Fig. 37.2

Case 38

History: 68-year-old female with otherwise noncontributory medical history presents with 3 days of fever and cough.

1. In which lobe of the lung is the abnormality located (Figs. 38.1 and 38.2)?
   A. Right upper lobe
   B. Right lower lobe
   C. Right middle lobe
   D. Left upper lobe
   E. Left lower lobe
2. Which imaging sign is demonstrated on the radiograph (Figs. 38.1 and 38.2)? (Choose all that apply.)
   A. Spine sign
   B. Halo sign
   C. Reverse halo sign
   D. Silhouette sign

3. Which of the following organisms is most likely responsible for these patterns?
   A. *Mycoplasma pnemoniae*
   B. *Bacillus anthracis*
   C. *Histoplasma capsulatum*
   D. *Streptococcus pneumoniae*

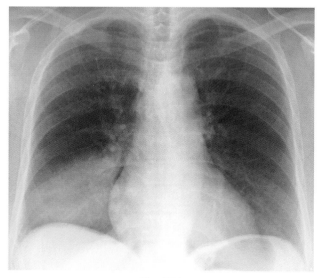

Fig. 38.1

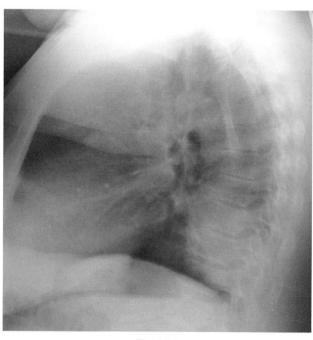

Fig. 38.2

Case 39

History: 33-year-old male smoker with progressive cough.

1. What is the most likely cause for the high-resolution computed tomography (HRCT) findings (Figs. 39.1 and 39.2)?
   A. Metastatic disease
   B. Usual interstitial pneumonia (UIP)
   C. Pulmonary Langerhans cell histiocytosis
   D. Sarcoidosis
2. Which pair of associations is typical of this entity?
   A. Skin folliculomas and renal cell carcinoma
   B. Intracranial subependymal tubers and renal angiomyolipomas
   C. Perilymphatic micronodules and hilar lymphadenopathy
   D. Smoking history and younger age

3. Which portion of the lung is typically spared in this disorder?
   A. Upper lobes
   B. Costophrenic sulci
   C. Apices
   D. Terminal bronchioles
4. Which of the following choices list the two most common complications of the disease?
   A. Emphysema and lung cancer
   B. Chylothorax and pneumothorax
   C. Pneumothorax and pulmonary hypertension
   D. Recurrent infections and bronchiectasis

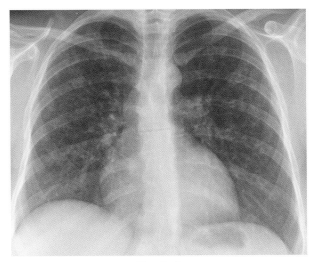

Fig. 39.1

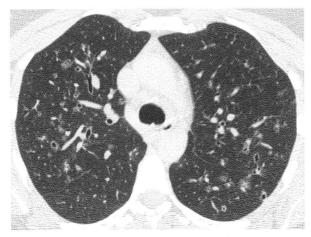

Fig. 39.2

Case 40

History: 62-year-old former smoker presents with dyspnea.

1. Based on the CT findings, what is the most likely diagnosis (Fig. 40.1)?
   A. Lymphangitic carcinomatosis
   B. Sarcoidosis
   C. Idiopathic pulmonary fibrosis
   D. Lymphoma
2. Which of the following is a high-resolution computed tomography (HRCT) feature of this condition? (Choose all that apply.)
   A. Smooth or nodular axial interstitial thickening
   B. Smooth or nodular interlobular septal thickening
   C. Smooth or nodular fissural thickening
   D. Preservation of normal lung architecture
   E. All the above

3. Which of the following primary malignant neoplasms is associated with lymphangitic carcinomatosis? (Choose all that apply.)
   A. Colon
   B. Lung
   C. Breast
   D. Stomach
   E. All of the above
4. Which of the following histologic subtypes of malignancy is most likely to exhibit a lymphangitic pattern?
   A. Squamous cell carcinoma
   B. Sarcoma
   C. Adenocarcinoma
   D. Neuroendocrine cell

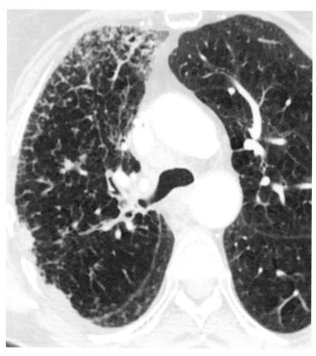

Fig. 40.1

Case 41

History: 57-year-old asymptomatic man.

1. What should be included in the differential diagnosis for the parenchymal abnormality (Fig. 41.1)?
   A. Pneumonia
   B. Pulmonary infarct
   C. Lung cancer
   D. Rounded pneumonia
   E. All of the above
2. Which computed tomography (CT) sign is demonstrated (Fig. 41.2)?
   A. Reverse halo sign
   B. Comet tail sign
   C. Bronchus cut-off sign
   D. Dark bronchus sign
3. What is the most likely diagnosis for the parenchymal abnormality?
   A. Pneumonia
   B. Rounded atelectasis

C. Lung cancer
D. Pulmonary infarct

4. Which of the following features must be present to make a definitive imaging diagnosis?
   A. Rounded, wedge-shaped, or lentiform morphology of mass-like opacity
   B. Pleural abnormality in contact with the subpleural mass-like opacity
   C. Signs of volume loss in the affected lobe
   D. Traction and convergence of adjacent bronchovascular structures
   E. All of the above

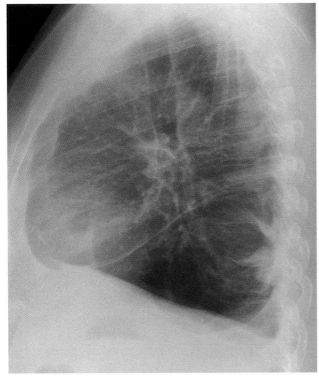

Fig. 41.1

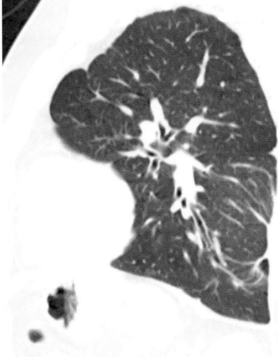

Fig. 41.2

Case 42

History: 44-year-old female with dyspnea on exertion.

1. Which of the following entities is associated with upper lung zone architectural distortion?
   A. Sarcoidosis
   B. Tuberculosis
   C. Pneumoconiosis (e.g., silicosis, berylliosis)
   D. Chronic hypersensitivity pneumonitis
   E. All of the above

2. Which radiographic stage of the diagnosis is depicted (Fig. 42.1)?
   A. Stage 0
   B. Stage I
   C. Stage II
   D. Stage III
   E. Stage IV

3. Which term is used to describe the airway abnormalities associated with pulmonary fibrosis?
   A. Traction bronchiectasis
   B. Honeycombing
   C. Bronchomalacia
   D. Bronchial stenosis
   E. Obliterative bronchiolitis

4. Which laboratory value is often elevated in patients with this condition?
   A. Alpha-1 antitrypsin
   B. Angiotensin converting enzyme (ACE)
   C. pCO_2
   D. Eosinophil count
   E. Cytoplasmic anti-neutrophil cytoplasmic antibody (c-ANCA)

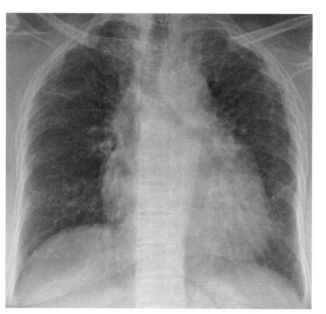

Fig. 42.1

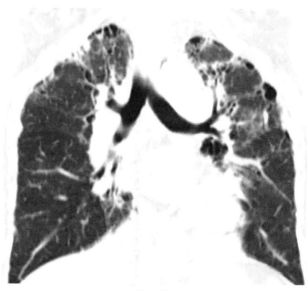

Fig. 42.2

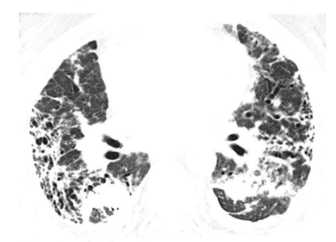

Fig. 42.3

Case 43

History: 66-year-old female smoker.

1. What is the anatomic distribution of the abnormality (Figs. 43.1 and 43.2)?
   A. Paraseptal
   B. Centrilobular
   C. Panlobular
   D. Paracicatricial
2. What is the most common cause of the abnormality?
   A. Autoimmune disease
   B. Drug reaction
   C. Smoking
   D. Positive airway pressure

3. What distribution is typical for this condition?
   A. Lower lobes
   B. Upper lobes
   C. Asymmetric
   D. Random
4. True or False? This condition is reversible with smoking cessation.
   A. True
   B. False

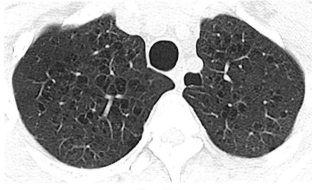

Fig. 43.1

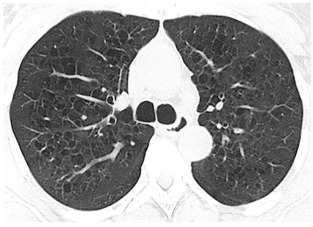

Fig. 43.2

Case 44

History: Asymptomatic 66-year-old female with incidental finding on routine imaging.

1. In what mediastinal compartment is the abnormality located (Figs. 44.1, 44.2 and 44.3)?
   A. Prevascular (anterior)
   B. Visceral (middle)
   C. Paravertebral (posterior)
   D. Superior
2. What is the most common primary neoplasm of the prevascular mediastinum?
   A. Thymoma
   B. Thymic carcinoma
   C. Thymic neuroendocrine tumor
   D. Lymphoma
   E. Germ cell neoplasm
3. At which age are thymomas typically encountered?
   A. 5 to 10 years
   B. 20 to 30 years
   C. 30 to 40 years
   D. >40 years
4. Which paraneoplastic syndrome is most commonly associated with thymoma?
   A. Myasthenia gravis
   B. Lambert-Eaton syndrome
   C. Syndrome of inappropriate antidiuretic hormone
   D. Serotonin syndrome

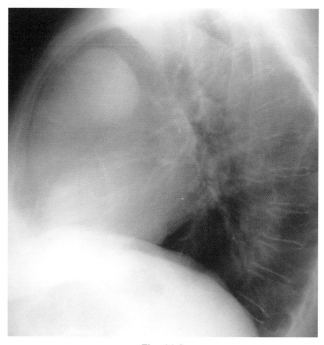

Fig. 44.2

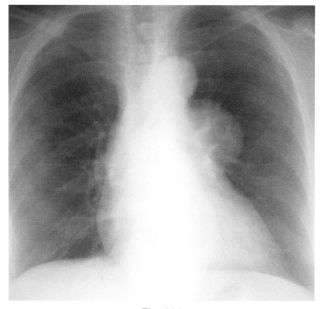

Fig. 44.1

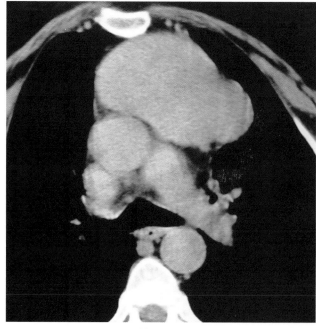

Fig. 44.3

Case 45

History: 67-year-old male smoker with weight loss.

1. What is the most likely diagnosis (Figs. 45.1A and 45.1B)?
   A. Bronchogenic cyst
   B. Hiatal hernia
   C. Mediastinal hematoma
   D. Lymphadenopathy
2. In which anatomic space is the abnormality located?
   A. Paraesophageal
   B. Subaortic
   C. Right paratracheal
   D. Subcarinal
3. In a patient with right upper lobe lung cancer, involvement of this level represents, at a minimum, which tumor, node, metastasis (TNM) nodal classification?
   A. N0
   B. N1
   C. N2
   D. N3

4. Which interventional staging procedure(s) can be used to access and sample abnormalities in this location?
   A. Bronchoscopy
   B. Endobronchial ultrasound (EBUS)
   C. Esophageal endoscopic ultrasound (EUS)
   D. Mediastinoscopy
   E. all of the above

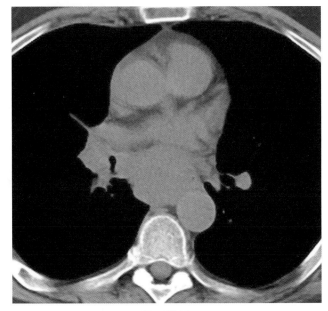

Fig. 45.1A

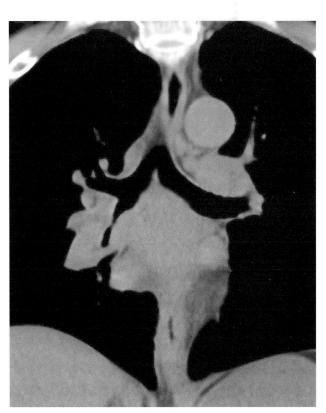

Fig. 45.1B

Case 46

History: Asymptomatic male.

1. What is the predominant imaging abnormality (Figs. 46.1A, 46.1B, 46.1C, 46.1D, and 46.1E)?
   A. Pleural plaques
   B. Nodules
   C. Masses
   D. Architectural distortion
2. Which of the following is most likely to have been the patient's occupation?
   A. Business executive
   B. Airplane pilot
   C. Fireman
   D. Quarry worker

3. In the simple form of this disease, which represents the typical temporal relationship from the exposure to the disease manifestation?
   A. 1 to 2 hours
   B. 1 to 2 weeks
   C. 1 to 2 years
   D. 10 to 20 years
4. The International Labor Office has established guidelines for the objective classification of this entity using which of the following?
   A. Pulmonary function test
   B. Whispered pectoriloquy
   C. Digital chest radiography
   D. Chest computed tomography

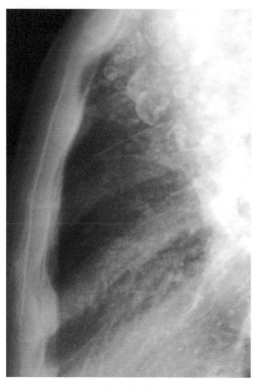

Fig. 46.1A

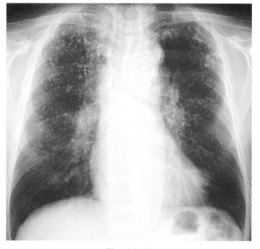

Fig. 46.1B

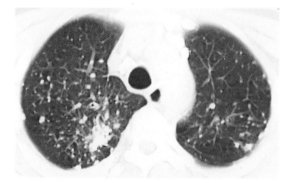

Fig. 46.1C

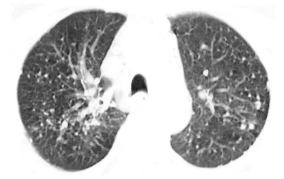

Fig. 46.1D

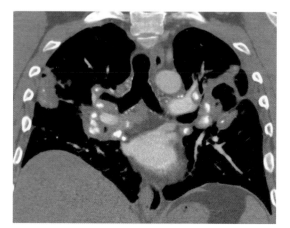

Fig. 46.1E

Case 47

History: 50-year-old woman with progressive decline in lung function.

1. Which of the following descriptors should be excluded as a predominant finding in this case (Fig. 47.1)?
   A. Peripheral
   B. Nodules
   C. Basilar predominant
   D. Ground-glass
   E. Subpleural sparing
2. Which of the following is the most likely cause for this computed tomography (CT) pattern in this patient?
   A. Cigarette smoking
   B. Connective tissue disease
   C. Hot tub use
   D. Asbestos exposure

3. Which of the following associated features shown may help narrow the differential diagnosis for the CT pattern in this patient?
   A. Traction bronchiectasis
   B. Coronary artery calcification
   C. Dilated pulmonary artery
   D. Esophageal dilation
4. Elevation of which serologic markers would be characteristic in this disease?
   A. Rheumatoid factor, anti-CCP
   B. Anti-ribonuclear protein
   C. Anti-centromere antibody, anti-SCL-70
   D. Anti-SS-A (Ro), anti-SS-B (La)

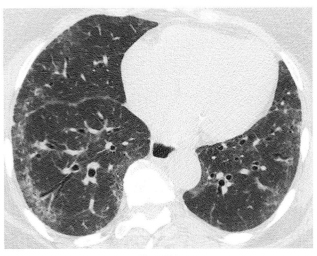

Fig. 47.1

Case 48

History: 44-year-old asymptomatic female with positive purified protein derivative (PPD) skin test during pre-employment physical.

1. What is the most likely cause of the imaging abnormality (Figs. 48.1A and 48.1B)?
   A. Asbestosis
   B. Broncholith
   C. Calcified metastasis
   D. Healed tuberculosis
2. Which historical eponym is given to the parenchymal finding?
   A. Fleischner sign
   B. Ghon focus
   C. S-sign of Golden
   D. Hampton hump

3. Which historical eponym is given to the combination of the parenchymal and hilar finding?
   A. Ranke complex
   B. Ghon focus
   C. Kerley's line
   D. Naclerio V-sign
4. Which of the following is included in the differential diagnosis for a calcified pulmonary nodule? (Choose all that apply.)
   A. Healed granulomatous disease
   B. Hamartoma
   C. Pneumoconiosis
   D. Carcinoid
   E. Calcific metastases
   F. Pulmonary ossification
   G. All of the above

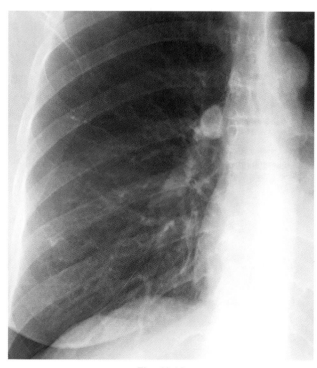

Fig. 48.1A

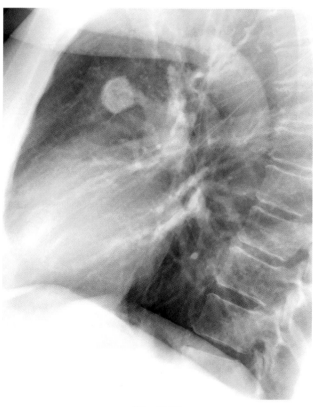

Fig. 48.1B

Case 49

History: 49-year-old woman with chronic cough.

1. What is the most prominent imaging abnormality (Fig. 49.1A)?
   A. Bronchiectasis
   B. Dilated pulmonary artery
   C. Middle lobe atelectasis
   D. Lingular atelectasis
2. Which of the following defines bronchiectasis by imaging criteria?
   A. Bronchoarterial ratio >0.5
   B. Bronchoarterial ratio >1.0
   C. Bronchoarterial ratio >1.5
   D. Greater than 70% luminal cross-sectional area collapse on expiration
   E. Greater anteroposterior airway diameter than transverse diameter
3. Which computed tomography (CT) imaging sign is associated with this condition (Fig. 49.1B)?
   A. Signet ring sign
   B. Three density sign
   C. Fallen viscera sign
   D. Reverse CT halo sign
4. Which of the following belong in the differential diagnosis? (Choose all that apply)
   A. Cystic fibrosis
   B. Allergic bronchopulmonary aspergillosis (ABPA)
   C. Chronic aspiration
   D. Chronic or recurrent infection
   E. Williams-Campbell syndrome
   F. Primary ciliary dyskinesia
   G. All of the above

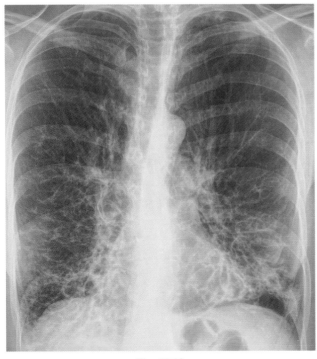

Fig. 49.1A

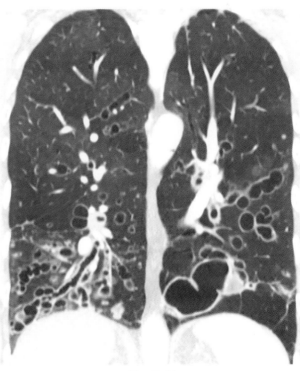

Fig. 49.1B

Case 50

History: 29-year-old woman with an incidental finding on chest radiography.

1. Which of the following should be included in the differential diagnosis of the chest radiographic finding (Figs. 50.1 and 50.2)? (Choose all that apply.)
   A. Lung cancer
   B. Septic embolus
   C. Arteriovenous malformation
   D. Pulmonary artery pseudoaneurysm
   E. All of the above
2. What percent of patients with this abnormality have the inherited disorder known as hereditary hemorrhagic telangiectasia?
   A. Less than 1%
   B. 1% to 20%
   C. 20% to 40%
   D. 40% to 60%
   E. 60% to 80%
   F. Greater than 80%
3. Which of the following is the most common presentation for persons with pulmonary arteriovenous malformation (AVMs)?
   A. Cerebral abscess
   B. Hemoptysis
   C. Cough
   D. Asymptomatic

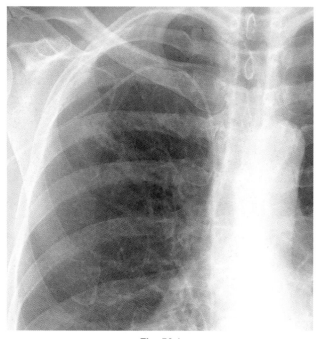

Fig. 50.1

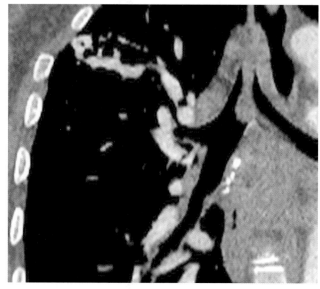

Fig. 50.2

Case 51

History: 52-year-old woman with an abnormal chest radiograph (Figs. 51.1A and 51.1B).

1. What is the most likely cause of the mediastinal mass?
   A. Mediastinal hematoma
   B. Lymphadenopathy
   C. Ascending aortic aneurysm
   D. Thymic neoplasm
2. What percentage of mediastinal masses are vascular in etiology?
   A. Less than 1%
   B. 10%
   C. 20%
   D. 50%
   E. 75%
3. In a patient with Marfan syndrome, what is the threshold dimension of luminal dilatation that prompts surgical repair of an aortic aneurysm?
   A. 4.0 cm
   B. 4.5 cm
   C. 5.0 cm
   D. 5.5 cm
   E. 6.0 cm

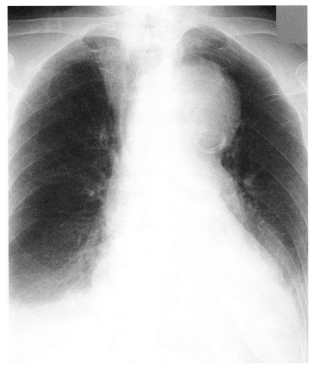

Fig. 51.1A

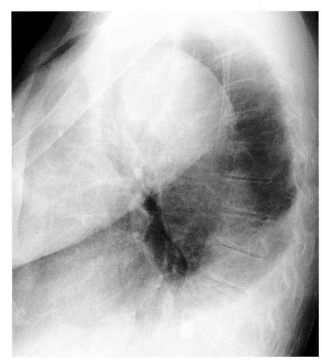

Fig. 51.1B

Case 52

History: 32-year-old man with right chest pain and dyspnea.

1. Which of the following should be included in the differential diagnosis of the chest radiographic finding (Fig. 52.1)? (Choose all that apply.)
   A. Lung cancer
   B. Pneumonia
   C. Pulmonary infarct
   D. Pulmonary contusion
   E. All of the above

2. Which of the following indicates a radiographic manifestation of pulmonary infarction?
   A. Wells score
   B. Hampton hump
   C. Westermark sign
   D. Knuckle sign
   E. Fleishner sign

3. Which of the following is a poor prognostic indicator in patients with acute pulmonary emboli?
   A. Pulmonary infarct
   B. Hemoptysis
   C. RV:LV ratio >1.0
   D. Subsegmental DECT perfusion defects

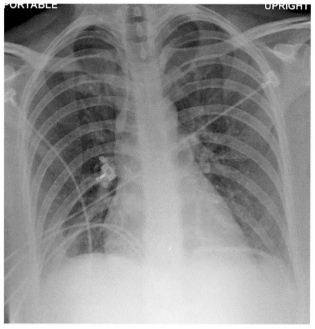

Fig. 52.1

Case 53

History: 25-year-old firefighter with fever, fatigue, and night sweats.

1. Which of the following should be included in the differential diagnosis of the chest radiographic finding (Fig. 53.1)? (Choose all that apply)
   A. Metastasis
   B. Lymphoma
   C. Germ cell neoplasm
   D. Thymic epithelial neoplasm
   E. All of the above
2. Which of the following is true regarding "bulky" disease for Hodgkin lymphoma (Figs. 53.2 and 53.3)?
   A. Portends a favorable prognosis
   B. Defined by chest radiograph extent
   C. Defined by a single nodal mass measuring greater than 3 cm on computed tomography (CT)
   D. Defined by a single nodal mass occupying greater than 1/3 of thoracic diameter
3. Which of the following is considered the gold standard imaging modality for initial, interim, and end-of-treatment assessment of lymphoma?
   A. Chest radiograph
   B. Non-contrast chest CT
   C. Fluorodeoxyglucose -positron emission tomography (^{18}FDG-PET)-CT
   D. Contrast-enhanced thoracic magnetic resonance imaging (MRI)

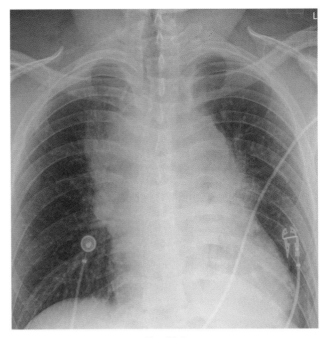

Fig. 53.1

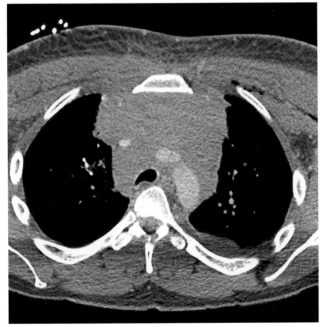

Fig. 53.2

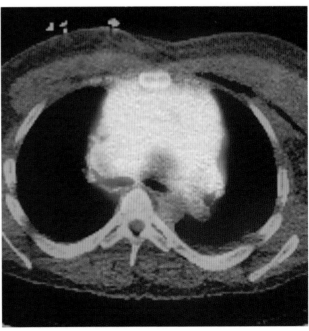

Fig. 53.3

Case 54

History: 35-year-old man after high-speed motorcycle accident.

1. Which of the following are the most common sites of traumatic aortic injury (TAI). (Choose all that apply.)
   A. Aortic root
   B. Aortic isthmus
   C. Sinotubular junction
   D. Branch vessel origins
   E. Diaphragmatic hiatus
2. Which of the following findings on the radiograph supports the diagnosis of TAI over other mimics (Fig. 54.1)?
   A. Atherosclerotic plaque
   B. Sinotubular junction dilation
   C. Rib notching
   D. Periaortic hemorrhage
3. What is the typical in-the-field mortality associated with TAI?
   A. 10% to 20%
   B. 20% to 30%
   C. 40% to 50%
   D. 50% to 60%
   E. 80% to 90%

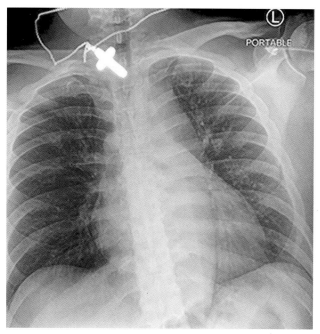

Fig. 54.1

Case 55

History: 88-year-old woman referred to CT for an abnormal chest radiograph (Figs. 55.1 and 55.2).

1. Which of the following should be included in the differential diagnosis for chronic airspace opacity? (Choose all that apply.)
   A. Lung adenocarcinoma
   B. Lymphoma
   C. Alveolar proteinosis
   D. Organizing pneumonia
   E. Lipoid pneumonia
2. Which of the following findings supports the diagnosis of lipoid pneumonia in the setting of a chronic consolidation?
   A. Spiculated margin
   B. Long-term stability

C. Macroscopic fat attenuation
D. Central cavitation
3. Which of the following may predispose a patient to developing lipoid pneumonia?
   A. Young age
   B. Smoking
   C. Positive pressure ventilation
   D. Zenker diverticulum
   E. Intravenous (IV) drug abuse

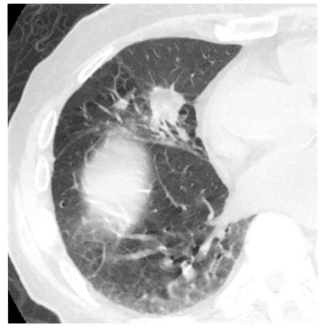

Fig. 55.1

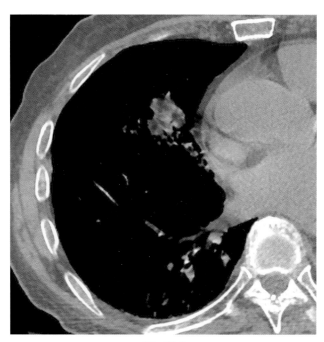

Fig. 55.2

Case 56

History: 33-year-old man referred for an abnormal chest radiograph (Fig. 56.1) and infertility.

1. What is the most likely diagnosis (Figs. 56.2 and 56.3)?
   A. Allergic bronchopulmonary Aspergillosis
   B. Kartagener syndrome
   C. Cystic fibrosis
   D. Recurrent aspiration
   E. Bronchial atresia
2. Which of the following comprise the triad associated with this entity? (Choose three.)
   A. Bronchiectasis
   B. Situs solitus
   C. Situs inversus
   D. Sinusitis
   E. Extralobar sequestration
3. Which of the following is the typical pattern of inheritance of this disorder?
   A. Autosomal dominant
   B. Autosomal recessive
   C. X-linked dominant
   D. X-linked recessive
   E. Mosaicism

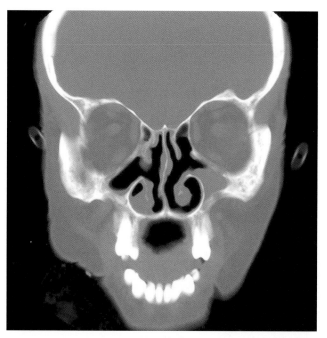

Fig. 56.2

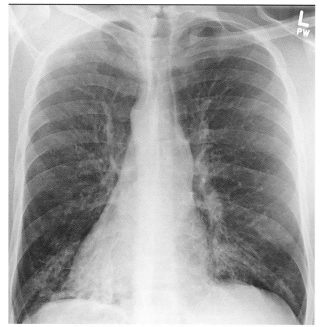

Fig. 56.1

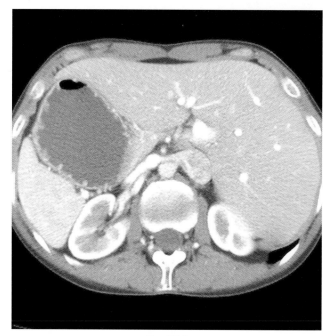

Fig. 56.3

Case 57

History: 59-year-old woman on chronic steroids for asthma presents with hemoptysis.

1. Which of the following should be included in the differential diagnosis for the radiographic findings (Fig. 57.1)? (Choose all that apply.)
   A. Pulmonary infarct
   B. Lung cancer
   C. Invasive aspergillus
   D. Rounded atelectasis
   E. Organizing pneumonia
2. What is the most likely diagnosis in this case?
   A. Pulmonary infarct
   B. Lung cancer
   C. Invasive aspergillus
   D. Rounded atelectasis
   E. Organizing pneumonia
3. What clinical information in this case supports the diagnosis?
   A. Female sex
   B. History of asthma
   C. Chronic steroid therapy
   D. Peripheral location
4. Which computed tomography (CT) sign is demonstrated (Fig. 57.2)?
   A. Signet ring
   B. Air bronchogram
   C. Comet tail
   D. Halo
   E. Reverse halo

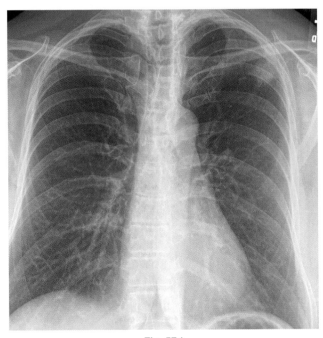

Fig. 57.1

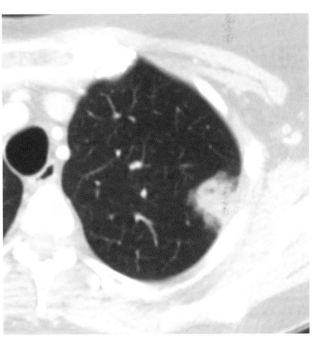

Fig. 57.2

Case 58

History: 75-year-old man with epistaxis.

1. What should be included in the differential diagnosis of the imaging findings (Figs. 58.1 and 58.2)? (Choose all that apply.)
   A. Septic emboli
   B. Lung abscess
   C. Multifocal pneumonia
   D. Metastatic disease
   E. Vasculitis
2. What is the most likely diagnosis in this case?
   A. Septic emboli
   B. Pulmonary abscesses
   C. Multifocal pneumonia
   D. Metastatic disease
   E. Vasculitis

3. What clinical information would support the diagnosis?
   A. Male sex
   B. Intravenous (IV) drug abuse
   C. Epistaxis
   D. Immunosuppression
4. What computed tomography (CT) sign is demonstrated?
   A. Signet ring
   B. Air bronchogram
   C. Comet tail
   D. CT halo
   E. Reverse CT halo

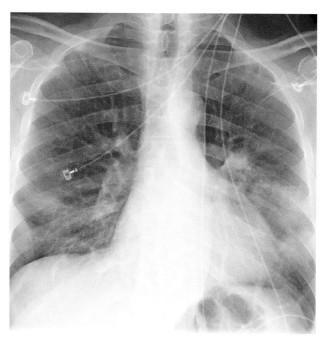

Fig. 58.1

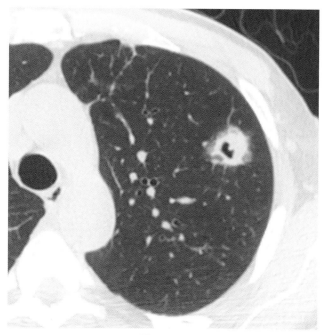

Fig. 58.2

Case 59

History: 52-year-old woman with chronic dyspnea (Figs. 59.1 and 59.2).

1. Which of the following should be included in the differential diagnosis for this patient? (Choose all that apply.)
   A. Langerhans cell histiocytosis
   B. Lymphangioleiomyomatosis
   C. Tuberous sclerosis
   D. Hermansky-Pudlak syndrome
2. What is a characteristic computed tomography (CT) finding in Langerhans cell histiocytosis?
   A. Ground-glass opacity
   B. Costophrenic angle sparing
   C. Consolidation
   D. Apical sparing

3. Which of the conditions listed is associated with chylous pleural effusions?
   A. Lymphangioleiomyomatosis
   B. Langerhans cell histiocytosis
   C. Amyloidosis
   D. Lymphocytic interstitial pneumonitis
4. Which of the following findings are not usually present in the setting of tuberous sclerosis?
   A. Fatty cardiac lesions
   B. Multinodular multifocal pneumocyte hyperplasia
   C. Hepatocellular carcinoma
   D. Angiomyolipomas

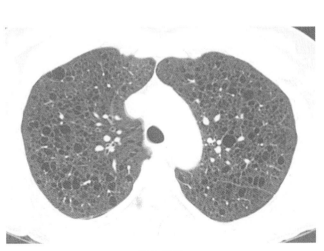

Fig. 59.1

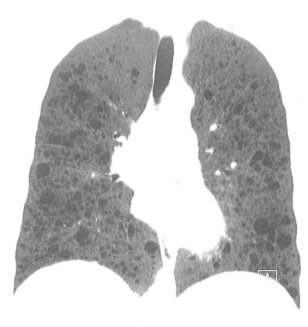

Fig. 59.2

Case 60

History: Young man with history of chest pain and cough (Fig. 60.1).

1. Which of the following should be included in the differential diagnosis for this patient? (Choose all that apply.)
   A. Lymphoma
   B. Tuberculosis
   C. Metastatic disease
   D. Sarcoidosis
2. In the setting of tuberculosis, which pulmonary finding is more common in children than adults?
   A. Fibrocavitary disease
   B. Ground-glass opacity
   C. Bronchiectasis
   D. Consolidation
3. Tuberculous lymphadenopathy is common in which of the following conditions?
   A. Acquired immune deficiency syndrome
   B. Rheumatoid arthritis
   C. Common variable immune deficiency
   D. Lymphocytic interstitial pneumonitis
4. In which demographic is tuberculous pleuritis least common?
   A. Infants
   B. Adolescents
   C. Young adults
   D. Elderly

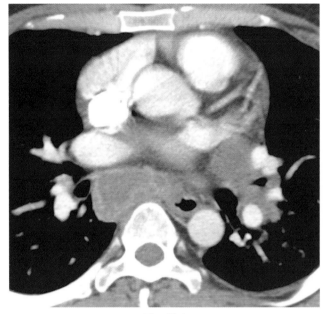

Fig. 60.1

Case 61

History: 49-year-old man with human immunodeficiency virus (HIV) and shortness of breath (Fig. 61.1).

1. Which of the following should be included in the differential diagnosis for this patient? (Choose all that apply.)
   A. Pulmonary edema
   B. Diffuse alveolar hemorrhage
   C. *Pneumocystis jirovecii* pneumonia
   D. Pulmonary alveolar proteinosis
2. Which of the following is another common computed tomography (CT) finding in patients with *Pneumocystis jirovecii* pneumonia?
   A. Pleural effusions
   B. Cysts
   C. Lymphadenopathy
   D. Tree-in-bud nodules
3. Which of the conditions listed below is associated with chylous pleural effusions?
   A. Lymphangioleiomyomatosis
   B. Langerhans cell histiocytosis
   C. Amyloidosis
   D. Lymphocytic interstitial pneumonitis
4. What is first-line therapy for *Pneumocystis jirovecii* pneumonia?
   A. Trimethoprim-sulfamethoxazole
   B. Amoxicillin/clavulanic acid
   C. Linezolid
   D. Azithromycin

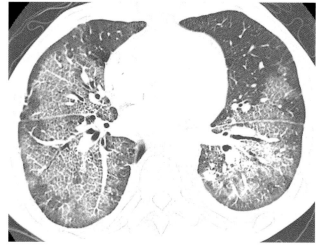

Fig. 61.1

Case 62

History: 25-year-old man; history withheld (Fig. 62.1).

1. Which of the following should be included in the differential diagnosis for the appearance of the mediastinum and hila? (Choose all that apply.)
   A. Silicosis
   B. Tuberculosis
   C. Histoplasmosis
   D. Sarcoidosis
2. Calcified lymphadenopathy following treatment is seen most frequently in which disease?
   A. Cat scratch disease
   B. Acquired immunodeficiency syndrome (AIDS)
   C. Systemic sclerosis
   D. Lymphoma

3. Which of the following conditions is *least* likely to cause egg-shell calcification in hilar and mediastinal lymphadenopathy?
   A. Silicosis
   B. Sarcoidosis
   C. Histoplasmosis
   D. Coal workers pneumoconiosis
4. Garland's triad is highly associated with which of the following diseases?
   A. Sarcoidosis
   B. Lymphoma
   C. Tuberculosis
   D. Leukemia

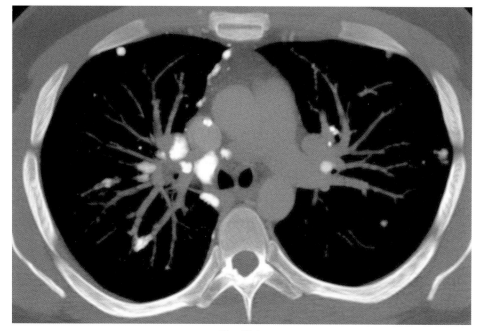

Fig. 62.1

Case 63

History: 52-year-old man with fever, chills, and pleuritic chest pain (Fig. 63.1).

1. Which of the following should be included in the differential diagnosis for this patient? (Choose all that apply.)
   A. Metastatic disease
   B. Septic infarcts
   C. Granulomatosis with polyangiitis
   D. Acute respiratory distress syndrome
2. What is the likely etiology for chronic cavitary lung nodules in a patient with joint pain and subcutaneous nodules?
   A. Tuberculosis
   B. Rheumatoid arthritis
   C. Granulomatosis with polyangiitis
   D. Invasive aspergillosis
3. Which the following is not a risk factor for development of septic infarcts?
   A. Central venous catheter
   B. Periodontal disease
   C. Pulmonary hypertension
   D. Intravenous drug use
4. What is the most common imaging manifestation of fat embolism?
   A. Ground-glass opacity
   B. Fatty attenuation pulmonary emboli
   C. Tree-in-bud nodules
   D. Consolidation

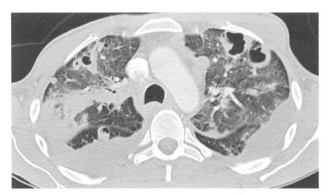

Fig. 63.1

Case 64

History: History of recent pneumonectomy. Two chest radiographs are shown acquired 2 days apart (Figs. 64.1 and 64.2).

1. What is the diagnosis?
   A. Extrapleural hematoma
   B. Hemothorax
   C. Bronchopleural fistula
   D. Expected postoperative evolution
2. What is likely underlying reason for a higher incidence of bronchopleural fistula after right pneumonectomy as compared to left pneumonectomy?
   A. Obtuse angle of the bronchial stump
   B. Shorter length of bronchial stump
   C. Technically more difficult surgery
   D. Greater frequency of right pneumonectomies

3. Which lobe is most prone to lobar torsion after ipsilateral lobectomy?
   A. Right middle lobe
   B. Right lower lobe
   C. Left upper lobe
   D. Left lower lobe
4. In the setting of suspected bronchopleural fistula after pneumonectomy, what is the next step in management?
   A. Chest tube drainage
   B. Watchful waiting
   C. Surgical exploration
   D. Bronchoscopy

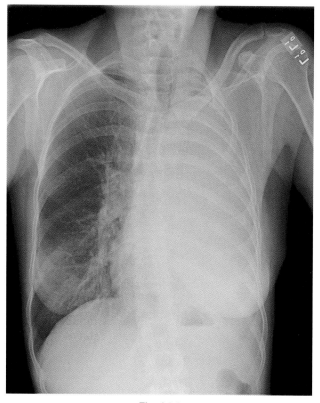

Fig. 64.1

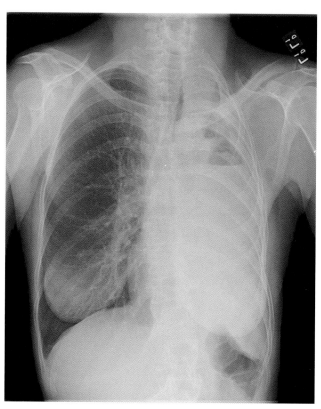

Fig. 64.2

Case 65

History: 59-year-old man with left shoulder pain and hand weakness.

1. The imaging findings in this case are most commonly associated with which cell type of lung cancer (Figs. 65.1, 65.2 and 65.3)?
   A. Small cell carcinoma
   B. Squamous cell carcinoma
   C. Large cell carcinoma
   D. Adenocarcinoma

2. If this tumor invaded the chest wall, what staging factor would make him an inoperable candidate?
   A. T3 disease
   B. N2 disease
   C. N3 disease
   D. Any nodal status

3. In the staging of lung cancer invasion of which of the following is considered T4 (non-operable)?
   A. Phrenic nerve
   B. Recurrent laryngeal nerve
   C. Diaphragm
   D. Parietal pericardium

4. What is the current standard therapy for most operable superior sulcus tumors?
   A. Chemotherapy
   B. Chemotherapy and radiotherapy
   C. Chemotherapy and radiotherapy with subsequent surgery
   D. Surgery with subsequent chemotherapy and radiotherapy

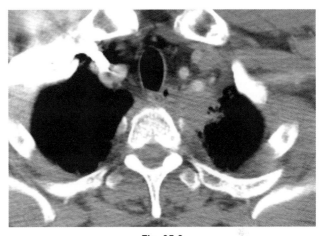

Fig. 65.3

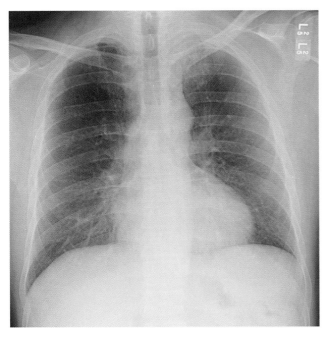

Fig. 65.1

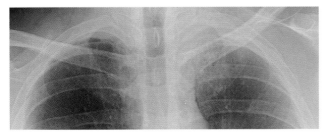

Fig. 65.2

Case 66

History: 26-year-old with fever, night sweats, and cough (Fig. 66.1).

1. Which of the following should be included in the differential diagnosis for this patient? (Choose all that apply.)
   A. Lung cancer
   B. Fungal pneumonia
   C. TB
   D. Pulmonary infarct
2. Which lung cancer cell type is associated most frequently with cavitation?
   A. Small cell lung cancer
   B. Adenocarcinoma
   C. Large cell carcinoma
   D. Squamous cell carcinoma
3. In adult patients with tuberculosis, tree-in-bud opacities indicate involvement in which anatomic structures?
   A. Arterioles
   B. Lymphatics
   C. Bronchioles
   D. Alveoli
4. In the setting of acute pulmonary embolism, which comorbid condition is most frequently associated with the development of pulmonary infarction?
   A. Congestive heart failure
   B. Asthma
   C. Pulmonary fibrosis
   D. Tricuspid regurgitation

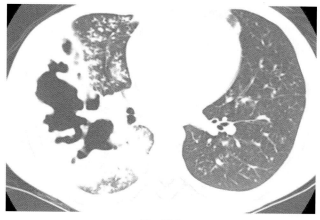

Fig. 66.1

Case 67

History: 63-year-old man with long history of smoking and chronic cough.

1. Which of the following lymph node stations demonstrate fluorodeoxyglucose (FDG) avidity in this patient with non-small cell lung cancer (Figs. 67.1, 67.2 and 67.3)? (Check all that apply.)
   A. Subaortic
   B. Low paratracheal
   C. High paratracheal
   D. Para-aortic
   E. Hilar
2. What finding makes this cancer unresectable?
   A. T3 disease
   B. N2 disease
   C. N3 disease
   D. M1 disease

3. What is the most common lobe affected by lung cancer?
   A. Right upper lobe
   B. Right middle lobe
   C. Right lower lobe
   D. Left lower lobe
4. What feature of lung cancer is least likely to be associated with a false negative result on positron emission tomography/computed tomography (PET/CT)?
   A. Small size
   B. Carcinoid histology
   C. Ground-glass attenuation
   D. Spiculated margins

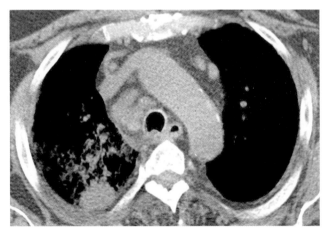

Fig. 67.1

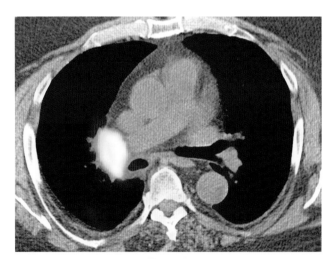

Fig. 67.3

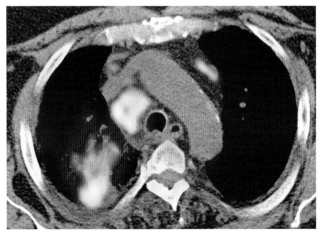

Fig. 67.2

Case 68

History: 57-year-old man with cough.

1. Which of the following should be included in the differential diagnosis for the nodule shown in (Fig. 68.1)? (Choose all that apply.)
   A. Pneumonia
   B. Aspiration
   C. Adenocarcinoma
   D. Scar or focal fibrosis
2. Which attenuation characteristic of a focal pulmonary nodule is most concerning for primary lung cancer?
   A. Ground-glass
   B. Part-solid
   C. Solid
   D. Solid with cavitation
3. A solitary 4 to 5 mm ground-glass nodule is identified incidentally on a chest computed tomography (CT) for evaluation of chronic dyspnea. According to current guidelines, what is the next step in management?
   A. CT follow-up in 3 months
   B. CT follow-up in 6 months
   C. CT follow-up in 12 months
   D. No CT follow-up
4. Which of the following is least likely to cause diffuse centrilobular ground-glass nodules throughout the lungs?
   A. Hypersensitivity pneumonitis
   B. Metastatic disease
   C. Pulmonary hemorrhage
   D. Respiratory bronchiolitis

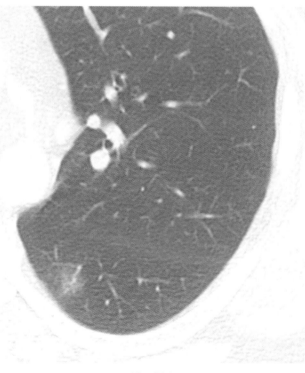

Fig. 68.1

Case 69

History: 45-year-old woman with chronic dyspnea.

1. Which of the following should be included in the differential diagnosis for this patient based solely on the radiograph (Fig. 69.1)? (Choose all that apply.)
   A. Lymphoma
   B. Azygos continuation of the inferior vena cava (IVC)
   C. Superior vena cava obstruction
   D. Partial anomalous pulmonary venous return
2. What is the most likely diagnosis based on all imaging available (Figs. 69.1, 69.2 and 69.3)?
   A. Lymphoma
   B. Azygos continuation of the inferior vena cava
   C. Superior vena cava obstruction
   D. Partial anomalous pulmonary venous return

3. In the setting of chronic superior vena cava obstruction, which collateral veins allow drainage of abdominal wall veins into the anterior aspect of the liver, which may produce enhancing pseudo-hepatic lesions?
   A. Veins of Sappey
   B. Veins of Marshall
   C. Veins of Galen
   D. Veins of Mayo
4. When compared to asplenia heterotaxy syndrome, polysplenia is more often associated with which of the following?
   A. Higher prevalence of cyanotic congenital heart disease
   B. Higher prevalence of midgut malrotation
   C. Lower prevalence of azygos continuation of IVC
   D. Lower prevalence of bilateral hyparterial bronchi

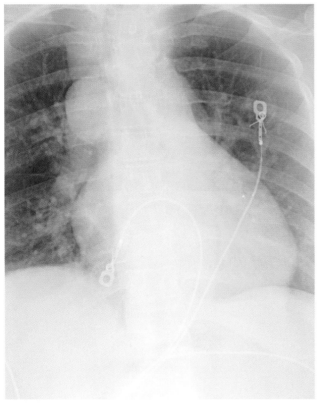 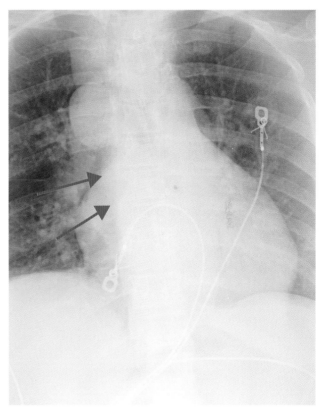

Fig. 69.1

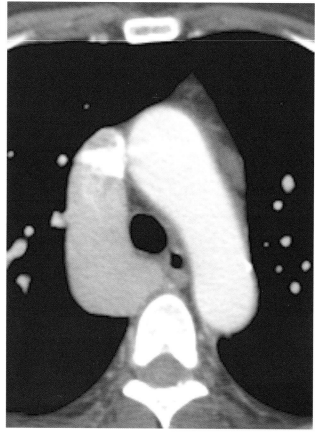

Fig. 69.2

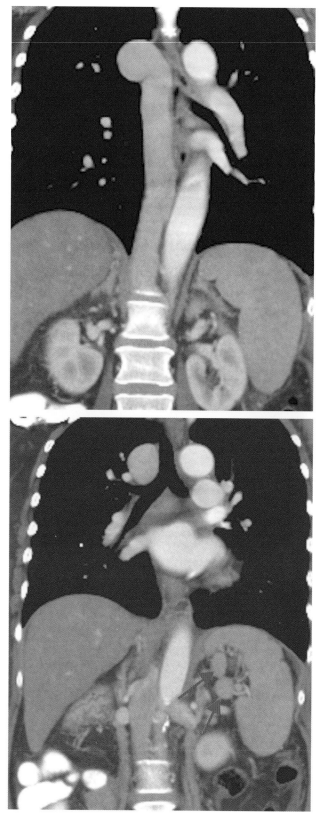

Fig. 69.3

Case 70

History: 75-year-old man with cough and dyspnea (Figs. 70.1 and 70.2).

1. Which of the following should be included in the differential diagnosis for this patient based solely on the radiograph? (Choose all that apply.)
   A. Pneumonia
   B. Aspiration
   C. Lung cancer
   D. Lymphoma
2. What imaging sign is demonstrated in this case?
   A. Flat-waist sign
   B. Hilar-overlay sign
   C. Ivory-heart sign
   D. S sign of Golden

3. What tumor is most likely in a young adult with lobar collapse associated with a calcified endobronchial lesion?
   A. Hamartoma
   B. Carcinoid tumor
   C. Adenoid cystic carcinoma
   D. Mucoepidermoid carcinoma
4. Based solely on the presence of postobstructive atelectasis present, what is the correct T (tumor) stage if the underlying lesion were a non–small cell lung cancer (NSCLC)?
   A. T1
   B. T2
   C. T3
   D. T4

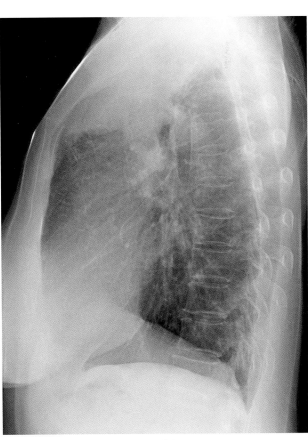

Fig. 70.1   **Fig. 70.2**

Case 71

History: 45-year-old man with history of falling off a ladder one-year ago.

1. Which of the following should be included in the differential diagnosis for this patient? (Choose all that apply.)
   A. Large pleural effusion
   B. Diaphragmatic rupture
   C. Diaphragmatic paralysis
   D. No abnormality
2. What imaging sign is present on the axial computed tomography (CT) images (Figs. 71.1 and 71.2)?
   A. Thoracoabdominal sign
   B. Cobweb sign
   C. Fleischner sign
   D. Dependent viscera sign
3. In diaphragmatic rupture from blunt trauma, what location of injury is most common?
   A. Anterolateral right hemidiaphragm
   B. Anterolateral left hemidiaphragm
   C. Posterolateral right hemidiaphragm
   D. Posterolateral left hemidiaphragm
4. A patient presents with marked elevation of the right hemidiaphragm on radiography after thoracic surgery. What is the most appropriate next imaging modality?
   A. Magnetic resonance imaging (MRI)
   B. CT
   C. Fluoroscopy
   D. Ultrasound

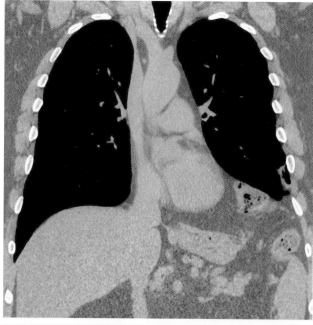

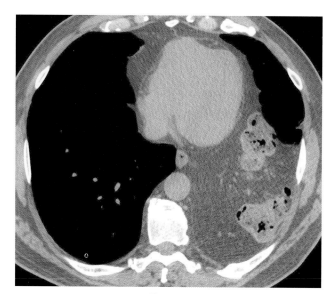

Fig. 71.1

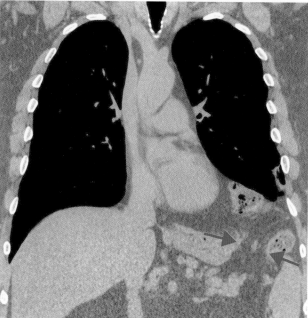

Fig. 71.2

Case 72

History: 38-year-old man with shortness of breath (Figs. 72.1 and 72.2).

1. Which of the following should be included in the differential diagnosis for this patient? (Choose all that apply.)
   A. Left superior vena cava (SVC)
   B. Azygos continuation of the inferior vena cava (IVC)
   C. Partial anomalous pulmonary venous return (PAPVR)
   D. Abnormal left superior intercostal vein
2. Into which vessel do most left-sided SVCs drain?
   A. Right SVC
   B. Hemiazygos vein
   C. Coronary sinus
   D. Right atrium
3. In the setting of right superior PAPVR, what is the most common associated anomaly?
   A. Left SVC
   B. Azygos continuation of the IVC
   C. Atrial septal defect (ASD)
   D. Patent ductus arteriosus (PDA)
4. An unroofed coronary sinus is a type of:
   A. Ventricular septal defect
   B. PAPVR
   C. PDA
   D. ASD

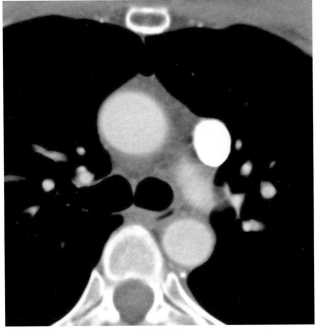

Fig. 72.1

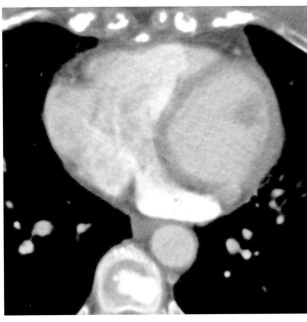

Fig. 72.2

Case 73

History: 56-year-old man with chronic cough (Fig. 73.1).

1. Which of the following should be included in the differential
   diagnosis for this patient? (Choose all that apply.)
   A. Aspiration
   B. Non-tuberculous mycobacterial infection
   C. Primary ciliary dyskinesia
   D. Diffuse panbronchiolitis
2. Which diffuse lung disease is *least* likely to be associated with
   aspiration?
   A. Usual interstitial pneumonitis
   B. Diffuse alveolar damage
   C. Lymphocytic interstitial pneumonitis
   D. Organizing pneumonia
3. Which of the following pulmonary segments is *least* likely to
   be affected by aspiration?
   A. Right upper lobe anterior
   B. Right upper lobe posterior
   C. Right lower lobe superior
   D. Right lower lobe basal posterior
4. Of the listed choices, which is the *least* common sequelae of
   foreign body aspiration?
   A. Pneumothorax
   B. Pneumonia
   C. Atelectasis
   D. Bronchiectasis

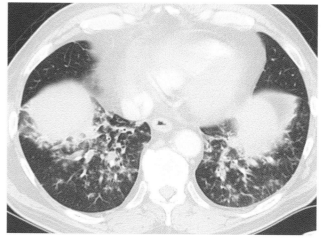

Fig. 73.1

Case 74

History: 48-year-old man with shortness of breath and crackles on physical examination (Figs. 74.1 and 74.2).

1. What is the most likely diagnosis?
   A. Usual interstitial pneumonitis (UIP)
   B. Nonspecific interstitial pneumonitis (NSIP)
   C. Acute interstitial pneumonitis (AIP)
   D. Desquamative interstitial pneumonitis (DIP)
2. Which finding is inconsistent with UIP?
   A. Lower lung zone preponderance
   B. Peripheral lung preponderance
   C. Honeycombing
   D. Predominant ground-glass opacity

3. What is the most specific differentiator of NSIP from UIP?
   A. Upper lung zone distribution
   B. Mid lung zone distribution
   C. Subpleural sparing
   D. Reticulation
4. What is the least common cause of NSIP pattern of lung disease?
   A. Collagen vascular disease
   B. Drugs
   C. Hypersensitivity pneumonitis
   D. Idiopathic

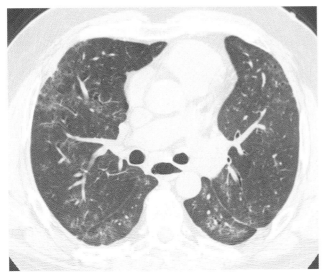

Fig. 74.1

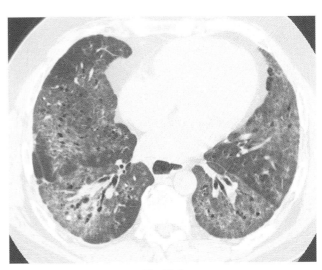

Fig. 74.2

Case 75

History: 42-year-old man with pleuritic chest pain (Fig. 75.1).

1. Which of the following are likely causes of the abnormal aorta? (Choose all that apply).
   A. Atherosclerosis
   B. Hypertension
   C. Marfan syndrome
   D. Ehlers Danlos syndrome
2. What is the size criteria for operative repair in ascending aortic aneurysms?
   A. >2.5 cm
   B. >3.5 cm
   C. >4.5 cm
   D. >5.5 cm
3. Which of the following is *least* often associated with bicuspid aortic valves?
   A. Aortic aneurysm
   B. Intracranial arterial aneurysm
   C. Turner syndrome
   D. Partial anomalous pulmonary venous return
4. There is an enlarged ascending aorta with loss of the normal concave junction between the sinus of Valsalva and tubular ascending aorta. This imaging finding is most specific for which condition?
   A. Syphilis
   B. Marfan syndrome
   C. Bicuspid aortic valve
   D. Atherosclerosis

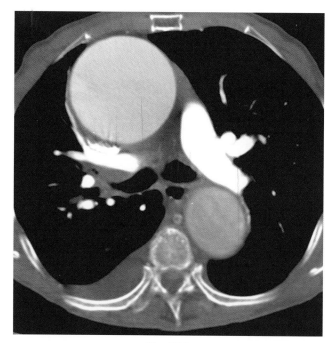

Fig. 75.1

Case 76

History: 30-year-old woman with chronic cough (Figs. 76.1, 76.2 and 76.3).

1. What is the most likely diagnosis?
   A. Small cell carcinoma
   B. Lymphoma
   C. Squamous cell carcinoma
   D. Carcinoid tumor
2. What is the most common benign pulmonary tumor?
   A. Lipoma
   B. Hamartoma
   C. Chondroma
   D. Papilloma
3. What percentage of carcinoid tumors are calcified?
   A. 10%
   B. 20%
   C. 30%
   D. 40%
4. What is a major finding in diffuse idiopathic pulmonary neuroendocrine cell hyperplasia (DIPNECH)?
   A. Consolidation
   B. Fibrosis
   C. Pneumothorax
   D. Air-trapping

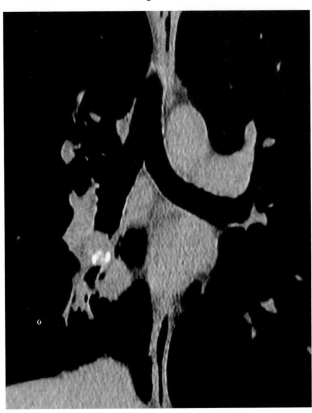

Fig. 76.2

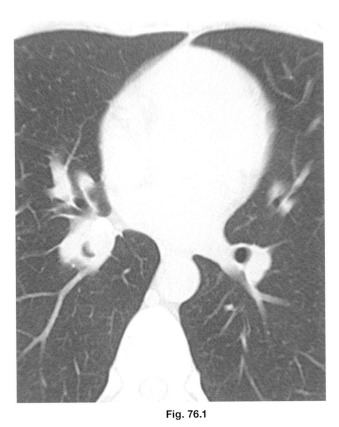

Fig. 76.1

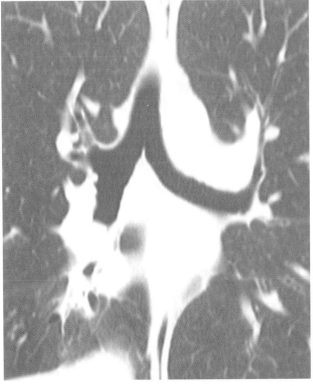

Fig. 76.3

Case 77

History: 58-year-old woman with acute chest pain (Figs. 77.1 and 77.2).

1. Which of the following etiologies should be considered? (Choose all that apply.)
   A. Childbirth
   B. Asthma
   C. Esophageal rupture
   D. Extension of pneumothorax
2. What condition is thought to be related to the development of asthma-related pneumomediastinum?
   A. Pneumothorax
   B. Pulmonary interstitial emphysema
   C. Honeycombing
   D. Centrilobular emphysema
3. In which anatomic area of the esophagus does rupture from vomiting usually occur?
   A. Left mid
   B. Right mid
   C. Right lower
   D. Left lower
4. What is the most serious complication of esophageal rupture?
   A. Pneumonia
   B. Pneumothorax
   C. Mediastinitis
   D. Empyema

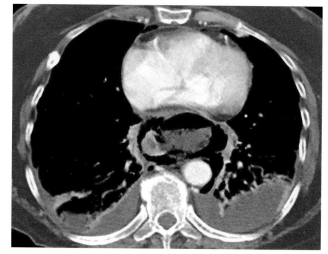

Fig. 77.2

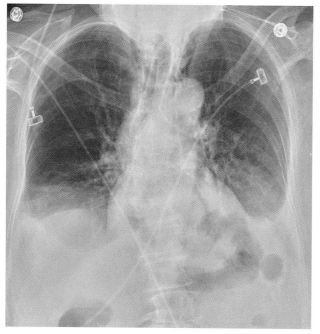

Fig. 77.1

Case 78

History: 67-year-old woman with chronic cough and malaise (Fig. 78.1).

1. Which of the following should be included in the differential diagnosis for this patient? (Choose all that apply.)
   A. Nontuberculous mycobacterial infection
   B. Allergic bronchopulmonary aspergillosis
   C. Cystic fibrosis
   D. Usual interstitial pneumonitis
2. Which computed tomography (CT) postprocessing tool is most helpful in differentiating bronchiectasis from cystic lung disease?
   A. Maximum intensity projection
   B. 3D volume rendering
   C. Surface rendering
   D. Minimum intensity projection
3. Which of the following is not an imaging subtype of bronchiectasis?
   A. Spherical
   B. Varicoid
   C. Cystic
   D. Cylindrical
4. Excluding the pancreas, which is the most frequently involved abdominal organ in cystic fibrosis?
   A. Kidneys
   B. Liver
   C. Spleen
   D. Stomach

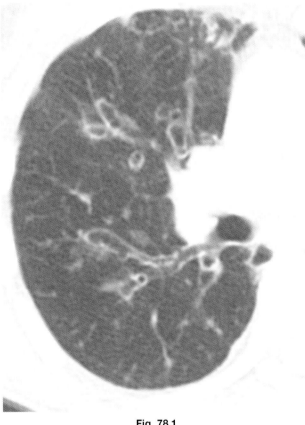

Fig. 78.1

Case 79

History: 43-year-old man with dyspnea.

1. Which of the following should be included in the differential diagnosis for this patient based on the chest radiograph (Fig. 79.1)? (Choose all that apply.)
   A. Pneumothorax
   B. Giant bulla
   C. Poland syndrome
   D. Langerhans cell histocytosis
2. What is the size criterion that distinguishes a bulla from a bleb?
   A. ≥0.5 cm
   B. ≥1 cm
   C. ≥1.5 cm
   D. ≥2 cm
3. Which of the following tests is most sensitive for the detection of early emphysema?
   A. Tomosynthesis
   B. Pulmonary function tests
   C. Hyperpolarized He magnetic resonance imaging (MRI)
   D. Chest computed tomography (CT)
4. Which illicit drug has been associated with basilar predominant panlobular emphysema?
   A. Smoked crack cocaine
   B. Smoked marijuana
   C. Intravenous (IV) heroin
   D. IV Ritalin

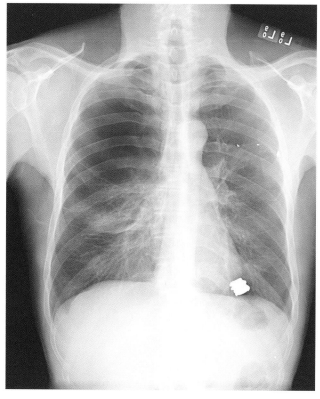

Fig. 79.1

Case 80

History: 61-year-old woman with history of breast cancer (Figs. 80.1 and 80.2).

1. Which is collapsed?
   A. Right upper lobe
   B. Right middle lobe
   C. Right lower lobe
   D. Combined right middle and lower lobes
2. Which bronchus is obstructed?
   A. Right upper lobe bronchus
   B. Right middle lobe bronchus
   C. Bronchus intermedius
   D. Right lower lobe bronchus

3. In a recently intubated patient, what is the most likely cause of complete right lung atelectasis?
   A. Foreign body aspiration
   B. Mucous plugging
   C. Endobronchial tumor
   D. Endotracheal tube misplacement
4. Which of the listed primary tumors are *least* likely to cause central airway metastases?
   A. Melanoma
   B. Renal cell carcinoma
   C. Breast cancer
   D. Hepatocellular carcinoma

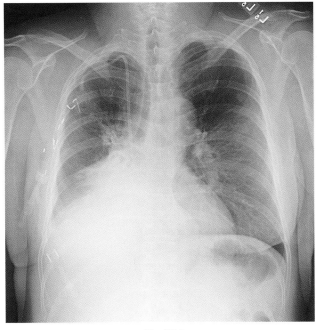

Fig. 80.1

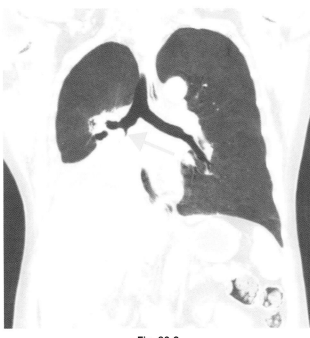

Fig. 80.2

Case 81

History: 41-year-old woman with chest asymmetry on examination (Figs. 81.1, 81.2 and 81.3).

1. Which of the following should be included in the differential diagnosis for this patient? (Choose all that apply.)
   A. Lipoma
   B. Hamartoma
   C. Liposarcoma
   D. Fat necrosis
2. Which of the following material is *not* inherently T1 hyperintense on magnetic resonance imaging (MRI)?
   A. Fat
   B. Melanin
   C. Methemoglobin
   D. Cerebral spinal fluid

3. Which of the follow-up findings is more suggestive of liposarcoma rather than lipoma?
   A. Larger size
   B. Amorphous shape
   C. Greater amount of soft tissue
   D. Greater T2 signal
4. A bilobed fat attenuation mass is noted in the interatrial septum with high fluorodeoxyglucose (FDG) uptake on positron-emission tomography–computed tomography (PET-CT). What is most likely diagnosis?
   A. Teratoma
   B. Liposarcoma
   C. Lipomatous hypertrophy
   D. Thymolipoma

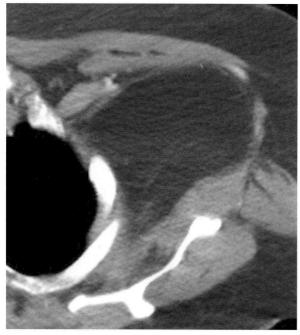

Fig. 81.1

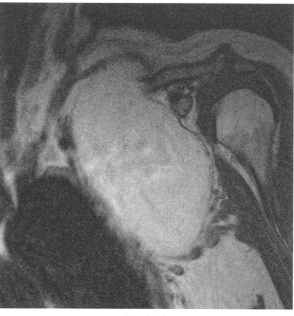

Fig. 81.3

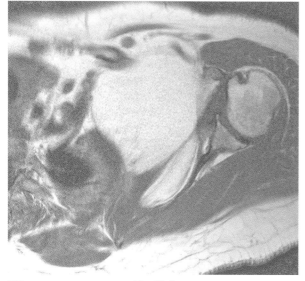

Fig. 81.2

Case 82

History: Found down and unresponsive (Figs. 82.1 and 82.2).

1. Which of the following should be included in the differential diagnosis for this patient? (Choose all that apply.)
   A. Extrapleural hematoma
   B. Pulmonary contusion
   C. Asbestos pleural thickening
   D. Hemothorax
2. Which of the following findings suggest primary lung cancer as the *most likely* cause of a unilateral apical cap?
   A. Hilar lymphadenopathy
   B. Pleural effusion
   C. Bone destruction
   D. Mediastinal widening

3. Which one of the following is the most likely to cause *bilateral* apical caps?
   A. Trauma associated with mediastinal hematoma
   B. Radiation for breast carcinoma
   C. Advancing age
   D. Head and neck carcinoma
4. Which one of the following is the *best next* step in the management of this patient?
   A. Computed tomography (CT)
   B. Magnetic resonance imaging (MRI)
   C. Ultrasound
   D. Fluorodeoxyglucose–positron emission tomography (FDG-PET) (FDG-PET)

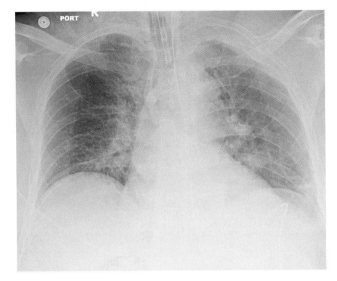

Fig. 82.1

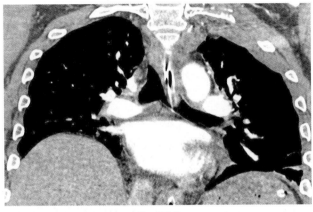

Fig. 82.2

Case 83

History: 35-year-old man with testicular cancer treated with chemotherapy.

1. Which of the following should be included in the differential diagnosis for this patient (Figs. 83.1 and 83.2)? (Choose all that apply.)
   A. Bleomycin lung toxicity
   B. Congestive heart failure
   C. Collagen vascular disease
   D. Fungal pneumonia
2. Approximately what percent of patients receiving bleomycin develop lung toxicity?
   A. < 5%
   B. 15%
   C. 25%
   D. 35%

3. Which one of the following *does not* increase the risk of developing bleomycin-related lung toxicity?
   A. Lymphoma
   B. Concurrent radiation therapy
   C. Renal insufficiency
   D. Advanced age
4. Which one of the following regarding treatment of bleomycin-related lung toxicity is *not* true?
   A. The drug must be discontinued.
   B. Corticosteroids are usually administered.
   C. Most patients improve within a few days.
   D. Some patients take up to 2 years to recover.

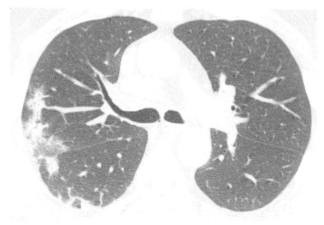

Fig. 83.1

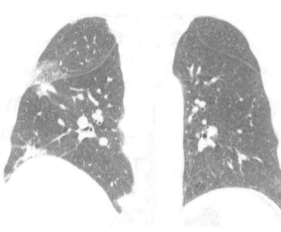

Fig. 83.2

Case 84

History: Hemoptysis.

1. Which of the following should be included in the differential diagnosis for this patient (Figs. 84.1, 84.2 and 84.3)? (Choose all that apply.)
   A. Lung Cancer
   B. Metastatic disease
   C. Silicosis
   D. Tuberculosis
2. Biopsy showed the left upper lobe mass to be primary lung adenocarcinoma. Which one of the following is the likely N staging of this patient based on the most recent tumor, node metastasis (TNM) staging system?
   A. N0
   B. N1
   C. N2
   D. N3

3. Which one of the following regarding lymph node metastases is true?
   A. Ipsilateral axillary lymph node metastases are staged as N3.
   B. N2 disease precludes surgical resection.
   C. Fluorodeoxyglucose–positron emission tomography (FDG-PET) is the standard for lymph node staging.
   D. N2 disease results in a minimal stage of IIIB.
4. Which one of the following findings is a contraindication for resection of non–small cell lung carcinoma?
   A. Chest wall invasion
   B. Tumor metastasis to the same lobe
   C. Ipsilateral pleural metastasis
   D. Post obstructive pneumonia involving the entire lung

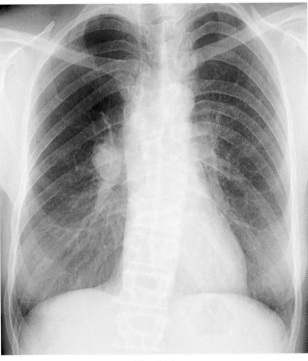

Fig. 84.1

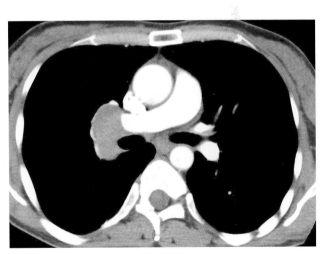

Fig. 84.2

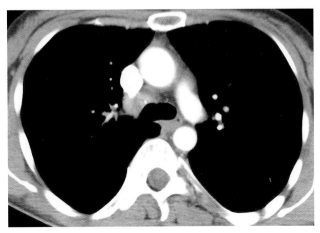

Fig. 84.3

Case 85

History: Swelling of the head and neck.

1. What is the most likely cause of the findings on the computed tomography (CT) scan (Fig. 85.1)?
   A. Superior vena cava syndrome
   B. Arteriovenous malformation
   C. Contrast extravasation
   D. None of the above
2. What is the most common cause of superior vena cava (SVC) syndrome?
   A. Long-term intravenous device
   B. Fibrosing mediastinitis
   C. Lung cancer
   D. Radiation therapy
3. Which one of the following is *not* a common clinical manifestation of SVC syndrome?
   A. Head and face edema
   B. Extremity edema
   C. Visual disturbances
   D. Dural venous sinus thrombosis
4. What is the *best initial treatment* for patients with non–small cell lung carcinoma who present with acute SVC syndrome?
   A. Chemotherapy
   B. Surgical resection
   C. SVC stenting
   D. Radiation therapy

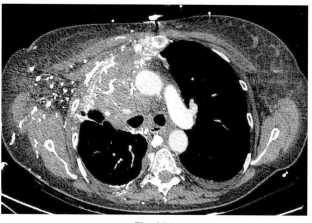

Fig. 85.1

Case 86

History: Acute onset dyspnea and hypoxia.

1. Which of the following should be included in the differential diagnosis for this patient (Figs. 86.1 and 86.2)? (Choose all that apply.)
   A. Pulmonary hemorrhage
   B. Langerhans cell histiocytosis
   C. Diffuse pneumonia
   D. Silicosis
2. What is the most common cause of diffuse alveolar hemorrhage?
   A. Hemophilia
   B. Drug toxicity
   C. Vasculitis
   D. Infection

3. Which of the following has the greatest association with diffuse alveolar hemorrhage?
   A. Granulomatosis with polyangiitis
   B. Microscopic polyangiitis
   C. Eosinophilic granulomatosis with polyangiitis
   D. Takayasu arteritis
4. What procedure best confirms the diagnosis of diffuse alveolar hemorrhage?
   A. Bronchoalveolar lavage
   B. Transbronchial biopsy
   C. Surgical biopsy
   D. Sputum analysis

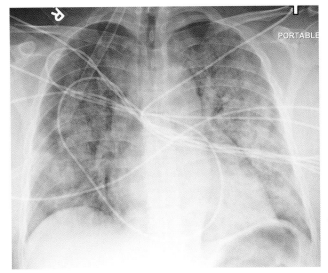

Fig. 86.1

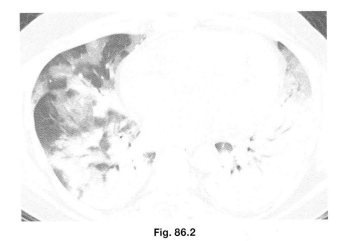

Fig. 86.2

Case 87

History: 72-year-old woman with progressive dyspnea on exertion.

1. Which of the following should be included in the differential diagnosis for this patient (Figs. 87.1, 87.2 and 87.3)? (Choose all that apply.)
   A. Desquamative interstitial pneumonia (DIP)
   B. Usual interstitial pneumonia (UIP)
   C. Nonspecific interstitial pneumonia (NSIP)
   D. Lymphoid interstitial pneumonia (LIP)
2. What is the next best approach to tissue diagnosis?
   A. Surgical lung biopsy
   B. Transbronchial biopsy
   C. Computed tomography (CT) guided needle biopsy
   D. No tissue sampling needed

3. Which of the following collagen vascular diseases has the highest association with usual interstitial pneumonia?
   A. Rheumatoid arthritis
   B. Progressive systemic sclerosis
   C. Polymyositis
   D. Sjögren syndrome
4. Which of the following occupational exposures has a strong association with usual interstitial pneumonia?
   A. Coal
   B. Silica
   C. Beryllium
   D. Asbestos

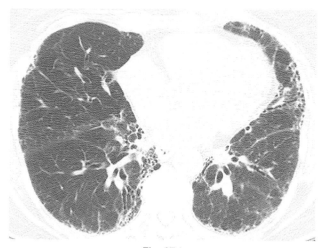

Fig. 87.1

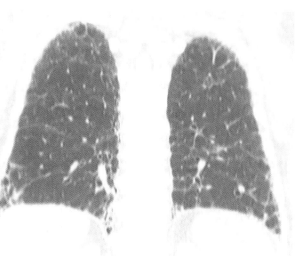

Fig. 87.3

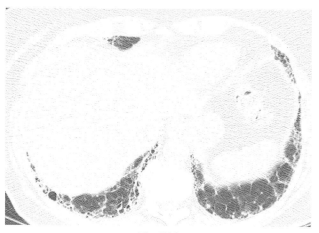

Fig. 87.2

Case 88

History: Chest pain. History of stroke.

1. Which of the following should be included in the differential diagnosis for this patient (Figs. 88.1 and 88.2)? (Choose all that apply.)
   A. Chest wall metastasis
   B. Abscess
   C. Hematoma
   D. Elastofibroma
2. The high-attenuation component of the mass on this computed tomography (CT) scan of a patient on warfarin most likely represents which one of the following?
   A. Tumor
   B. Blood
   C. Calcium
   D. Fat

3. Which one of the following is *not* a potential complication of intramuscular hemorrhage?
   A. Malignant degeneration
   B. Ischemic myopathy
   C. Neuropathy
   D. Pressure necrosis of adjacent bone
4. Which of the following is a common cause of spontaneous intramuscular hematoma?
   A. Aspirin therapy
   B. Intravenous (IV) contrast administration
   C. Vitamin K supplements
   D. Hemophilia

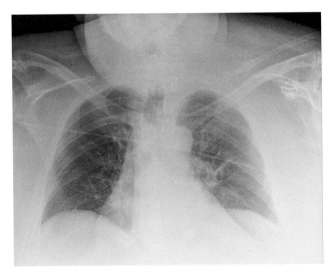

Fig. 88.1

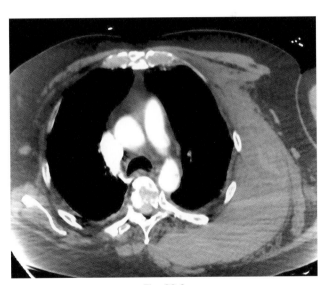

Fig. 88.2

Case 89

History: Occupational screening. Patient is asymptomatic.

1. Which of the following should be included in the differential diagnosis for this patient (Figs. 89.1 and 89.2)? (Choose all that apply.)
   A. Scimitar syndrome
   B. Congenital pulmonary airway malformation
   C. Pulmonary arteriovenous malformation
   D. Bronchial atresia
2. What type of shunt is most likely present?
   A. Left-to-left
   B. Left-to-right
   C. Right-to-right
   D. Right-to-left

3. What other findings are associated with this diagnosis?
   A. Hypoplastic lung with abnormal airway branching
   B. Lung cancer
   C. Kidney agenesis
   D. Muscular dystrophy
4. Which of the following is the best management for this patient?
   A. Right lower lobectomy
   B. Endovascular coiling
   C. Bronchoscopy
   D. Observation

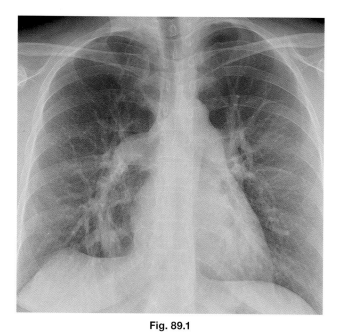

Fig. 89.1

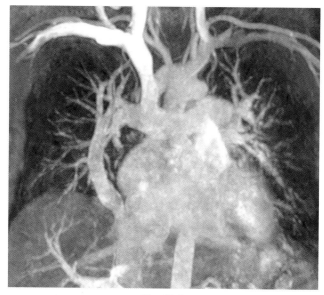

Fig. 89.2

Case 90

History: Chest pain and pericardial rub on auscultation.

1. Which of the following should be included in the differential diagnosis of pericardial effusion (Figs. 90.1, 90.2 and 90.3)? (Choose all that apply.)
   A. Myocardial infarction
   B. Systemic lupus erythematosus
   C. Relapsing polychondritis
   D. Acute pulmonary thromboembolism
2. The lateral view shows (Figs. 90.2) which of the following?
   A. "Oreo cookie sign"
   B. Myocardial fat stripe
   C. Epicardial fat stripe
   D. A and C

3. Which of the following is *most* sensitive for detecting a pericardial effusion?
   A. Chest radiograph
   B. Transthoracic echocardiogram
   C. Cardiac magnetic resonance imaging (MRI)
   D. Transesophageal echocardiogram
4. Which of the following defines Dressler syndrome?
   A. Rheumatoid arthritis-associated pleural and pericardial effusions
   B. Viral myocarditis-related pleural and pericardial effusions
   C. Radiation-induced pleural and pericardial effusions
   D. Myocardial infarction-related pleural and pericardial effusions

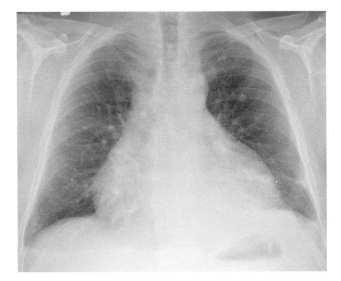

Fig. 90.1

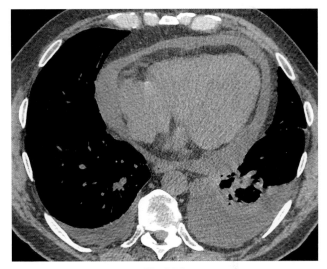

Fig. 90.3

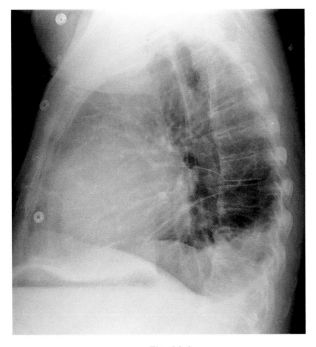

Fig. 90.2

Case 91

History: Chronic cough and recurrent pneumonia.

1. Which of the following should be included in the differential diagnosis for this patient (Figs. 91.1 and 91.2)? (Choose all that apply.)
   A. Ciliary dyskinesia
   B. Allergic bronchopulmonary aspergillosis
   C. Idiopathic pulmonary fibrosis
   D. Lymphangioleiomyomatosis
2. What is the *most common* cause of this abnormality?
   A. Congenital condition
   B. Interstitial pneumonia
   C. Cigarette smoking
   D. Infection

3. Which of the following is *not* a specific sign of bronchiectasis on high-resolution computed tomography (HRCT)?
   A. Bronchial diameter greater than that of the adjacent artery
   B. Lack of normal bronchial tapering
   C. Bronchial wall thickening
   D. Bronchus visible in peripheral 1 cm of lung
4. Which of the following is *not* a complication of bronchiectasis?
   A. Hemoptysis
   B. Atelectasis
   C. Pneumonia
   D. Pleural effusion

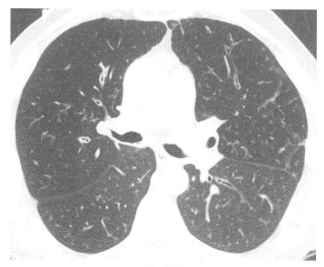

Fig. 91.1

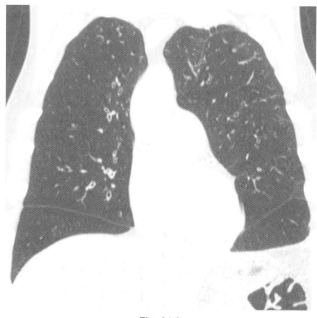

Fig. 91.2

Case 92

History: Dysphagia.

1. Which of the following should be included in the differential diagnosis for this patient (Fig. 92.1)? (Choose all that apply.)
   A. Esophageal duplication cyst
   B. Achalasia
   C. Esophageal diverticulum
   D. Esophageal carcinoma
2. Which one of the following structures is most likely responsible for displacement of the azygoesophageal contour in this patient?
   A. Esophagus
   B. Azygos vein
   C. Right atrium
   D. Left atrium
3. Which one of the following imaging studies would be most helpful for further evaluation of this finding?
   A. Computed tomography (CT) scan
   B. Magnetic resonance imaging (MRI)
   C. Esophagram
   D. Lateral radiograph
4. Which one of the following does not result in a chronically constricted lower esophageal sphincter?
   A. Progressive systemic sclerosis (scleroderma)
   B. Achalasia
   C. Chagas disease
   D. Pseudoachalasia

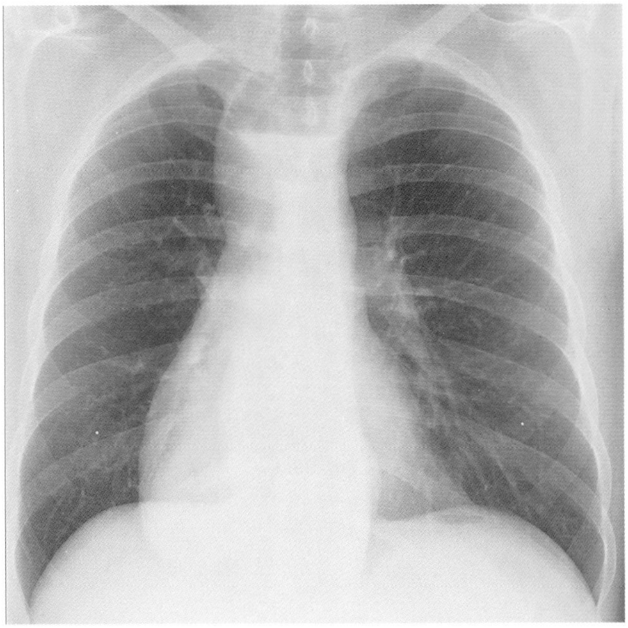

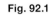

Fig. 92.1

Case 93

History: Cough.

1. Which of the following should be included in the differential diagnosis for this patient (Figs. 93.1 and 93.2)? (Choose all that apply.)
   A. Granulomatosis with polyangiitis
   B. Sarcoidosis
   C. Coccidioidomycosis
   D. Septic infarct
2. In which geographic location is *Coccidioides* endemic?
   A. New England
   B. Mississippi River valley
   C. Pacific Northwest
   D. American Southwest

3. Which one of the following regarding coccidioidomycosis is *true*?
   A. Most affected patients are symptomatic.
   B. Cavities are typical of chronic infection.
   C. Disseminated disease is common.
   D. The pneumonic form requires antifungal therapy.
4. What pattern is most associated with disseminated coccidioidomycosis?
   A. Multifocal lung consolidation
   B. Numerous small nodules
   C. Diffuse ground-glass opacity
   D. Septic pulmonary infarcts

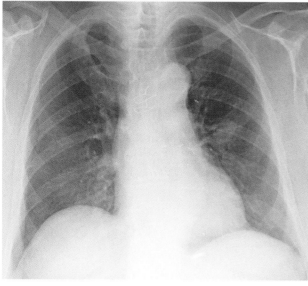

Fig. 93.1

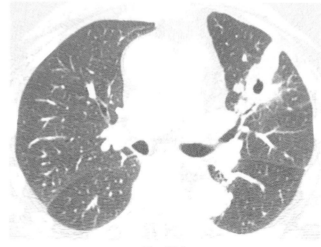

Fig. 93.2

Case 94

History: Dyspnea.

1. Which of the following should be included in the differential diagnosis for this patient (Fig. 94.1)? (Choose all that apply.)
   A. Hydrostatic pulmonary edema
   B. Usual interstitial pneumonia
   C. Lymphangitic carcinomatosis
   D. Sarcoidosis
2. Which one of the following chest radiographic finding correlates with the computed tomography (CT) finding of thickened interlobular septa?
   A. Kerley B lines
   B. Thickened fissures
   C. Bronchovascular bundle thickening
   D. Lung consolidation
3. Which one of the following are required components of high-resolution computed tomography (HRCT) imaging?
   A. Thin collimation (≤1.5 mm)
   B. Prone imaging
   C. Multiplanar reformations
   D. Smoothing reconstruction kernel
4. Which of the following is the best next step in management of this patient in whom congestive heart failure is not suspected?
   A. Fluorodeoxyglucose–positron emission tomography (FDG-PET)
   B. Repeat chest imaging after diuresis
   C. Transbronchial biopsy
   D. Surgical lung biopsy

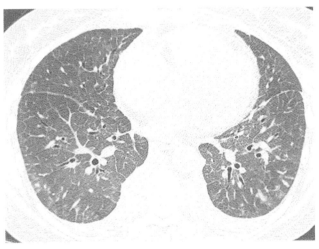

Fig. 94.1

Case 95

History: Chest pain (Figs. 95.1 and 95.2).

1. Based on the lateral chest radiograph (Fig. 95.1), which of the following should be included in the differential diagnosis for this patient? (Choose all that apply.)
   A. Aortic coarctation
   B. Lymphoma
   C. Breast carcinoma
   D. Tuberculosis
2. Which one of the following is the most common site of lymph node metastases in patients with breast carcinoma?
   A. Internal mammary
   B. Axillary
   C. Hilar
   D. Subcarinal

3. True or false? A normal chest radiograph excludes internal mammary lymphadenopathy.
   A. True
   B. False
4. Which type of lymphoma is most commonly associated with neoplastic tissue confined to the anterior mediastinum?
   A. Classical Hodgkin lymphoma
   B. Follicular lymphoma
   C. Diffuse large B cell lymphoma
   D. Small lymphocytic lymphoma

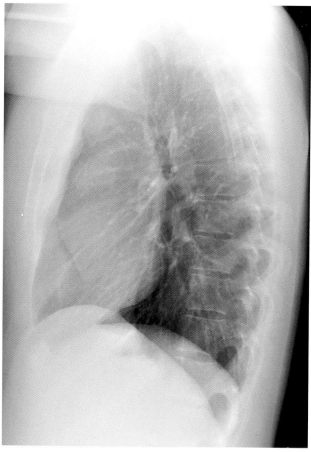

Fig. 95.1

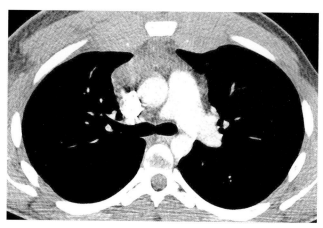

Fig. 95.2

Case 96

History: Lung nodule (Fig. 96.1).

1. Which of the following is the greatest risk factor for developing pneumothorax as a result of needle biopsy?
   A. Older age
   B. Emphysema
   C. Lower lobe location
   D. Subpleural location
2. What is the sensitivity of transthoracic needle biopsy (TTNB) for *malignant* nodules?
   A. 50%
   B. 70%
   C. 80%
   D. >90%

3. Which one of the following is the most common complication of TTNB?
   A. Hemoptysis
   B. Pneumothorax
   C. Air embolism
   D. Seeding of biopsy track
4. Which one of the following improves the diagnostic yield of TTNB for *benign* lesions?
   A. Use two needles to increase volume of aspirate.
   B. Have a cytopathologist on-site.
   C. Use a cutting needle to obtain core needle biopsy specimens.
   D. Use CT fluoroscopy.

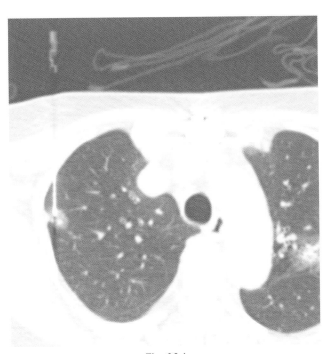

Fig. 96.1

Case 97

History: Abnormal chest radiograph.

1. Which of the following should be included in the differential diagnosis for this patient (Figs. 97.1 and 97.2)? (Choose all that apply.)
   A. Carcinoid tumor
   B. Constrictive bronchiolitis
   C. Bronchial atresia
   D. Lung abscess
2. What allows aeration of lung distal to a bronchocele?
   A. Bronchopleural fistula
   B. Incomplete obstruction
   C. Anomalous bronchus
   D. Collateral air flow through adjacent lung
3. What is the most common site of bronchial atresia?
   A. Left upper lobe
   B. Left lower lobe
   C. Right upper lobe
   D. Right lower lobe
4. Which of the following is the best treatment for bronchial atresia?
   A. Surgical resection
   B. Endobronchial stenting
   C. Observation
   D. Endobronchial laser ablation

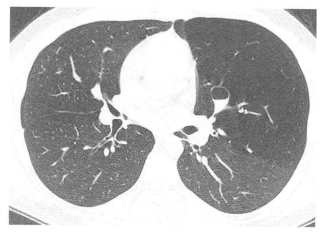

Fig. 97.1

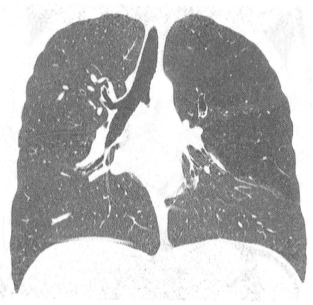

Fig. 97.2

Case 98

History: Dyspnea on exertion and intermittent fever.

1. Which of the following should be included in the differential diagnosis for this patient (Figs. 98.1 and 98.2)? (Choose all that apply.)
   A. Sarcoidosis
   B. Silicosis
   C. Hypersensitivity pneumonitis
   D. Respiratory bronchiolitis

2. What anatomic structures are located in the central core of the pulmonary lobule?
   A. Pulmonary artery and vein
   B. Pulmonary artery and bronchiole
   C. Pulmonary vein and bronchiole
   D. Pulmonary vein and lymphatics

3. Which of the following *is not* associated with cigarette smoking?
   A. Respiratory bronchiolitis
   B. Pulmonary Langerhans cell histiocytosis
   C. Desquamative interstitial pneumonia
   D. Chronic eosinophilic pneumonia

4. Which type of immunologic reaction is most strongly associated with hypersensitivity pneumonitis?
   A. Type 1 (IgE mediated)
   B. Type 2 (cytotoxic: IgG or IgM mediated)
   C. Type 3 (immune complex)
   D. Type 4 (delayed-type hypersensitivity)

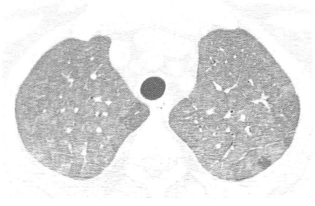

Fig. 98.1

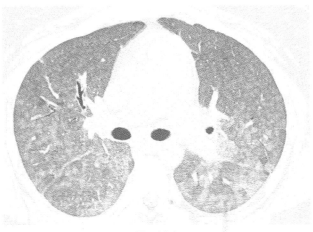

Fig. 98.2

Case 99

History: Baseline lung cancer screening.

1. Which of the following should be included in the differential diagnosis for this patient (Fig. 99.1)? (Choose all that apply.)
   A. Lung carcinoma
   B. Metastasis
   C. Granuloma
   D. Streptococcal pneumonia
2. What is the appropriate Lung-RADS category for this patient?
   A. Lung-RADS 1
   B. Lung-RADS 2
   C. Lung-RADS 3
   D. Lung-RADS 4a

3. What is the next best management?
   A. Computed tomography (CT) follow-up in 6 months
   B. Fluorodeoxyglucose–positron emission tomography (FDG-PET)/CT
   C. Transthoracic needle biopsy
   D. Resection
4. What is the probability that this nodule is malignant?
   A. <5%
   B. 5% to 10%
   C. 11% to 20%
   D. >20%

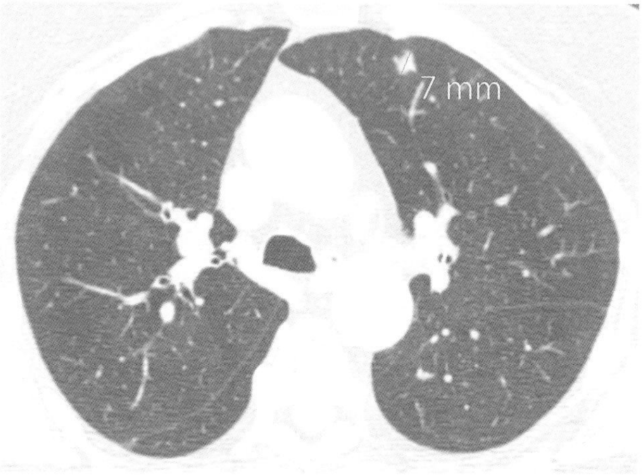

Fig. 99.1

Case 100

History: Stridor and cough.

1. Which of the following should be included in the differential diagnosis for this patient (Figs. 100.1 and 100.2)? (Choose all that apply.)
   A. Double aortic arch
   B. Previous intubation
   C. Granulomatosis with polyangiitis
   D. Mounier-Kuhn syndrome
2. Which of the following *is not* a risk factor for tracheal stenosis?
   A. Prolonged intubation
   B. Tracheostomy
   C. Balloon cuff overdistention
   D. Tracheal bronchus
3. Which of the following causes of tracheal stenosis characteristically *spares* the posterior tracheal wall?
   A. Relapsing polychondritis
   B. Inflammatory bowel disease
   C. Granulomatosis with polyangiitis
   D. Amyloidosis
4. Which of the following is *the least* common sign or symptom of central airway stenosis?
   A. Cough
   B. Stridor
   C. Wheeze
   D. Hemoptysis

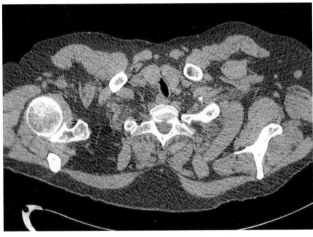

Fig. 100.1

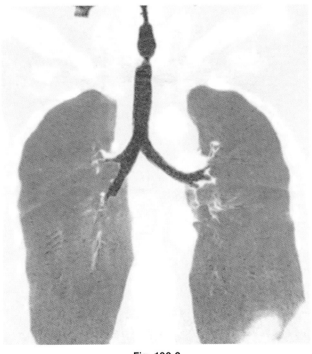

Fig. 100.2

Case 101

History: Fatigue.

1. Based on the computed tomography (CT) image (Fig. 101.1), which of the following should be included in the differential diagnosis for this patient? (Choose all that apply.)
   A. Thymoma
   B. Thymolipoma
   C. Thymic hyperplasia
   D. Thymic cyst
2. Which of the following CT attenuation values is *not* typical of normal thymus?
   A. Soft tissue
   B. Fat and soft tissue
   C. Fatty replacement
   D. Calcification

3. Pure red cell aplasia is most commonly associated with which of the following thymic lesions?
   A. Thymic carcinoma
   B. Thymoma
   C. Thymic carcinoid
   D. Thymolipoma
4. Which imaging examination is most useful for distinguishing thymic hyperplasia from thymic neoplasia?
   A. Fluorodeoxyglucose–positron emission tomography (FDG-PET)/CT
   B. Magnetic resonance imaging
   C. Contrast-enhanced CT
   D. Gallium scan

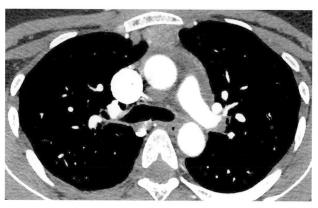

Fig. 101.1

Case 102

History: Cough.

1. Which of the following should be included in the differential diagnosis for this patient (Fig. 102.1)? (Choose all that apply.)
   A. Respiratory bronchiolitis
   B. Focal fibrosis
   C. Lung carcinoma
   D. Histoplasmoma

2. For nodules smaller than 10 mm, which of the following is *most likely* to be malignant?
   A. Solid nodule
   B. Ground-glass nodule
   C. Solid and ground-glass nodule
   D. Calcified nodule

3. What type of lung cancer most commonly presents as a ground-glass attenuation or part solid nodule?
   A. Adenocarcinoma
   B. Squamous cell carcinoma
   C. Small cell carcinoma
   D. Large cell carcinoma

4. Which of the following is the next best step in the follow-up of this patient?
   A. Fluorodeoxyglucose–positron emission tomography (FDG-PET)/CT
   B. Follow-up computed tomography (CT)
   C. Left upper lobectomy
   D. Bronchoscopy

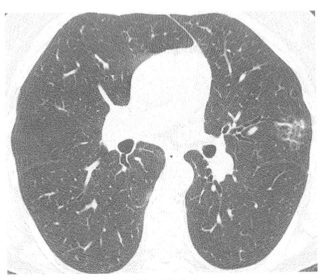

Fig. 102.1

Case 103

History: Patient with chronic cough and an abnormality on chest radiography.

1. What should be included in the differential diagnosis of the imaging abnormalities (Figs. 103.1 and 103.2)? (Choose all that apply.)
   A. Pulmonary edema
   B. *Pneumocystic jirovecii* pneumonia
   C. Diffuse alveolar hemorrhage
   D. Diffuse alveolar damage
   E. Pulmonary alveolar proteinosis
2. What is the most likely diagnosis in this case?
   A. Pulmonary edema
   B. *Pneumocystic jirovecii* pneumonia
   C. Diffuse alveolar hemorrhage
   D. Diffuse alveolar damage
   E. Pulmonary alveolar proteinosis
3. What computed tomography (CT) sign is demonstrated?
   A. Signet ring
   B. Crazy-paving
   C. Comet tail
   D. CT halo
   E. Reverse CT halo
4. What clinical information would support the diagnosis?
   A. Female sex
   B. Intravenous (IV) drug abuse
   C. Chronicity
   D. Immunosuppression

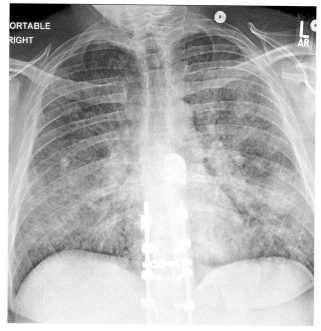

Fig. 103.1

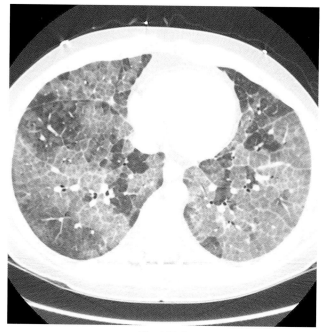

Fig. 103.2

Case 104

History: Patient with asthma and an abnormality on chest radiography (Fig. 104.1).

1. What imaging sign is demonstrated (Figs. 104.1 and 104.2)?
   A. Signet ring
   B. Crazy-paving
   C. Finger-in-glove
   D. Computed tomography (CT) halo
   E. Reverse CT halo
2. Which of the following organisms is often implicated in this condition?
   A. Human papillomavirus type 6
   B. *Mycobacterium tuberculosis*
   C. *Staphylococcus aureus*
   D. *Aspergillus fumigatus*
3. Patients with which of the following diseases are predisposed to develop this condition?
   A. Tracheobronchopathia osteochondroplastica
   B. Primary lung cancer
   C. Cystic fibrosis
   D. Carcinoid tumor
4. What clinical information would support the diagnosis?
   A. Recurrent aspiration
   B. Asthma
   C. Smoking
   D. Immunosuppression

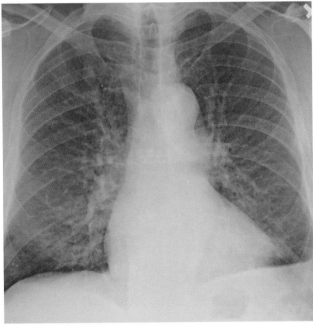

Fig. 104.1

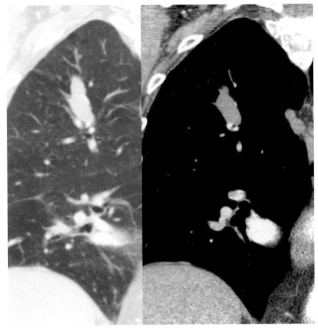

Fig. 104.2

Case 105

History: 60-year-old woman with cough and dyspnea.

1. What is the salient radiographic abnormality (Fig. 105.1)?
   A. Right-sided pneumothorax
   B. Left lower lobe pneumonia
   C. Left upper lobe atelectasis
   D. Left pneumonectomy
2. What is the most likely cause of the branching low-attenuation opacities within the collapsed left upper lobe (Fig. 105.2)?
   A. Obstruction by tumor
   B. Bronchial atresia
   C. Allergic bronchopulmonary aspergillosis
   D. Cystic fibrosis

3. Which of the following would favor a benign cause for the computed tomography (CT) findings?
   A. Smoking history
   B. Hemoptysis
   C. Enhancing mass
   D. Mediastinal infiltration
   E. Macroscopic fat and calcium

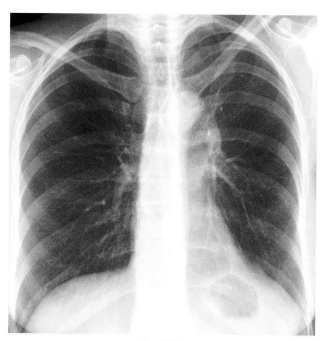

Fig. 105.1

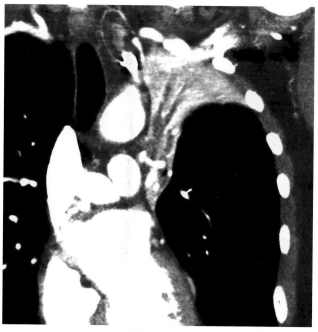

Fig. 105.2

Case 106

History: 22-year-old female with abnormality on chest radiograph.

1. In which anatomic compartment is the lesion arising (Figs. 106.1 and 106.2)?
   A. Parenchyma
   B. Pleura
   C. Chest wall
   D. Lymphatics
2. Which of the following imaging features may help determine lesion location?
   A. Ipsilateral pleural effusion
   B. Obtuse angles with parenchyma
   C. Chest wall invasion
   D. Rib erosion
3. Which of the following extrathoracic manifestations might occur in conjunction with this lesion?
   A. Digital clubbing
   B. Hypertrophic osteoarthropathy
   C. Episodic hypoglycemia
   D. Galactorrhea
   E. All of the above
4. Which of the following reflects typical magnetic resonance imaging (MRI) features of small, uncomplicated lesions with this histology?
   A. Hyperintense signal on T1- and T2-weighted images, no enhancement
   B. Heterogeneous signal on T1- and T2-weighted images, no enhancement
   C. Hypointense signal on T1- and T2-weighted images, no enhancement
   D. Hypointense signal on T1- and T2-weighted images, progressive enhancement

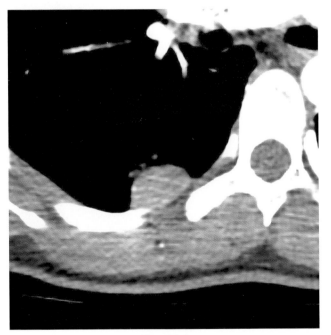

Fig. 106.1

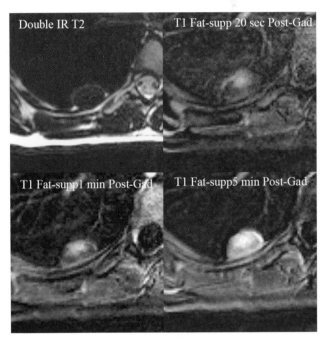

Fig. 106.2

Case 107

History: 85-year-old man with weight loss undergoes outpatient evaluation.

1. What is the most likely cause of this radiographic abnormality (Fig. 107.1)?
   A. Right-sided pneumothorax
   B. Left pleural effusion
   C. Left lung collapse
   D. Left pneumonectomy
2. Which of the following would be the most likely cause for this pattern in an intubated patient in the intensive care unit?
   A. Left-sided infusothorax
   B. Left lung re-expansion edema
   C. Left lung hemorrhage
   D. Left main bronchus mucus plug
3. What term is applied to the preservation of enhancing vessels within the collapsed lung (Figs. 107.2 and 107.3)?
   A. Computed tomography (CT) halo sign
   B. Air bronchogram sign
   C. CT angiogram sign
   D. Juxtaphrenic peak sign
4. Which of the following would raise suspicion for a malignant etiology of the abnormality? (Choose all that apply.)
   A. Smoking history
   B. Weight loss
   C. Age of 85
   D. Outpatient setting
   E. Lymphadenopathy

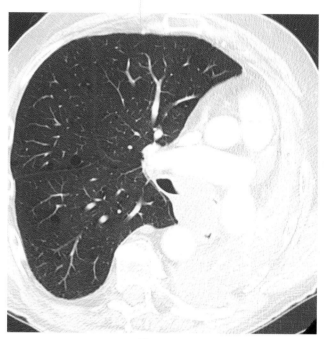

Fig. 107.2

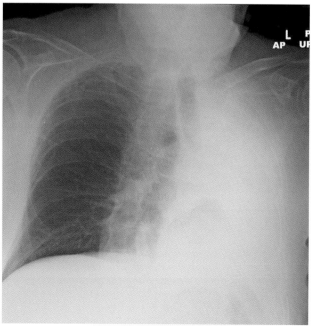

Fig. 107.1

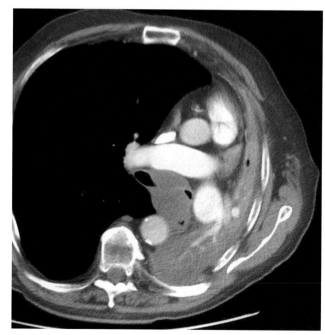

Fig. 107.3

Case 108

History: 79-year-old female never smoker with chronic cough.

1. In which anatomic compartment is the computed tomography (CT) abnormality predominantly located (Fig. 108.1)?
   A. Trachea
   B. Bronchi
   C. Parenchyma
   D. Lymphatics
2. Which organism is most likely responsible for the clinical and imaging abnormalities?
   A. Influenza-A
   B. Mucormycosis
   C. *Aspergillus fumigatus*
   D. *Mycobacterium avium complex* (MAC)
3. Which form of this disease is most likely in this case?
   A. Cavitary (classic)
   B. Bronchiectatic (non-classic)
   C. Immunocompromised host
   D. Nodular
   E. Hypersensitivity

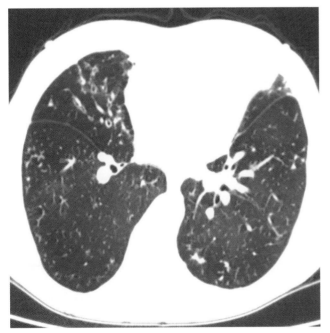

Fig. 108.1

Case 109

History: 47-year-old asymptomatic man.

1. Which of the following best describes the pattern of nodules shown (Figs. 109.1 and 109.2)?
   A. Random, diffuse
   B. Centrilobular, branching
   C. Centrilobular, non-branching
   D. Perilymphatic
2. Which of the following should be included in the differential diagnosis for this pattern?
   A. Sarcoidosis
   B. Lymphangitic carcinomatosis
   C. Silicosis
   D. Lymphoma
   E. Miliary tuberculosis

3. Which term is used to describe computed tomography (CT) finding of confluent perilymphatic sarcoid granulomas organized into a focal nodule with surrounding smaller nodules and reticulation?
   A. Comet tail sign
   B. Mosaic attenuation
   C. Reverse CT halo sign
   D. Galaxy sign
4. Which is the most common clinical presentation of patients with this disease?
   A. Asymptomatic
   B. Bird fancier with chronic cough
   C. Profound weight loss
   D. History of malignancy

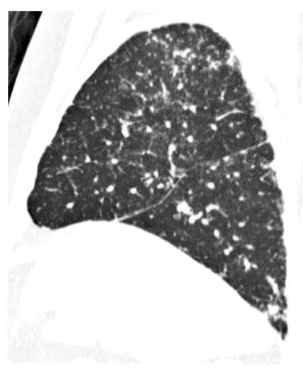

Fig. 109.1

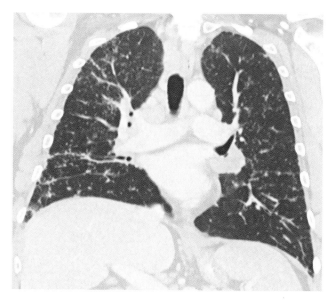

Fig. 109.2

Case 110

History: 22-year-old male presents with cough and fever.

1. Which computed tomography (CT) pattern is shown (Fig. 110.1)?
   A. Interstitial
   B. Centrilobular, nonbranching
   C. Centrilobular, branching
   D. Perilymphatic
2. Which anatomic structure(s) may be abnormal?
   A. Alveolar septae
   B. Interlobular septae
   C. Centrilobular arteriole
   D. Centrilobular bronchiole

3. What is the most common cause of this imaging pattern?
   A. Infectious bronchiolitis
   B. Aspiration bronchiolitis
   C. Diffuse panbronchiolitis
   D. Excipient lung disease
   E. Cellulose granulomatosis

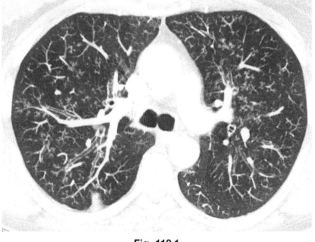

Fig. 110.1

Case 111

History: 42-year-old male with chronic cough.

1. Which computed tomography (CT) pattern is shown (Fig. 111.1)? (Choose all that apply.)
   A. Crazy paving
   B. Mosaic attenuation
   C. Air trapping
   D. Tree-in-bud
2. Which anatomic structure may be abnormal? (Choose all that apply.)
   A. Alveolar septae
   B. Interlobular septae
   C. Centrilobular arteriole
   D. Centrilobular bronchiole
3. What is the most common cause of this imaging pattern?
   A. Infectious bronchiolitis
   B. Aspiration bronchiolitis
   C. Diffuse panbronchiolitis
   D. Excipient lung disease
   E. Chronic thromboembolism

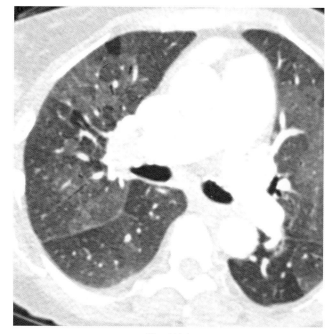

Fig. 111.1

Case 112

History: 90-year-old male former lightbulb assembly worker with dyspnea.

1. Which indirect sign(s) of volume loss are demonstrated on the radiographs (Figs. 112.1 and 112.2)? (Choose all that apply.)
   A. Superior hilar displacement
   B. Increased retrosternal clear space
   C. Juxtaphrenic peak
   D. Reticulonodular opacities
2. What is the primary distribution of abnormality?
   A. Upper lung zone
   B. Lower lung zone
   C. Diffuse
   D. Subpleural
3. Which of the following should be included in the differential diagnosis? (Choose all that apply.)
   A. Tuberculosis
   B. Chronic (cluster 2) hypersensitivity pneumonitis
   C. Sarcoidosis (stage IV)
   D. Coal worker's pneumoconiosis
   E. Silicosis
4. Which descriptor is given for the lymph node calcifications (Fig. 112.3)?
   A. Popcorn
   B. Toothpaste
   C. Stippled
   D. Onion skin
   E. Egg shell

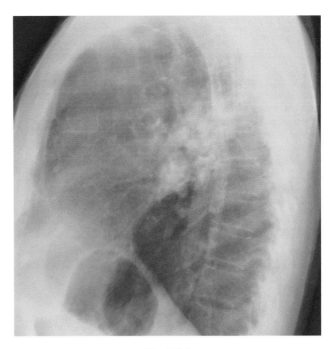

Fig. 112.2

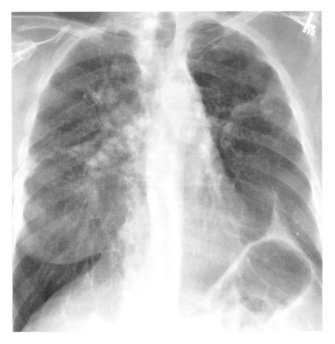

Fig. 112.1

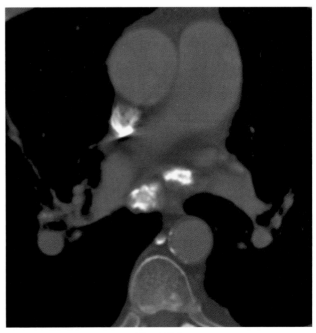

Fig. 112.3

Case 113

History: 56-year-old woman asthmatic patient with fevers and cough (Figs. 113.1, 113.2 and 113.3).

1. Which entities may manifest with a peripheral consolidation pattern? (Choose all that apply.)
   A. Cryptogenic organizing pneumonia
   B. Chronic eosinophilic pneumonia
   C. Granulomatosis with polyangiitis
   D. Pulmonary infarcts
   E. Simple pulmonary eosinophilia
2. Which cell type is implicated in this disorder?
   A. Neutrophil
   B. Erythrocyte
   C. Langerhans cell
   D. Eosinophil
3. More than 50% of patients with this disorder will have what associated condition?
   A. Rheumatoid arthritis
   B. Takayasu arteritis
   C. Asthma
   D. Sarcoidosis
4. What is the most appropriate treatment for the airspace opacities in this condition?
   A. Doxycycline
   B. Oseltamivir
   C. Corticosteroids
   D. Pembrolizumab
   E. Montelukast

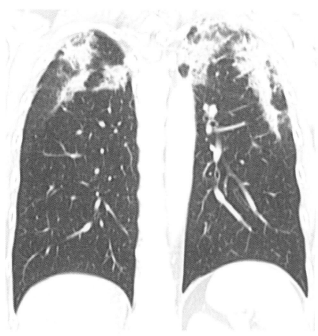

Fig. 113.2

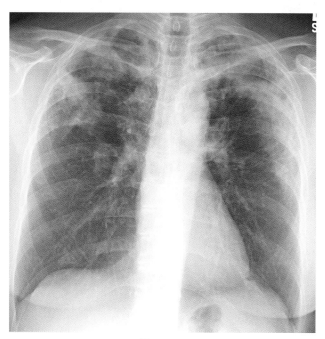

Fig. 113.1

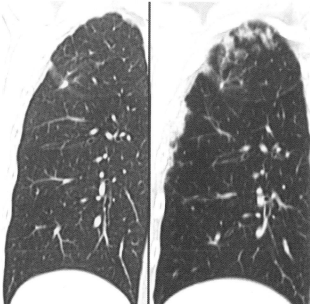

5 months after treatment   8 months after treatment

Fig. 113.3

Case 114

History: 77-year-old man with chronic obstructive pulmonary disease (COPD) and incidental finding on computed tomography (CT).

1. What is the salient CT abnormality (Fig. 114.1)?
   A. Tracheal diverticulum
   B. Apical paraseptal emphysema
   C. Tracheal rupture
   D. Pneumomediastinum
2. What is the most common location of this finding?
   A. Left paratracheal, T1-T2
   B. Left paratracheal, T10-T11
   C. Right paratracheal, T1-T2
   D. Right paratracheal, T10-T11
3. With which clinical scenario is this finding most commonly associated?
   A. Recurrent aspiration
   B. Reduced forced expiratory volume/forced vital capacity (FEV1/FVC) ratio
   C. Smoking
   D. Histoplasmosis infection

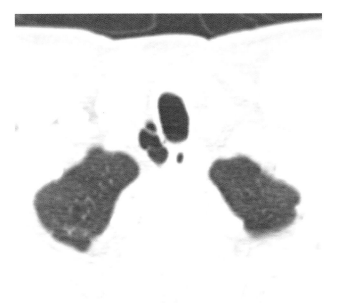

114.1

Case 115

History: 66-year-old man undergoing standard postoperative evaluation after coronary artery bypass.

1. What is the salient radiographic abnormality (Figs. 115.1 and 115.2)?
   A. Sternal wire fracture
   B. Sternal wire unraveling
   C. Sternal wire displacement
   D. Mediastinal hematoma
2. The detection of "wandering wires" implies what underlying sternotomy complication?
   A. Sternal hematoma
   B. Mediastinitis
   C. Sternal dehiscence
   D. Sternal non-union

3. During which postoperative time period may this complication be detected?
   A. First week
   B. First month
   C. 6 months to 1 year
   D. Greater than 1 year
   E. Any
4. Which of the following may increase the risk for this complication?
   A. Reoperation
   B. Internal mammary bypass graft
   C. Diabetes mellitus
   D. Chronic obstructive pulmonary disease
   E. All of the above

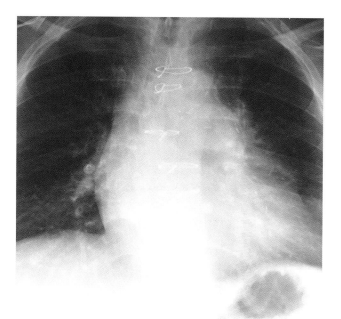

Fig. 115.1

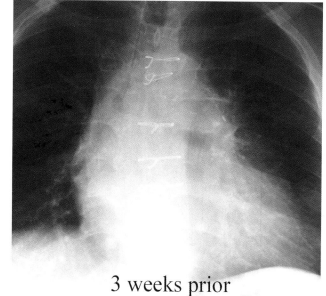

3 weeks prior

Fig. 115.2

Case 116

History: 61-year-old male with prior tonsillar abscess and worsening fevers.

1. What is the concerning abnormality depicted on computed tomography (CT) (Figs. 116.1 and 116.2)?
   A. Malpositioned endotracheal tube
   B. Malpositioned enteric tube
   C. Mediastinal fat inflammation
   D. Aortic dissection
2. Which of the following are potential causes for the imaging findings? (Choose all that apply.)
   A. Sternal osteomyelitis
   B. Mediastinal hemorrhage
   C. Mediastinal radiation
   D. Esophageal perforation
   E. Retropharyngeal infection
3. What is the most likely diagnosis?
   A. Post-traumatic mediastinal hemorrhage
   B. Diffuse lymphangiomatosis
   C. Acute descending mediastinitis, retropharyngeal extension
   D. Acute mediastinitis after median sternotomy
   E. Acute mediastinitis after esophageal trauma

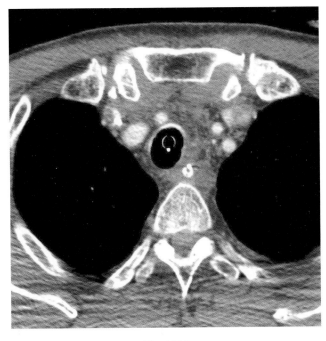

Fig. 116.1

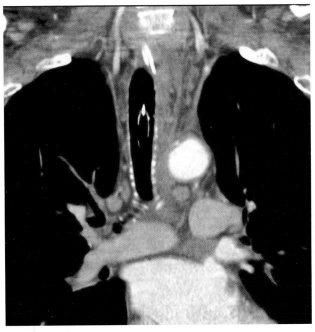

Fig. 116.2

Case 117

History: 56-year-old otherwise healthy, afebrile woman with cough.

1. What is the distribution of the parenchymal abnormalities in the first image (Fig. 117.1)?
   A. Peribronchovascular, focal
   B. Peripheral, focal
   C. Peribronchovascular, diffuse
   D. Peripheral, diffuse
2. What imaging sign is demonstrated in the second image after the patient was treated with corticosteroids (Fig. 117.2)?
   A. Computed tomography (CT) halo sign
   B. Reverse CT halo sign
   C. Air bronchogram sign
   D. Random

3. What is the most likely diagnosis in this case?
   A. Bacterial pneumonia
   B. Aspiration pneumonia
   C. Pulmonary infarcts
   D. Cryptogenic organizing pneumonia
   E. Multifocal mucinous adenocarcinoma
4. What clinical entities may be associated with this imaging pattern? (Choose all that apply.)
   A. Drug reaction
   B. Collage vascular disorders
   C. Vasculitis
   D. Aspiration pneumonia
   E. Eosinophilic pneumonia

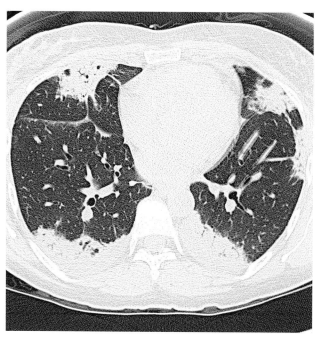

Fig. 117.1

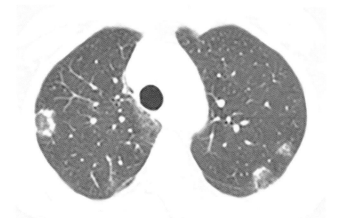

Fig.117.2

Case 118

History: 53-year-old male with history of asthma, restrictive cardiomyopathy, and incidental finding on chest computed tomography (CT) (Fig. 118.1).

1. What of the following entities affect only the cartilaginous portions of the tracheal wall?
   A. Relapsing polychondritis
   B. Tracheobronchopathia osteochondroplastica
   C. Granulomatosis with polyangiitis
   D. Chondrosarcoma
   E. Amyloidosis
2. What is a possible complication of this condition?
   A. Hemoptysis
   B. Reduced diffusing capacity for carbon monoxide (DLCO)
   C. Swelling of ears
   D. Protein-losing enteropathy
3. What is the histopathologic abnormality?
   A. Submucosal deposition of abnormal protein
   B. Cartilage inflammation and destruction
   C. Necrotizing granulomatosis vasculitis
   D. Non-caseating granulomas in airway wall
4. What is the most likely diagnosis in this case?
   A. Tracheobronchial amyloidosis
   B. Relapsing polychondritis
   C. Granulomatosis with polyangiitis
   D. Adenoid cystic carcinoma
   E. Endobronchial metastases

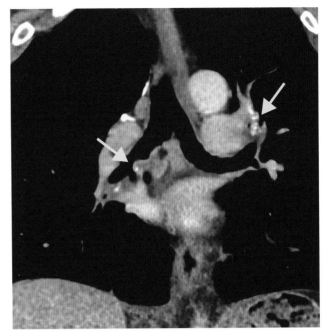

Fig. 118.1

Case 119

History: 43-year-old otherwise healthy man with recurrent episodes of dyspnea (Figs. 119.1 and 119.2).

1. What should be included in the differential diagnosis for a unilateral hyperlucent hemithorax? (Choose all that apply.)
   A. Pneumothorax
   B. Mastectomy
   C. Endobronchial obstruction
   D. Bronchial atresia
   E. Fibrosing mediastinitis
2. What is the most likely underlying pathophysiology of the imaging findings in this case?
   A. Autosomal recessive mutation in cystic fibrosis transmembrane conductance regulator (CFTR) gene
   B. X-linked agammaglobulinemia
   C. Constrictive bronchiolitis, post-infectious
   D. Constrictive bronchiolitis, transplant-related
3. Which feature of clinical history is typically associated with these findings?
   A. Acute chest pain
   B. Childhood viral bronchiolitis
   C. Chest wall radiation
   D. Inhabitation of Ohio River Valley
4. By which eponym is this condition known?
   A. Poland syndrome
   B. Swyer-James-MacLeod syndrome
   C. Westermark
   D. Williams-Campbell

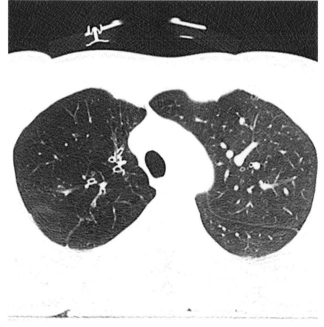

Fig. 119.1

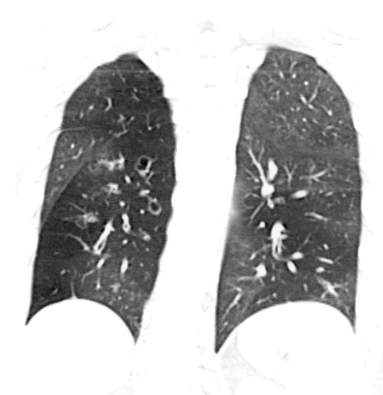

Fig. 119.2

Case 120

History: 53-year-old woman with remote history of hysterectomy.

1. Based on the chest radiographic findings (Fig. 120.1), what is the distribution pattern of the pulmonary nodules?
   A. Peripheral predominant
   B. Upper lung zone predominant
   C. Lower lung zone predominant
   D. Central predominant
2. What is the anatomic distribution of nodules on the corresponding computed tomography (CT) (Fig. 120.2)?
   A. Centrilobular, branching
   B. Centrilobular, non-branching

C. Perilymphatic
D. Random
3. What is the most common cause of this imaging pattern?
   A. Hematogenous metastases
   B. Lymphatic metastases
   C. Aspiration bronchiolitis
   D. Respiratory bronchiolitis
   E. Excipient lung disease

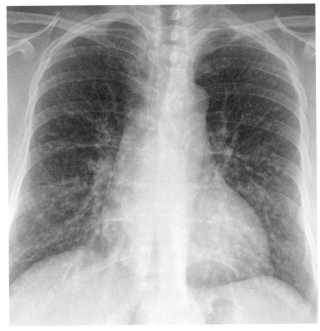

Fig. 120.1

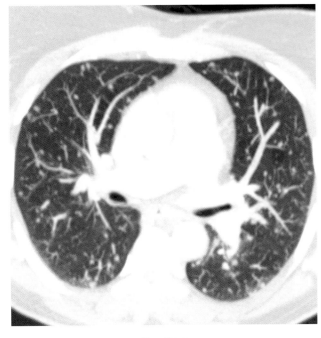

Fig. 120.2

Case 121

History: 68-year-old man with crackles on auscultation (Figs. 121.1 and 121.2).

1. What is the best diagnosis?
   A. Idiopathic pulmonary fibrosis
   B. Asbestosis
   C. Hypersensitivity pneumonitis (HP)
   D. Sarcoidosis
2. What proportion of usual interstitial pneumonia (UIP) cases can be confidently diagnosed solely on chest computed tomography (CT)?
   A. 20%
   B. 30%
   C. 50%
   D. 70%

3. What is the most helpful findings in differentiating fibrotic HP from UIP and nonspecific interstitial pneumonitis (NSIP)?
   A. Subpleural sparing
   B. Basilar sparing
   C. Reticulation
   D. Traction bronchiectasis
4. Which of the following features occurs with equal frequency in chronic beryllium disease and sarcoidosis?
   A. Isolated lymphadenopathy
   B. Pulmonary nodularity
   C. Pulmonary fibrosis
   D. Airway involvement

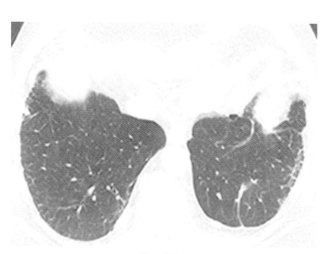

Fig. 121.1

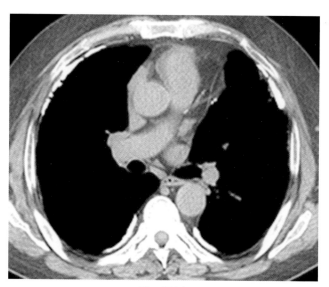

Fig. 121.2

Case 122

History: 45-year-old woman with chronic cough and sputum production.

1. What is the best diagnosis (Figs. 122.1 and 122.2)?
   A. Mounier-Kuhn syndrome
   B. Tracheomalacia
   C. Tracheobronchopathia osteochondroplastica
   D. Relapsing polychondritis
2. Which of the following is not a common finding in Mounier-Kuhn syndrome?
   A. Bronchiectasis
   B. Tracheal diverticula
   C. Hyperinflation
   D. Nodules
3. What is the treatment for tracheobronchopathia osteochondroplastica?
   A. Surgical resection
   B. Laser ablation
   C. Immunotherapy
   D. No treatment
4. What portion of the tracheal wall is free of cartilaginous support?
   A. Anterior wall
   B. Lateral walls
   C. Posterior wall
   D. Trachea has circumferential cartilaginous rings

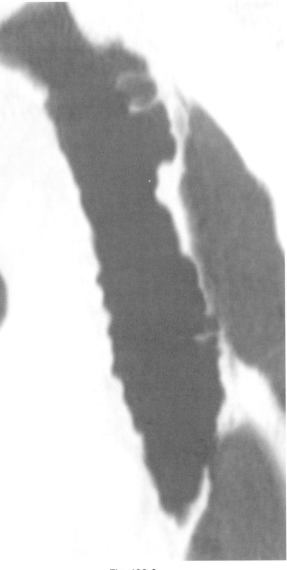

Fig. 122.2

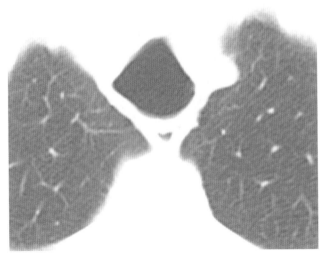

Fig. 122.1

Case 123

History: 59-year-old woman with chronic dyspnea and history of "asthma."

1. What is the best diagnosis (Figs. 123.1 and 123.2)?
   A. Saber sheath trachea
   B. Tracheomalacia
   C. Relapsing polychondritis
   D. Tracheal rupture
2. During which phase of the respiratory cycle is tracheomalacia most evident?
   A. Dynamic inspiration
   B. Dynamic expiration
   C. End-inspiration
   D. End-expiration
3. If the tracheal wall is thickened circumferentially but the posterior wall is spared what other condition (other than relapsing polychondritis) should be considered in the differential diagnosis?
   A. Amyloidosis
   B. Tuberculosis
   C. Granulomatosis with polyangiitis
   D. Tracheobronchopathia osteochondroplastica
4. What is the name ascribed to a trachea in which the transverse diameter is wider than the anterior-posterior diameter?
   A. Bowed trachea
   B. Parabolic trachea
   C. Lunate trachea
   D. Quadrilateral trachea

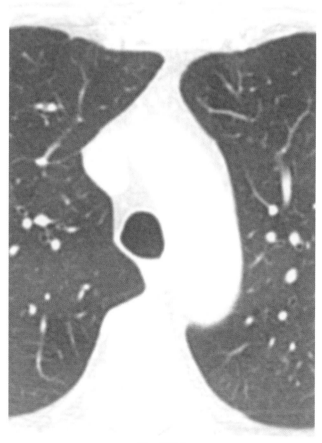

Fig. 123.1

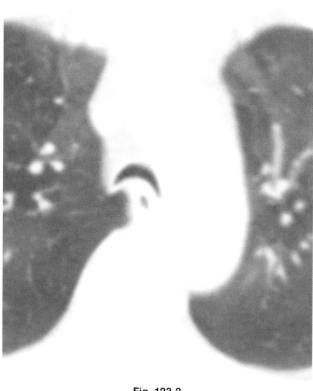

Fig. 123.2

Case 124

History: Middle-aged man with shortness of breath and wheezing.

1. Which of the following diagnoses should be included on the differential diagnosis (Figs. 124.1 and 124.2)? (Choose all that apply.)
   A. Metastasis
   B. Squamous cell carcinoma
   C. Adenoid cystic carcinoma
   D. Leiomyoma
2. What degree of tracheal narrowing is typically present before airway symptoms develop in primary tracheal malignancy?
   A. 25%
   B. 50%
   C. 75%
   D. 90%

3. Which of the listed primary malignancies is most likely to spread hematogenously to the trachea?
   A. Melanoma
   B. Testicular cancer
   C. Thyroid cancer
   D. Pancreatic cancer
4. In addition to lipomas, what benign airway tumor commonly contains fat?
   A. Leiomyoma
   B. Hamartoma
   C. Adenoma
   D. Papilloma

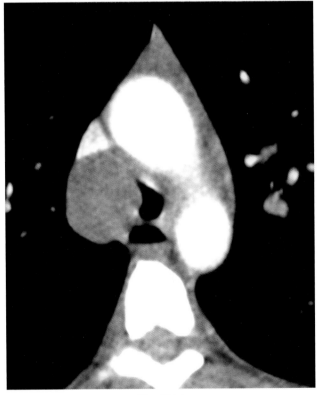

Fig. 124.1

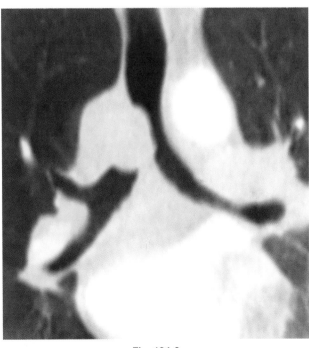

Fig. 124.2

Case 125

History: 53-year-old man with history of heart transplant with new fever (Fig. 125.1).

1. Which of the following diagnoses infectious etiologies are most likely in this setting?
   A. Histoplasmosis
   B. Nocardiosis
   C. Tuberculosis
   D. Aspergillosis
2. What is the most common cause of death in the first 30 days after cardiac transplant?
   A. Graft failure
   B. Infection
   C. Acute allograft rejection
   D. Cardiac allograft vasculopathy
3. Which of the following entities is least likely to manifest with a tree-in-bud pattern on computed tomography (CT)?
   A. Acute tuberculosis
   B. Invasive aspergillosis
   C. Chronic aspiration
   D. Cystic fibrosis

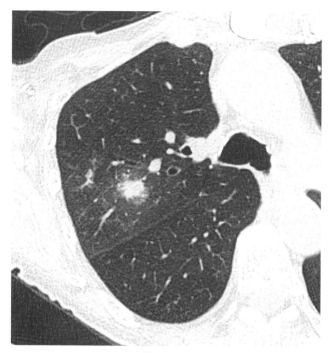

Fig. 125.1

Case 126

History: 69-year-old man with chronic shortness of breath (Figs. 126.1 and 126.2).

1. What is the most likely diagnosis?
   A. Proximal interruption of the pulmonary artery
   B. Pulmonary artery sarcoma
   C. Primary pulmonary hypertension
   D. Chronic thromboembolic disease
2. Which of the following is the likely cause of mosaic attenuation?
   A. Air-trapping
   B. Left-sided heart failure
   C. Vasculitis
   D. Infection

3. Which of the following computed tomography (CT) findings is specific for chronic as opposed to acute thromboembolic disease?
   A. Mosaic attenuation
   B. Ground-glass opacity
   C. Central arterial filling defect
   D. Decreased arterial caliber
4. What pulmonary finding is invariably present in long-standing proximal interruption of pulmonary artery?
   A. Mosaic attenuation
   B. Consolidation
   C. Bronchiectasis
   D. Fibrosis/scarring

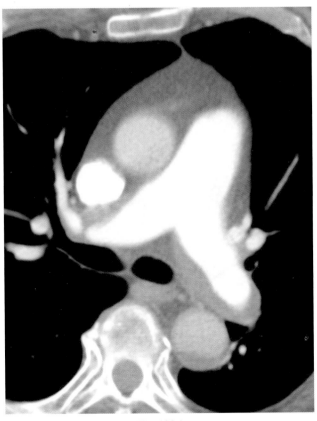

Fig. 126.1

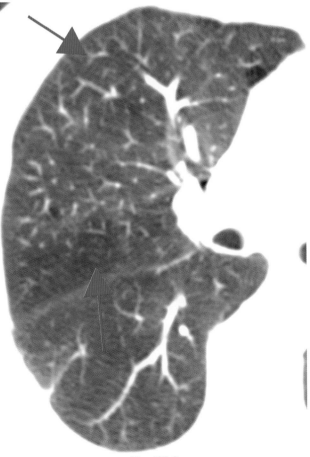

Fig. 126.2

Case 127

History: Middle-aged man with shortness of breath (Figs. 127.1 and 127.2).

1. What is the most likely diagnosis?
   A. Sarcoidosis
   B. Silicosis
   C. Langerhans cell histiocytosis
   D. Metastatic disease
2. Which of the following disease processes most commonly present with a random pattern of diffuse nodular lung disease on computed tomography (CT)?
   A. Disseminated infection
   B. Silicosis
   C. Hypersensitivity pneumonitis
   D. Chronic beryllium disease
3. What is the typical zonal distribution for silicosis?
   A. Upper
   B. Mid
   C. Lower
   D. Diffuse
4. A woman with an occupational history of nuclear reactor manufacturing presents with chronic shortness of breath. What is the next step in management?
   A. Purified protein derivative (PPD) skin test
   B. Chest CT
   C. Beryllium lymphocyte proliferation test (BeLPT)
   D. Ventilation/perfusion scan

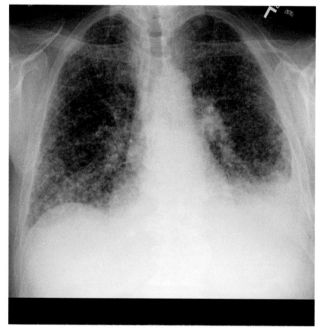

Fig. 127.1

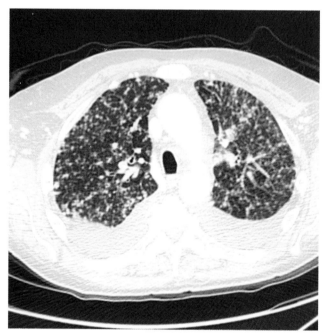

Fig. 127.2

Case 128

History: 35-year-old woman with an incidental computed tomography (CT) finding (Fig. 128.1).

1. What should be included in the differential diagnosis?
   A. Sarcoidosis
   B. Tuberculosis
   C. Castleman's disease
   D. Hypervascular metastasis
2. Lymph node metastases from which of the following primary malignancies are typically *not* hypervascular?
   A. Melanoma
   B. Renal cell carcinoma
   C. Colon cancer
   D. Thyroid cancer
3. Which of the following is not common in the plasma cell variant of Castleman's disease?
   A. Avid nodal enhancement
   B. Systemic symptoms
   C. Multicentric involvement
   D. Progression to lymphoma
4. Which chronic infection predisposes to the development of human herpesvirus 8 (HHV-8) associated Castleman's disease?
   A. Tuberculosis
   B. Human immunodeficiency virus (HIV)
   C. Hydatid disease
   D. Nocardiosis

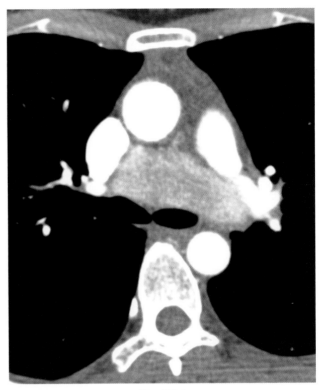

Fig. 128.1

Case 129

History: 37-year-old man with chest tightness and dyspnea.

1. What is the diagnosis (Figs. 129.1 and 129.2)?
   A. Penetrating aortic ulceration
   B. Intramural hematoma
   C. Aortic dissection
   D. Motion artifact
2. What is the next step in management?
   A. Surgery
   B. Watchful waiting
   C. Blood pressure control
   D. B and C
3. Which portion of the aorta is most commonly affected by penetrating aortic ulcerations?
   A. Sinus of Valsalva
   B. Ascending thoracic aorta
   C. Aortic arch
   D. Descending thoracic aorta
4. In the setting of ascending aortic intramural hematoma, into which other vessel wall can hematoma extend?
   A. Right pulmonary artery
   B. Superior vena cava
   C. Left pulmonary vein
   D. Azygous vein

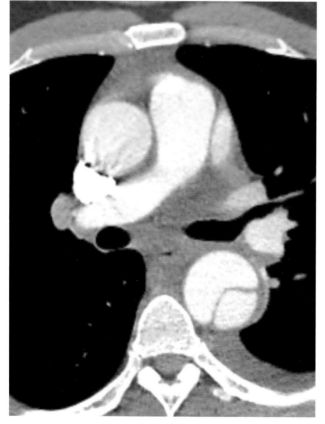

Fig. 129.1

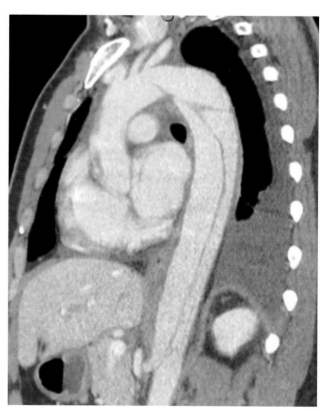

Fig. 129.2

Case 130

History: 53-year-old woman with chronic dyspnea.

1. What is the best diagnosis (Fig. 130.1)?
   A. Granulomatosis with polyangiitis
   B. Relapsing polychondritis
   C. Sarcoidosis
   D. Amyloidosis
2. What portion of the central airways is usually involved in the setting of granulomatosis with polyangiitis?
   A. Subglottic
   B. Carina
   C. Mid-trachea
   D. Proximal bronchi
3. Which of the following can present with nodular hyperdense foci within the tracheal walls?
   A. Sarcoidosis
   B. Relapsing polychondritis
   C. Amyloidosis
   D. Granulomatosis with polyangiitis
4. Which of the following conditions can lead to diffuse tracheal dilation?
   A. Emphysema
   B. Asthma
   C. Pulmonary fibrosis
   D. Pleural thickening

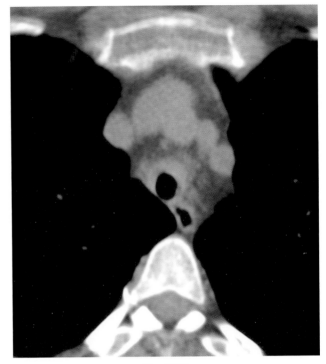

Fig. 130.1

Case 131

History: 23-year-old man with shortness of breath and chronic cough. History of severe childhood pulmonary infection.

1. What of the following should be included in the differential diagnosis (Figs. 131.1 and 132.2)?
   A. Congenital lobar emphysema
   B. Swyer-James-Macleod syndrome
   C. Bronchial atresia
   D. Obliterative bronchiolitis
2. Hyperdense bronchial mucus plugging is typical of which condition?
   A. Bronchial atresia
   B. Obliterative bronchiolitis
   C. Williams-Campbell syndrome
   D. Allergic bronchopulmonary aspergillosis
3. Computed tomography (CT) performed in expiration is characterized by inward bowing of which?
   A. Posterior wall of the trachea
   B. Anterior wall of the trachea
   C. Posterior wall of the bronchus intermedius
   D. Anterior wall of the bronchus intermedius
4. In an older female patient with long history of asthma, a chest CT showed severe air-trapping and multiple, well-defined pulmonary nodules. Biopsy of the dominant nodule was diagnostic of a well-differentiated carcinoid tumor. What is the best diagnosis?
   A. Granulomatous lymphocytic interstitial lung disease
   B. Carney complex
   C. Erdheim-Chester disease
   D. Diffuse idiopathic pulmonary neuroendocrine cell hyperplasia

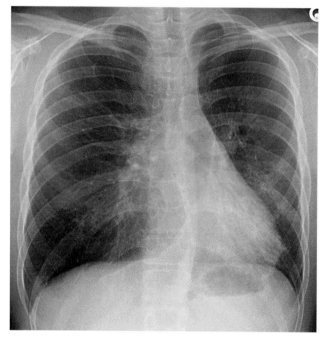

Fig. 131.1

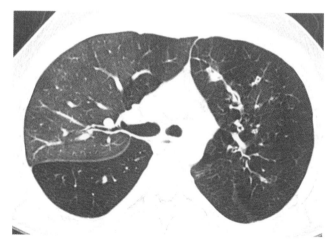

Fig. 131.2

Case 132

History: Middle-aged man with chronic shortness of breath.

1. What is the correct diagnosis (Figs. 132.1 and 132.2)?
   A. Tracheal bronchus
   B. Bridging bronchus
   C. Bronchial atresia
   D. Cardiac bronchus
2. Which condition is associated with a bridging bronchus?
   A. Right pulmonary artery atresia
   B. Interruption of the right pulmonary artery
   C. Pulmonary artery sling
   D. Patent ductus arteriosus

3. Which lobe is most commonly affected by bronchial atresia?
   A. Left upper lobe
   B. Right upper lobe
   C. Left lower lobe
   D. Right lower lobe
4. In the setting of a tracheal bronchus (arising from the distal trachea), an endotracheal tube position close to the carina would most likely lead to atelectasis of which pulmonary lobe?
   A. Left upper lobe
   B. Right upper lobe
   C. Left lower lobe
   D. Right lower lobe

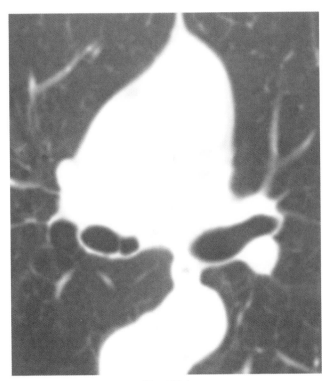

Fig. 132.1

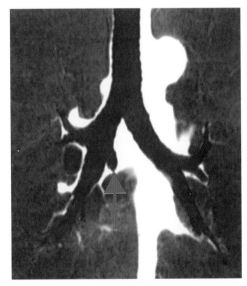

Fig. 132.2

Case 133

History: Young adult with recurrent pneumonia.

1. What is the most likely diagnosis (Figs. 133.1 and 133.2)?
   A. Pulmonary sequestration
   B. Congenital pulmonary airway malformation
   C. Bronchogenic cyst
   D. Pneumatocele
2. Patients with extralobar sequestrations typically present at which age?
   A. Infancy
   B. Adolescence
   C. 20 to 30 years of age
   D. 30 to 40 years of age

3. What is the typical treatment for congenital pulmonary airway malformations that have come to clinical attention?
   A. Long-term antibiotics
   B. Surgical resection
   C. Annual imaging surveillance
   D. No treatment
4. Which pulmonary lobe is most commonly affected by bronchogenic cysts?
   A. Upper lobes
   B. Right middle lobe/lingula
   C. Lower lobes
   D. All lobes are equally affected

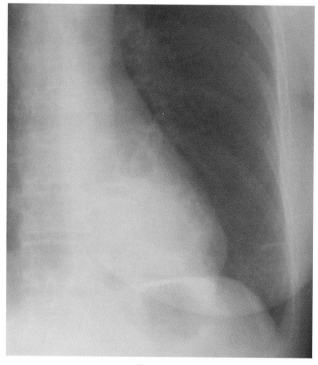

Fig. 133.1

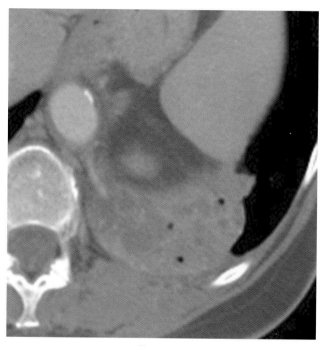

Fig. 133.2

Case 134

History: Dyspnea.

1. Which of the following should be included in the differential diagnosis for this patient (Figs. 134.1 and 134.2)? (Choose all that apply.)
   A. Acute pulmonary embolism
   B. Flow artifact
   C. Pulmonary artery sarcoma
   D. Pulmonary artery pseudoaneurysm
2. Which other important finding is present?
   A. Pulmonary infarct
   B. Pulmonary hemorrhage
   C. Right heart strain
   D. Aortic dissection
3. What is the radiographic sign used to describe oligemia distal to an obstructing embolus?
   A. S sign of Golden
   B. Hampton hump
   C. Fleischner sign
   D. Westermark sign
4. What finding on magnetic resonance imaging (MRI) *best* distinguishes pulmonary thromboembolism from pulmonary artery sarcoma?
   A. High T2 signal intensity
   B. Enhancement with gadolinium
   C. Shape of filling defect
   D. High T1 signal intensity

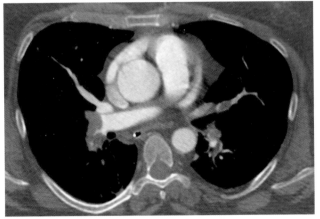

Fig. 134.1

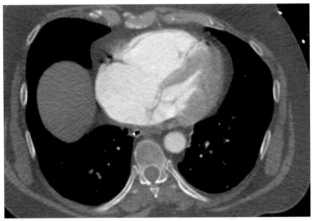

Fig. 134.2

Case 135

History: Dyspnea.

1. Which of the following should be included in the differential diagnosis for this patient (Figs. 135.1, 135.2 and 135.3)? (Choose all that apply.)
   A. Coal-worker's pneumoconiosis
   B. Alpha-1 Antitrypsin deficiency
   C. Intravenous drug abuse
   D. Nontuberculous mycobacterial infection
2. What type of emphysema predominates in this patient?
   A. Centrilobular
   B. Paraseptal
   C. Panlobular
   D. Paracicatricial
3. What is the pattern of inheritance of alpha-1 antitrypsin deficiency?
   A. Autosomal dominant
   B. Autosomal recessive
   C. X-linked dominant
   D. X-linked recessive
4. Which of the following is another established complication of alpha-1 antitrypsin deficiency?
   A. Liver cirrhosis
   B. Pancreatitis
   C. Renal cell carcinoma
   D. Aortic aneurysm

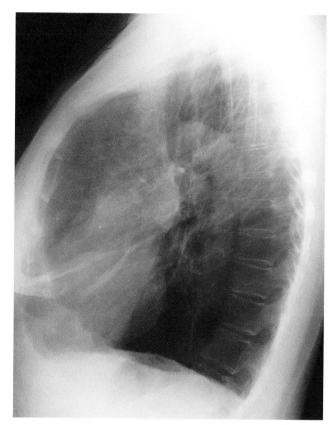

Fig. 135.2

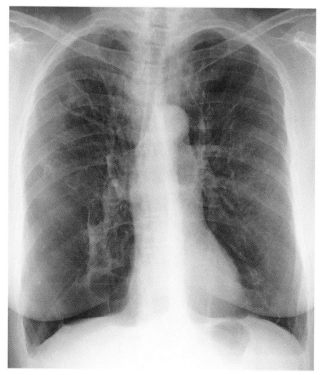

Fig. 135.1

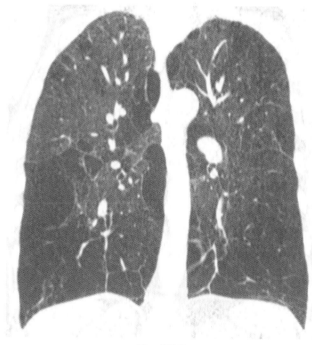

Fig. 135.3

Case 136

History: Abnormal chest radiograph.

1. Based on the computed tomography (CT) findings (Fig. 136.1), which of the following should be included in the differential diagnosis for this patient. (Choose all that apply.)
   A. Thymoma
   B. Lymphoma
   C. Thymic cyst
   D. Normal thymus
2. Which of the following *is not* a common cause of mixed solid and cystic anterior mediastinal mass?
   A. Thymoma
   B. Germ cell neoplasm
   C. Hodgkin lymphoma
   D. Pericardial cyst

3. Which of the following is the most common cause of a thymic mass?
   A. Thymic cyst
   B. Thymolipoma
   C. Thymic carcinoid
   D. Thymoma
4. If a thymic cyst has been complicated by hemorrhage, how would it most likely appear on T1-weighted magnetic resonance imaging (MRI)?
   A. Low T1 signal intensity
   B. High T1 signal intensity
   C. No T1 signal intensity
   D. Intermediate T1 signal intensity

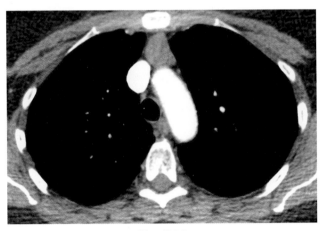

Fig. 136.1

Case 137

History: Lung nodule.

1. What congenital abnormality is present (Figs. 137.1 and 137.2)?
   A. Pulmonary sling
   B. Tracheal bronchus
   C. Cardiac bronchus
   D. Complete tracheal rings
2. What portion of the lung does a tracheal bronchus usually supply?
   A. Right upper lobe
   B. Right middle lobe
   C. Left upper lobe
   D. Left lower lobe
3. What is the most common clinical presentation of a tracheal bronchus?
   A. Recurrent infection
   B. Hemoptysis
   C. Stridor
   D. Incidental finding
4. What term describes a tracheal bronchus supplying *the entire right upper lobe*?
   A. Cow bronchus
   B. Pig bronchus
   C. Sheep bronchus
   D. Horse bronchus

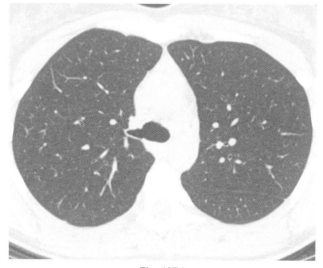

Fig. 137.1

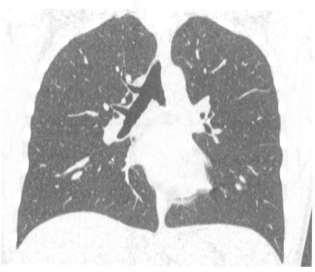

Fig. 137.2

Case 138

History: Dyspnea, heart disease.

1. Which of the following should be included in the differential diagnosis for this patient (Figs. 138.1, 138.2 and 138.3)? (Choose all that apply.)
   A. Amiodarone toxicity
   B. Renal cell carcinoma
   C. Talcosis
   D. Bleomycin toxicity
2. Considering the high-attenuation liver parenchyma, what is the most likely cause of these nodules?
   A. Amiodarone toxicity
   B. Renal cell carcinoma
   C. Talcosis
   D. Bleomycin toxicity
3. What disorder is amiodarone used to treat?
   A. Acute respiratory distress syndrome (ARDS)
   B. Cardiac dysrhythmia
   C. Myocarditis
   D. Congestive heart failure
4. Approximately what percentage of patients treated with amiodarone develop pulmonary toxicity?
   A. <25%
   B. 25% to 50%
   C. 51% to 75%
   D. >75%

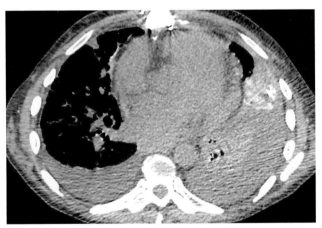

Fig. 138.1

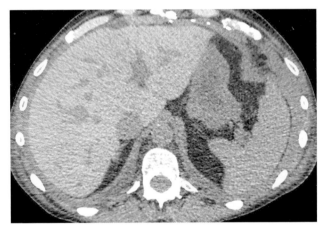

Fig. 138.3

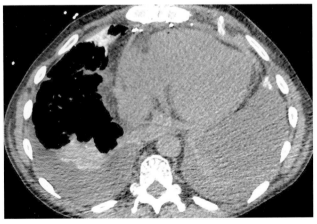

Fig. 138.2

Case 139

History: Chest pain.

1. Which of the following should be included in the differential diagnosis for this patient (Fig. 139.1)? (Choose all that apply.)
   A. Lymphoma
   B. Aneurysm
   C. Pseudoaneurysm
   D. Thymoma
2. What is the *most severe* complication of this abnormality?
   A. Rupture
   B. Myocardial ischemia
   C. Fistula formation
   D. Compression of the superior vena cava (SVC)

3. Approximately what percent of patients with venous graft aneurysms contain thrombus?
   A. 5%
   B. 15%
   C. 25%
   D. 50%
4. What is the *best next* step in the management of this patient?
   A. Follow-up radiograph in 3 months
   B. Cardiac magnetic resonance imaging (MRI)
   C. Surgical repair
   D. Coil embolization

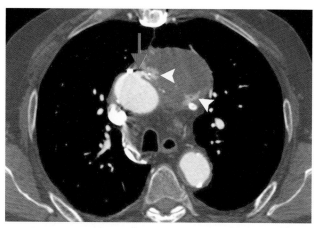

Fig. 139.1

Case 140

History: Cough and fever.

1. Which of the following should be included in the differential diagnosis for this patient (Figs. 140.1 and 140.2)? (Choose all that apply.)
   A. *Mycoplasma* infection
   B. *Staphylococcus aureus* infection
   C. Respiratory syncytial virus (RSV) infection
   D. *Streptococcus pneumoniae* infection
2. Which of the following terms describes the nodular and linear branching centrilobular opacities due to small airways disease?
   A. Acinar nodule
   B. Tree-in-bud opacity
   C. Ring shadow
   D. Mosaic attenuation

3. Which of the following regarding bronchioles is *true*?
   A. Bronchioles contain cartilage.
   B. Normal bronchioles are visible on computed tomography (CT).
   C. Respiratory bronchioles communicate directly with alveoli.
   D. Terminal bronchioles participate in gas exchange.
4. Where in the pulmonary lobule are bronchioles located?
   A. Center
   B. Interlobular septa
   C. Subpleural interstitium
   D. Adjacent to the pulmonary vein

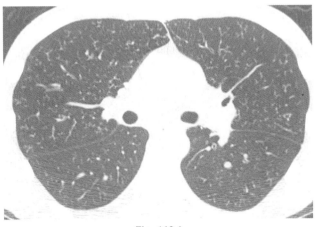

Fig. 140.1

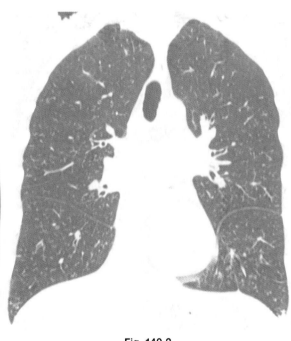

Fig. 140.2

Case 141

History: Lung transplantation 2 months ago. Low-grade fever and nonproductive cough.

1. Which of the following should be included in the differential diagnosis for this patient (Figs. 141.1 and 141.2)? (Choose all that apply.)
   A. Tuberculosis
   B. Drug reaction
   C. Viral pneumonia.
   D. Post-transplant lymphoproliferative disorder (PTLD)
2. True or false? *Pneumocystis jiroveci* pneumonia a common opportunistic infection in transplant recipients.
   A. True
   B. False
3. Which of the following is the most common viral pneumonia in solid organ transplant recipients?
   A. Epstein-Barr virus (EBV)
   B. Cytomegalovirus (CMV) pneumonia

C. Respiratory syncytial virus (RSV) pneumonia
D. Adenovirus pneumonia

4. Which of the following regarding renal transplantation is *not* true?
   A. Opportunistic infections are uncommon during the first month after transplant.
   B. *Streptococcus pneumoniae* is a common cause of pneumonia after the sixth month following transplant.
   C. T-cell mediated immunity is most severely depressed during the second through sixth months after transplant.
   D. Fungal pneumonia is uncommon after the sixth month following transplant.

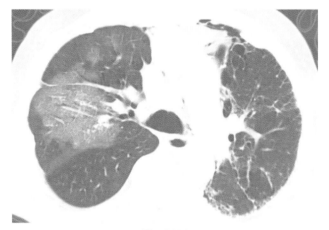

Fig. 141.1

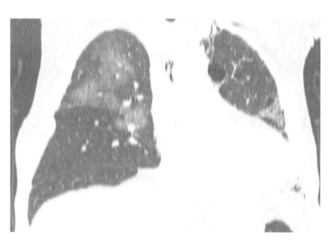

Fig. 141.2

Case 142

History: Severe pulmonary hypertension.

1. Which of the following should be included in the differential diagnosis for this patient (Figs. 142.1, 142.2 and 142.3)? (Choose all that apply.)
   A. Diffuse alveolar hemorrhage
   B. Usual interstitial pneumonia
   C. Pulmonary veno-occlusive disease (PVOD)
   D. Noncardiogenic pulmonary edema
2. What is the most likely diagnosis based on the findings of severe pulmonary hypertension and pulmonary edema?
   A. PVOD
   B. Chronic pulmonary thromboembolic disease
   C. Chronic obstructive pulmonary disease (COPD)
   D. Primary pulmonary hypertension
3. Which one of the following is *true* regarding PVOD?
   A. Prognosis is excellent.
   B. Most patients are asymptomatic at diagnosis.

C. Venous and venule obstruction results from intimal fibrosis.
D. Central pulmonary veins are dilated on computed tomography (CT).

4. Which of the following is the best next step in the management of this patient with suspected PVOD?
   A. Cardiac magnetic resonance imaging (MRI)
   B. Surgical biopsy
   C. Bronchoalveolar lavage (BAL)
   D. Fluorodeoxyglucose–positron emission tomography (FDG-PET)/CT

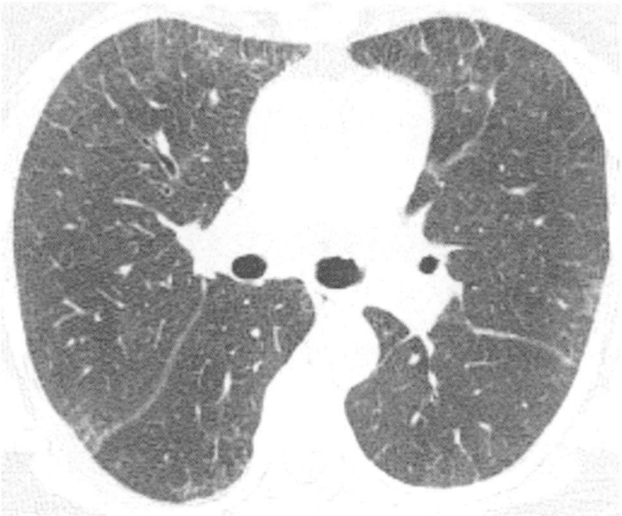

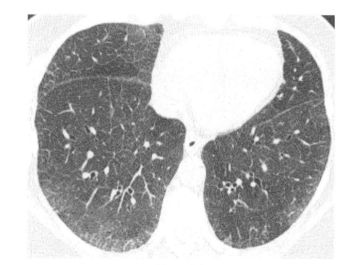

Fig. 142.1

Fig. 142.2

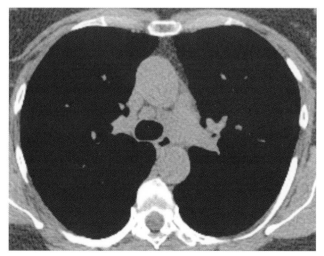

Fig. 142.3

Case 143

History: Cough.

1. Which of the following should be included in the differential diagnosis for this patient (Figs. 143.1 and 143.2)? (Choose all that apply.)
   A. Tracheobronchial papillomatosis
   B. Relapsing polychondritis
   C. Bacterial tracheitis
   D. Amyloidosis
2. How can magnetic resonance imaging (MRI) help distinguish amyloid from other causes of tracheal masses?
   A. Amyloid has high signal intensity on both T1- and T2-weighted images.
   B. Amyloid has low signal intensity on both T1- and T2-weighted images.
   C. Amyloid has low signal intensity on T1- and high signal intensity on T2-weighted images.
   D. Amyloid has high signal intensity on T1- and low signal intensity on T2-weighted images.

3. Which virus is *most* associated with this condition?
   A. Human immunodeficiency virus
   B. Human papilloma virus (HPV)
   C. Epstein-Barr virus (EBV)
   D. Cytomegalovirus (CMV)
4. Which of the following *is not* a complication of respiratory papillomatosis?
   A. Life-threatening airway obstruction
   B. Hemoptysis
   C. Adenocarcinoma
   D. Recurrent infection

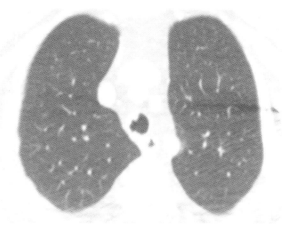

Fig. 143.1

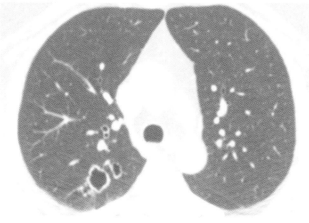
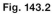

Fig. 143.2

Case 144

History: Abnormal chest radiograph. Cough.

1. What infection is associated with a mass within a cyst, as shown in the figure (Figs. 144.1 and 144.2)?
   A. Aspergillosis
   B. Nocardiosis
   C. Echinococcosis
   D. Mucormycosis
2. Which term is used to describe air collection within the cyst in the first figure?
   A. Crescent sign
   B. Water lily sign
   C. Tip-of-the-iceberg sign
   D. Collar sign
3. What is the significance of the crescent sign in the first figure?
   A. Secondary infection
   B. Impending rupture
   C. Healing
   D. Hemorrhage
4. Which of the following is the *most common* site of hydatid cysts in humans?
   A. Lung
   B. Brain
   C. Liver
   D. Spleen

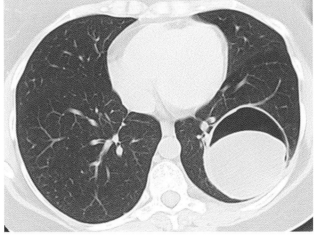

Fig. 144.1

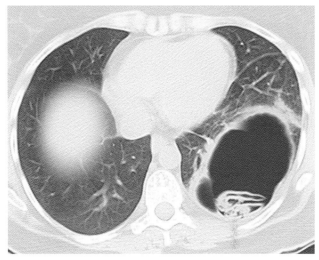

Fig. 144.2

Case 145

History: Cough.

1. Which of the following should be included in the differential diagnosis for this patient (Figs. 145.1 and 145.2)? (Choose all that apply.)
   A. Lung abscess
   B. Lymphangioleiomyomatosis
   C. Congenital pulmonary airway malformation
   D. Bronchogenic cyst
2. Which of the following congenital lung lesions is characterized by systemic arterial supply?
   A. Bronchogenic cyst
   B. Congenital pulmonary airway malformation
   C. Pulmonary sequestration
   D. Congenital lobar overinflation

3. What is the most common location of a bronchogenic cyst?
   A. Right lower lobe
   B. Left lower lobe
   C. Anterior mediastinum
   D. Middle mediastinum
4. Patients with congenital pulmonary airway malformations are at increased risk for developing which of the following tumors?
   A. Lymphoma
   B. Pleuropulmonary blastoma
   C. Adenocarcinoma
   D. Small cell lung carcinoma

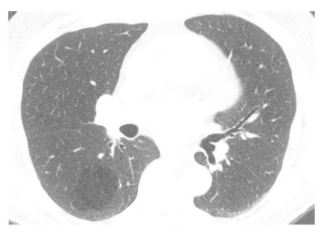

Fig. 145.1

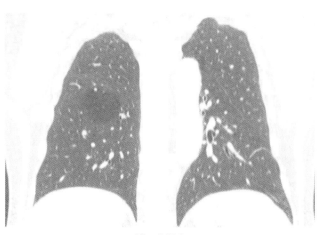

Fig. 145.2

Case 146

History: Xerostomia and facial swelling.

1. Which of the following should be included in the differential diagnosis for this patient (Figs. 146.1 and 146.2)? (Choose all that apply.)
   A. Usual interstitial pneumonia (UIP)
   B. Lymphangioleiomyomatosis
   C. Pulmonary Langerhans cell histiocytosis
   D. Lymphocytic interstitial pneumonia
2. Lymphocytic interstitial pneumonia is *most commonly* associated with which of the following?
   A. Systemic lupus erythematosus
   B. Sjögren syndrome
   C. Idiopathic pulmonary fibrosis
   D. Acute interstitial pneumonia

3. What is the *predominant* computed tomography (CT) finding of *Pneumocystis jirovecii* pneumonia?
   A. Ground-glass opacity
   B. Consolidation
   C. Lung cysts
   D. Lymphadenopathy
4. Which of the following is *not* associated with lung cysts?
   A. Lymphangioleiomyomatosis
   B. Pulmonary Langerhans cell histiocytosis
   C. Respiratory bronchiolitis–associated interstitial lung disease
   D. Birt-Hogg-Dubé syndrome

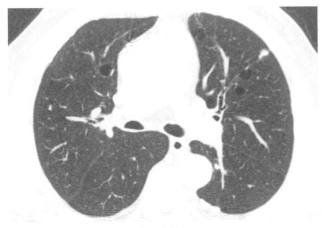

Fig. 146.1

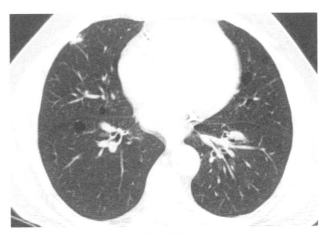

Fig. 146.2

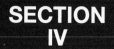

Opening Round

CASE 1

Squamous Cell Carcinoma of the Lung

1. **A and B**. The most common causes of a solitary lung nodule or mass are neoplasms and infection. The most likely neoplastic cause is primary lung carcinoma. Infections that present as large nodules or masses include lung abscesses, nocardiosis, actinomycosis, and fungal infection such as blastomycosis or invasive aspergillosis. Occasionally, community-acquired bacterial infections can present as a round mass during the early stages of infection (round pneumonia). Although pulmonary sequestrations can present as medially located lower lobe masses on chest radiography, lymphadenopathy is not a typical finding unless the sequestration is infected.
2. **A**. Adenocarcinoma is the most common histopathologic type of lung cancer. Squamous cell carcinoma and small cell carcinoma are somewhat less common. Carcinoid accounts for approximately only 1% of all lung malignancies.
3. **C**. Cigarette smoking is the signal largest risk factor for developing lung carcinoma. Other risk factors include occupational and environmental exposures such as asbestos and silica. Radon may be a factor contributing to lung cancer in some patients. Obesity has not been shown to be an independent risk factor for lung carcinoma.
4. **D**. Stage at diagnosis is the best predictor of 5-year survival with lung carcinoma. The current staging system follows the T(umor), N(ode), M(etastasis) model and describes local, regional, and systemic extent of malignancy.

Comment

Differential Diagnosis

Primary lung carcinoma is the leading diagnostic consideration. Other entities to consider include infections particularly fungal or bacterial conditions such as actinomycosis or nocardiosis.

Lung Cancer

Lung cancer remains the leading cause of cancer-related death in both males and females. Adenocarcinoma is the most common histopathologic type of lung cancer, followed by squamous cell and small cell carcinoma. Other histopathologic types are much less common. Cigarette smoking remains the leading cause of lung cancer, as 85% of lung cancers develop in current or former smokers. Most lung cancers are detected at later stages when patients become symptomatic. Chest radiography has not been shown to reduce mortality when used as a screening test in patients at risk of lung cancer. However, the National Lung Screening Trial showed a 20% reduction in all-cause mortality with low-dose computed tomography (CT) screening in patients deemed at highest risk for developing lung cancer. Earlier stage lung cancer is associated with higher survival rates.

Imaging Findings

PA and lateral chest radiographs (Fig. 1.1, Fig. 1.2) show a right lower lobe mass. The mass and right hilar lymphadenopathy were confirmed on CT (Fig. 1.3, Fig. 1.4). Primary lung carcinoma most commonly presents as a solitary lung nodule or mass. Associated hilar and mediastinal lymphadenopathy may be apparent on chest radiographs, although CT is superior to radiography for detecting thoracic lymphadenopathy. Other associated findings can include bone destruction (chest wall invasion or metastasis), pleural effusion, lung metastases, and septal thickening from lymphangitic carcinomatosis. Patients with radiographs suggestive of lung carcinoma should undergo chest CT for further evaluation. Fluorodeoxyglucose–positron emission tomography/CT (FDG-PET/CT) is used to stage patients with lung cancer and is particularly valuable in detecting occult metastases. Such upstaging of lung cancer occurs frequently after PET imaging and can often alter therapy. Because of the intrinsically high level of FDG uptake in the brain, magnetic resonance imaging (MRI) is used to evaluate for brain metastasis in patients with lung cancer.

REFERENCES
Maldonado F, Jett JR. Invasive and noninvasive advances in the staging of lung cancer. *Semin Oncol.* 2014 Feb;41(1):17–27.
Thoracic Radiology: The Requisites, 3rd ed, 405–427.

CASE 2

Spontaneous Pneumothorax

1. **C**. Playing basketball does not involve sufficient trauma to produce a traumatic pneumatocele. There is no radiographic evidence of pneumomediastinum. Spontaneous pneumothorax typically occurs in healthy young individuals, often during athletic activities. Swyer-James-McLeod syndrome is characterized on radiography by a hyperlucent lung with slightly decreased lung volume and a small ipsilateral hilum.
2. **B**. A traumatic pneumatocele results from compression-decompression trauma of the chest during partial airway closure, causing rupture of small airways.
3. **B**. Swyer-James-McLeod syndrome results from postinfectious constrictive bronchiolitis, most commonly a result of childhood infection that is usually viral. There is reduced blood flow to the affected lung and air trapping on expiratory imaging, which manifests as unilateral hyperlucency of the affected hemithorax.
4. **D**. Tension pneumothorax manifests with characteristic displacements that result from increased intrathoracic pressure in the affected hemithorax, shifting the mediastinum toward the opposite side, displacing the ipsilateral hemidiaphragm inferiorly, and widening the ipsilateral intercostal spaces.

Comment

Differential Diagnosis

Unilateral hyperlucent lung (hemithorax) may result from pneumothorax, Swyer-James-McLeod syndrome, endobronchial tumor or foreign body, mastectomy, or Poland syndrome.

Discussion

PA chest radiograph (Fig. 2.1 and 2.2) shows abnormal lucency in the left hemithorax, with atelectasis of the left lung, shift of mediastinal structures to the right, downward displacement of the left hemidiaphragm, and widening of left intercostal spaces.

Pneumothorax is defined as the presence of air or gas in the pleural space. Although there is a wide variety of causes, spontaneous pneumothorax is the most common etiology. Affected patients are typically in their third or fourth decade of life.

Spontaneous pneumothoraces are almost always secondary to rupture of an apical bleb, which represents an air pocket within the elastic fibers of the visceral pleura. Such blebs have been reported to be detectable on chest radiographs in approximately 15% of cases of spontaneous pneumothorax. However, blebs are rarely evident on chest radiographs following resolution of the pneumothorax. Computed tomography (CT) is much more sensitive than radiography for detecting blebs and has been shown to detect blebs in approximately 80% of patients following resolution of spontaneous pneumothoraces. The size and number of apical blebs detected on CT have been shown to correlate with the risk for recurrent pneumothoraces and the need for surgical intervention. The ipsilateral and contralateral rates of recurrence of spontaneous pneumothorax is approximately 30% and 10%, respectively.

Tension pneumothorax is a life-threatening condition. Affected patients present with clinical signs of tachypnea, tachycardia, cyanosis, sweating, and hypotension. Radiographic findings may include contralateral mediastinal shift, downward displacement of the ipsilateral hemidiaphragm, widening of intercostal spaces. In severe cases, there may be flattening of the contours of the right heart border and/or vena cavae.

REFERENCES
Sahn SA, Heffner JE. Spontaneous pneumothorax. *N Engl J Med.* 2000;342:868–874.
Thoracic Radiology: The Requisites, 3rd ed, 159–192.

CASE 3

Pleural Plaques

1. **C.** Based on the characteristic radiographic and computed tomography (CT) findings, the most likely diagnosis is C, asbestos-related pleural plaques. Fibrothorax is typically a unilateral process and the pleural thickening and calcification are characteristically continuous rather than discontinuous, and often involve and obscure the cardiophrenic sulcus. Talc pleurodesis may be performed to treat intractable pleural effusion or chronic pneumothorax and often results in focal or multifocal areas of smooth or nodular pleural thickening that often exhibit high attenuation or calcification. The findings typically involve the posterior and basilar aspects of the treated hemithorax. Calcified pleural metastases are uncommon but do occur in patients with osteosarcomatous malignancies and may mimic pleural plaques.

2. **C.** Approximately 25% of patients with the primary pleural malignant mesothelioma will also exhibit pleural plaques, an imaging marker of their previous asbestos exposure.

3. **D.** The characteristic latency period is 30 to 40 years between the time of a person's occupational exposure to asbestos and the development of mesothelioma.

4. **E. All of the above.** Asbestos was once an ingredient in many different construction materials. In the mid-1960s, scientists confirmed that breathing airborne asbestos fibers can cause a variety of lung diseases, including mesothelioma, lung cancer and asbestosis. Many buildings built before 1980 were constructed with asbestos-containing materials including roofing materials, cement, floor and ceiling tiles, pipe and duct insulation. Asbestos was once considered a critical element in the shipbuilding industry, especially in the military, because it could resist heat and prevent fires that would be disastrous for a vessel at sea. It was also recognized as a great insulator and was resistant to corrosion. Many of the goods that were produced and processed in textile mills from the 1940s to the 1970s were made with asbestos fibers, which put many textile workers at risk of asbestos exposure.

Comment

Differential Diagnosis

Pleural thickening resulting from infection, primary or secondary neoplasia, or pleurodesis.

Pleural plaques are the most common manifestation of asbestos exposure and typically occur after a latency period of approximately 15 to 20 years. They do not cause symptoms and are usually discovered incidentally, as in this case. Pathologically, pleural plaques are composed of dense bands of avascular collagen.

Pleural plaques may be detected in patients whose occupation or other activities involved exposure to asbestos fibers (e.g., construction, boat building). They are typically found in chest radiographic and CT examinations performed 15 to 20 years after such exposure and have characteristic imaging features. Pleural plaques are not premalignant lesions, but affected individuals are at increased risk for lung cancer, mesothelioma, and asbestosis (pulmonary fibrosis) due to their asbestos exposure. Plaques serve as a signpost of asbestos exposure.

On chest imaging, detection of bilateral calcified pleural plaques along the diaphragmatic pleura (S3.1 and S3.2) is considered diagnostic of asbestos-related pleural disease. They manifest as bilateral multifocal areas of discontinuous pleural thickening, with or without calcification, and typically occur adjacent to the 6th to 9th ribs, along the diaphragmatic pleura, and along the right lower paravertebral pleura (Fig. 3.1). When more extensive, the larger plaques may have a distinctive *en face* radiographic appearance resembling the fringes of a holly leaf. Pleural plaques may also exhibit incomplete borders on chest radiography, an imaging feature that often occurs in pleural and chest wall lesions.

REFERENCES
Jamrozik E, et al. Clinical Review: Asbestos-related Disease. *Intern Med J.* 2011;Feb 10 https://doi.org/10.1111/j.1445-5994. 2011.
Thoracic Radiology: The Requisites, 3rd ed, 159–192.

CASE 4

Emphysema

1. **A, C, and D.** Fibrotic (chronic) hypersensitivity pneumonitis is characterized by imaging signs of fibrosis, namely volume loss that often involves the mid and upper lung zones. The chest radiograph may be normal in patients with mild

centrilobular emphysema and in early cases of lymphangi-oleiomyomatosis (LAM), but in moderate to advanced cases the lungs may appear hyperinflated. Most patients with asthma have normal chest radiographs, but hyperinflation of the lungs does occur in patients with severe disease and may be transient or fixed.

2. **B.** Swyer-James-McLeod syndrome is associated with post-infectious bronchiolitis occurring in childhood, usually at <8 years of age. Microscopic findings include constrictive bronchiolitis, bronchiectasis, and parenchymal destruction. Follicular bronchiolitis is a chronic cellular bronchiolitis associated with hyperplasia of bronchus-associated lymphoid tissue (BALT), typically in association with collagen vascular disease or immunodeficiency. Bronstitis occurs second-ary to calcified endobronchial material that typically extends from adjacent calcified lymph nodes that have eroded into the airway lumen. Bronchial atresia is a developmental disorder characterized by focal bronchus atresia with resultant for-mation of a distal mucocele that is surrounded by an area of hyperinflated lung that occurs through collateral ventilation.

3. **C.** Panlobular emphysema is associated with alpha-1-anti-trypsin deficiency and is not always secondary to smoking. It manifests as lower lobe predominant emphysema with "sim-plification of lung structure and progressive loss of tissue." Advanced cases of centrilobular emphysema may involve the entire secondary pulmonary lobule and mimic panlobular emphysema. The other listed entities are associated with smoking.

4. **A, B, C, and D.** Hyperinflation is a characteristic finding of advanced centrilobular emphysema, with widening of the retrosternal air space (>2.5 cm) on lateral chest radiography. Hyperlucency of the upper lung zones occurs as result of moderate to severe lung destruction with decreased perfu-sion. Rapid tapering and attenuation of pulmonary vessels is a characteristic radiographic finding in the upper lung zones of affected patients. Flattened hemidiaphragms occur because of hyperinflation and air trapping and are usually most apparent on the lateral view

Comment

PA and lateral views of the chest show hyperinflation, with flat-tened hemidiaphragms and widening of the retrosternal space (Fig. 4.1). On the PA view, the upper lung zones appear hyperlu-cent, with a paucity of pulmonary vessels that demonstrate rapid tapering and attenuation as they emanate from the hila. The central pulmonary arterial structures appear dilated, consistent with associated pulmonary hypertension.

Emphysema is defined as permanent, abnormal enlargement of airspaces distal to the terminal bronchiole, accompanied by destruction of their walls.

Radiographic abnormalities in patients with emphysema are related to overinflation of the lungs and lung destruction. The latter is characterized by reduced vascularity or the presence of bullae. Overinflation of the lungs may be characterized by several findings, most notably flattening of the hemidiaphragms best appreciated on the lateral view and an increase in the ret-rosternal air space diameter. Chest radiographic abnormalities are usually evident in moderate to severe cases of emphysema, but radiographs are frequently normal in patients with early emphysema. Thin-section computed tomography (CT) is supe-rior to chest radiographs in detecting and characterizing emphy-sema and has a high sensitivity and specificity for establishing the diagnosis. Other conditions that may result in overinflation of the lungs are asthma and cystic fibrosis.

REFERENCES

Gietema HA, et al. Quantifying the extent of emphysema: factors associated with radiologists' estimations and quantitative indices of emphysema severity using the ECLIPSE cohort. *Acad Radiol.* 2011;18(6):661–671.
Raghu G, Remy-Jardin M, Ryerson CJ, et al. Diagnosis of Hyper-sensitivity Pneumonitis in Adults. An Official ATS/JRS/ALAT Clinical Practice Guideline. *Am J Respir Crit Care Med.* 2020 Aug 1;202(3):e36–e69.
Thoracic Radiology: The Requisites, 3rd ed, 391–404.

CASE 5

Sarcoidosis (Stage I)

1. **C.** Mediastinal and hilar lymphadenopathy may occur in sarcoidosis, lymphoma, metastatic disease, infection, and pneumoconiosis. In a young patient with no systemic symp-toms, as in this case, the presence of symmetric bilateral hilar and mediastinal lymphadenopathy is most characteristic of sarcoidosis.

2. **E.** Head and neck malignancies, melanoma, breast can-cer, and genitourinary malignancies are all associated with metastases to mediastinal and hilar lymph nodes. Other causes of bilateral symmetric hilar lymphadenopathy include lymphoma, other metastases (e.g., renal cell carcinoma, tes-ticular cancer) and pneumoconiosis (i.e., silicosis) in occupa-tionally exposed individuals.

3. **C.** Patients infected by histoplasmosis may be asymptomatic or suffer from progressive pulmonary disease and possible dissemination; and mediastinal lymphadenopathy is com-mon in both acute and subacute cases. Blastomycosis may manifest as acute or chronic pulmonary disease mimicking community-acquired pneumonia and malignancy, and may ultimately progress to disseminated disease with cutaneous, genitourinary, and bony lesions. Primary coccidioidomycosis manifests with pulmonary involvement and affected patients are often asymptomatic. Symptomatic patients usually pres-ent with fever, cough, and chest pain, features that mimic community-acquired pneumonia. Chest radiographs may show consolidation, nodules, or peripheral, solitary thin-walled cavities and parapneumonic effusion.

4. **D.** Bilateral asymmetric hilar lymphadenopathy may occur in lymphoma, sarcoidosis, and metastatic disease (e.g., renal cell carcinoma, testicular cancer, breast cancer, lung cancer).

Comment

Differential Diagnosis

Sarcoidosis, lymphoma, metastatic disease

Discussion

Composite image of PA chest radiograph and axial contrast-en-hanced computed tomography (CT) (Fig. 5.1). The chest radiograph shows right paratracheal and bilateral hilar lymph-adenopathy, forming the radiographic "1,2,3 sign" that is char-acteristic of sarcoidosis (Stage I). CT images confirm those areas of lymphadenopathy and reveals additional involvement of prevascular and subcarinal lymph node stations.

Sarcoidosis is a multisystem chronic inflammatory disease of unknown etiology, characterized by widespread noncaseating granulomas. Because this pathologic finding may also be seen in a variety of other conditions, a diagnosis of sarcoidosis requires con-cordant radiologic, clinical, laboratory, pathologic findings, and exclusion of other entities (especially granulomatous infections).

The chest radiograph is abnormal in approximately 90% of patients with sarcoidosis. Bilateral, symmetric hilar lymph node enlargement is the most common radiographic abnormality and is frequently accompanied by bilateral mediastinal lymph node enlargement. Lung parenchymal disease is usually nodular or reticulonodular in appearance, with a predilection for the upper and mid-lung zones.

On thin-section CT, sarcoid granulomas typically manifest as small (2–3 mm) nodules, with a characteristic perilymphatic distribution that includes the peribronchovascular lymphatics, the interlobular septa, and subpleural lymphatics (peripherally and along the fissures). Approximately 20% of patients with sarcoidosis may progress to have pulmonary fibrosis with upper lung architectural distortion, volume loss, and cystic changes.

REFERENCES

Little BP. Sarcoidosis: overview of pulmonary manifestations and imaging. *Semin Roentgenol*. 2015 Jan;50(1):52–64.

Thoracic Radiology: The Requisites, 3rd ed, pp 355–376.

CASE 6

Mesothelioma

1. **A, B, C, D**. The computed tomography (CT) imaging features of pleural thickening that suggest the presence of malignancy include the following: >1 cm in thickness, nodularity, circumferential growth pattern within the involved hemithorax, and involvement of the mediastinal pleural.
2. **C**. Pleural metastasis is the most common form of pleural malignancy, whereas mesothelioma and pleural involvement by lymphoma are much less common.
3. **B**. Although pleural plaques may be present in the setting of mesothelioma, their presence is not required for a diagnosis of mesothelioma. The earliest manifestation of mesothelioma is unilateral diffuse pleural thickening and a pleural effusion.
4. **A**. Epithelioid is the most common histologic subtype of mesothelioma. Although all are associated with a poor prognosis, the sarcomatoid subtype is typically most aggressive albeit least common.

Comment

Differential Diagnosis

Pleural metastases, mesothelioma, lymphoma, invasive thymoma.

Discussion

Although relatively rare, malignant mesothelioma is the most common primary neoplasm of the pleura. Most affected individuals (80% of cases) have a history of asbestos exposure 30 to 40 years before the diagnosis, typically through their occupation. Males are affected more commonly than females, likely reflecting a gender disparity in the occupations associated with asbestos exposure (e.g., construction and shipyard workers, fire fighters).

Affected patients typically present with complaints of chest pain and dyspnea. The most common radiographic finding is the presence of diffuse pleural thickening that is typically nodular and irregular in configuration and often circumferential within the involved hemithorax (Figs. 6.1A and B). In some cases, diffuse pleural thickening may be accompanied by a reduction in the size of the affected hemithorax, with associated ipsilateral shift of the mediastinum. Pleural effusion is often present.

CT and magnetic resonance imaging (MRI) are superior to radiography in assessing the extent of disease. In many cases, the two modalities play complementary roles in the evaluation of resectability and may be useful in assessing for transdiaphragmatic extension, diffuse chest wall invasion, invasion of vital mediastinal structures, vertebral body invasion, direct extension of tumor to the contralateral pleura, and the presence of distant metastases. The presence of any one or more of these findings precludes surgical resection. Patients with limited disease may be considered candidates for attempted surgical cure by extrapleural pneumonectomy. Regardless of therapy, however, malignant mesothelioma is almost always fatal.

REFERENCES

Leung AN, Müller NL, Miller RR. CT in differential diagnosis of diffuse pleural disease. *AJR Am J Roentgenol*. 1990 Mar;154(3):487–492.

Miller BH, Rosado-de-Christenson ML, Mason AC, et al. Malignant pleural mesothelioma: radiologic pathologic correlation. *Radiographics*. 1996;16:613–644.

Thoracic Radiology: The Requisites, 3rd ed, 159–192

CASE 7

Junction Lines

1. **D**. The structures indicated by the arrow and arrowhead are the anterior and posterior junction lines, respectively.
2. **A, B, C, and D**. Pneumomediastinum may develop in individuals who engage in inhalational substance abuse and is also known to occur in the setting of a sustained Valsalva maneuver (e.g., vomiting, straining, weightlifting). It is also associated with obstructive lung disease and occurs in up to 15% of patients with pulmonary fibrosis.
3. **B**. The concept of radiologic mediastinal compartments was introduced by Dr. Benjamin Felson in the 1970s using the lateral chest radiograph to evaluate a detected mediastinal mass and help formulate a differential diagnosis. In his method, the mediastinum was divided into anterior, middle, and posterior compartments using anatomic landmarks visible on the lateral chest radiograph. Felson's anterior compartment extends from the sternum to a line drawn along the anterior aspect of the trachea and along the posterior aspect of the heart, and the middle compartment extended from that same line to a posterior line drawn along the anterior third of each thoracic vertebral body. The posterior compartment extends posteriorly from that line and includes the paravertebral region. This designation differs from the definition of mediastinal compartments used by anatomists and pathologists in which the heart occupies the middle mediastinum.
4. **B**. Total atelectasis of either lung is associated with increased compensatory mechanisms as compared to lobar atelectasis. The anterior junction line is typically displaced ipsilaterally toward the atelectatic lung, and the contralateral lung hyperinflates in a compensatory fashion and often crosses the midline toward the atelectatic lung. The ipsilateral hemidiaphragm may be elevated, particularly in total atelectasis of the left lung, and there is often marked ipsilateral shift of the mediastinum, particularly of the anterior mediastinal components since the posterior mediastinal structures are relatively tethered to paraspinal structures.

Comment

Differential Diagnosis

None.

Discussion

The coned-down frontal radiograph demonstrates the normal appearance of the anterior (arrow) and posterior (arrowhead) junction lines (Fig. 7.1), formed by the close apposition of visceral and parietal layers of pleura of both lungs as they approximate in the anterior and posterior aspects of the mediastinum, respectively. The anterior and posterior junction lines may be seen on 24.5% to 57% and 32% of chest radiographs, respectively.

The anterior portion of the thorax begins at the thoracic inlet and the superior aspect of the anterior junction line begins at the undersurface of the clavicles and typically courses obliquely from right to left but may appear more vertical in alignment as demonstrated in this case. The posterior portion of the thorax extends more superiorly than the anterior portion and thus the posterior junction line may be seen to extend above the level of the clavicles, as in this illustration. It typically appears as a straight vertical line, often visible through the tracheal air column.

Obliteration or abnormal convexity of the anterior junction line suggests underlying anterior mediastinal disease (e.g., thyroid or thymic mass, lymphadenopathy, lipomatosis) whereas similar findings related to the posterior junction line suggest a posterior mediastinal abnormality (e.g., esophageal mass, lymphadenopathy, aortic disease, or neurogenic tumor). Either junction line may also be displaced by volume loss or hyperinflation of the surrounding lung

A line typically measures <1 mm in width and is formed by normal anatomic structures. Stripes are recognized as thicker lines, typically formed by air outlining thicker intervening soft tissues (e.g., paratracheal stripe, posterior tracheal stripe). An interface, (or edge) is a third component of the "lines, stripes and interfaces" concept and are formed when structures of different densities are in contact with each another. Examples include the left paraspinal line and the azygoesophageal recess, both of which may be useful in detecting mediastinal abnormalities.

REFERENCES

Gibbs JM, et al. Lines and stripes: where did they go? From conventional radiography to CT. *Radiographics*. 2007;27:33–48.

Zylak CM, et al. Pneumoediastinum revisited. *Radiographics*. 2000;20:1043–1057.

Thoracic Radiology:The Requisites, 3rd ed, 19–60.

CASE 8

Hamartoma

1. **C.** The sharp, spherical morphology of this fat-containing nodular lesion is most consistent with a hamartoma. The nodule abuts an airway, an imaging feature often seen in bronchial carcinoid tumors. Lepidic adenocarcinoma typically manifests as nodular ground-glass opacity. On the mediastinal window image (right), there is clear demonstration of fat attenuation within the nodule, a characteristic feature of hamartoma. Lipoid pneumonia is characterized by fat attenuation within focal or multifocal areas of consolidation, typically in the lower lobes and dependent areas of lung parenchyma.
2. **E.** All the listed entities have the potential of exhibiting FDG-avidity to varying degrees. Lepidic adenocarcinoma, typically detected as nodular ground-glass opacity, may be non-avid on PET imaging, but larger nodular lesions may show low-level FDG uptake. Bronchial carcinoid tumors are variable in their degree of FDG-avidity, typically ranging from little or none to moderate degrees of FDG uptake. Lipoid pneumonia may exhibit moderate to intense FDG avidity, and hamartomas may manifest with low-level or moderate FDG uptake.
3. **C.** The range of fat attenuation on the Hounsfield scale of CT numbers is -100 to -50.
4. **C.** Thin-section CT is the optimal imaging modality for detection and characterization of pulmonary hamartomas, and approximately 59% of hamartomas will exhibit fat

attenuation, 39% with focal fat and no calcification, and 21% with both fat attenuation and calcification. An additional 36% of hamartomas will exhibit no fat attenuation or calcification, and 4% may appear as diffusely calcified nodules. Occasionally, a hamartoma will manifest with focal calcification and no fat.

Comment

Differential Diagnosis

Hamartoma, lipoid pneumonia, metastasis (e.g., liposarcoma).

Discussion

Composite image of same CT image in lung window (left) and mediastinal window (right) shows a spherical, well-defined nodule that abuts an airway along its posterior aspect (left image) and exhibits internal fat attenuation (right image Fig. 8.1). The nodule contains areas of low attenuation that represent focal deposits of fat. The identification of fat deposits (–50 to –150 Hounsfield units) within a pulmonary nodule is diagnostic of a hamartoma, the most common benign pulmonary neoplasm.

A hamartoma represents a focus of disorganized growth of tissue normally found within the lung. Histologically, the tumors may be comprised of varying amounts of cartilage, fibrous tissue, and mature fat cells. Other mesenchymal elements such as bone, vessels, and smooth muscle may also be present. Affected patients range in age from 30 to 70 years, with a peak incidence observed in the sixth decade of life. There is a slight female predominance. Most lesions are detected incidentally on routine chest radiographs of asymptomatic patients but may also be detected on lung cancer screening CT studies. Approximately 10% of hamartomas may occur as endobronchial lesions and affected patients may present with symptoms of airway obstruction. Hamartomas may grow slowly over time.

REFERENCES

Erasmus JJ, Connolly JE, McAdams HP, Roggli VL. Solitary pulmonary nodules: Part I. Morphologic evaluation for differentiation of benign and malignant lesions. *Radiographics*. 2000;20:43–58.

Gaerte SC, et al. Fat-containing lesions of the chest. *Radiographics*. 2002;22(Spec No):61–78.

Thoracic Radiology: The Requisites, 3rd ed, 405–427.

CASE 9

Cystic Fibrosis

1. **B.** On chest radiography, cystic fibrosis is characterized by hyperinflation, bronchiectasis, and bronchial wall thickening with predominance of findings in the upper lobes. The chest radiograph in patients with lymphangioleiomyomatosis may appear normal or exhibit reticular or reticulonodular opacities that reflect underlying diffuse parenchymal cysts. The lungs appear hyperinflated and hyperlucent on radiography in 50% of patients with moderate centrilobular emphysema, and in virtually all patients with severe disease. Pulmonary Langerhans cell histiocytosis manifests on chest radiography with reticulonodular opacities, nodules, and cysts with an upper to mid lung zone predominance.
2. **C.** CT images reformatted in the coronal and/or sagittal planes aid in the detection of bronchiectasis by displaying the tubular and branching morphology of dilated airways. MIPs optimize detection of pulmonary nodules. MinIPs emphasize

areas of low lung attenuation and regional heterogeneity, whereas expiratory images optimize detection of air-trapping.
3. **E.** Bronchiectasis, cavitary infection, cavitary sarcoidosis, and lung cancer are among the conditions associated with bronchial artery dilatation. However, inflammatory conditions such as bronchiectasis and cavitary infection produce the most severe dilation and occasionally life-threatening hemoptysis. Additional causes are chronic thromboembolic disease, fibrosing mediastinitis, and congenital anomalies of the thorax (e.g., proximal interruption of the pulmonary artery, bronchial artery malformations). Patients affected by these conditions may present with hemoptysis.
4. **E.** In patients with cystic fibrosis, reactive mediastinal/hilar lymphadenopathy occurs as a result of chronic infection, involvement of the respiratory epithelium often leads to pansinusitis, and biliary cirrhosis may result from plugging of liver bile ducts by dehydrated bile. Most men (98%) affected by cystic fibrosis are infertile because of failure of the vas deferens to form properly. Bone demineralization is also a common clinical feature of patients with cystic fibrosis.

Comment

Differential Diagnosis

Cystic fibrosis, allergic bronchopulmonary aspergillosis, primary ciliary dyskinesia, post-infectious bronchiectasis.

Discussion

The chest radiograph and magnified views in this case demonstrate cylindrical bronchiectasis, manifested by bronchial dilatation, airway wall thickening, tram-tracking, and ring-like shadows (Fig. 9.1). Although the distribution is diffuse, the bronchiectasis is most severe in the upper lobes. The lungs appear hyperinflated, with occasional nodular opacities that likely represent mucoid impaction. The findings are typical of cystic fibrosis (CF), an autosomal recessive hereditary disorder characterized by abnormal secretions from exocrine glands, including the airways, pancreas, large bowel, and salivary and sweat glands.

The major clinical manifestations of this disorder are chronic pulmonary disease caused by bronchiectasis and pancreatic insufficiency. The thick mucus, resulting from abnormal chloride transport, in turn causes reduced mucociliary clearance and associated airway obstruction that leads to recurrent infections and destruction of airway walls. The most characteristic imaging feature is extensive upper lobe predominant cylindrical bronchiectasis that, in some cases, may progress to varicose and cystic morphologies.

Although CF is usually diagnosed during infancy or childhood, milder forms of the disease are occasionally first diagnosed in adults. Affected patients are at increased risk for pulmonary infections with a variety of organisms, including *Staphylococcus aureus*, *Pseudomonas aeruginosa*, *Haemophilus influenzae*, and *Pseudomonas cepacia*. The last organism is a major cause of infection late in the course of CF. Presenting symptoms of CF are related to recurrent pulmonary infections and include productive cough, wheezing, dyspnea, and hemoptysis. The diagnosis of CF may be confirmed by an abnormal sweat test or by detection of faulty Cystic Fibrosis Transmembrane Conductance Regulator (CFTR) genes. CFTR protein functions as a channel for movement of chloride ions and out of cells, thereby affecting salt and water balance on epithelial surfaces in the lungs and pancreas.

REFERENCES
Brody AS, et al. High-resolution computed tomography in young patients with cystic fibrosis: distribution of abnormalities and correlation with pulmonary function tests. *J Pediatr.* 2004;145:32–38.
Cantin L, et al. Bronchiectasis. *AJR Am J Roentgenol.* 2009;193(3): W158–W171.
Thoracic Radiology: The Requisites, 3rd ed, 137–158.

CASE 10
Mediastinal Mass (Vascular)

1. **B.** Felson used a line coursing anterior to the trachea and posterior to the heart to separate the anterior mediastinum from the middle mediastinum. In Felson's system, the posterior mediastinum includes the paravertebral region, and its anterior border extends along a vertical line that courses along the anterior thirds of the thoracic vertebral bodies.
2. **C.** The radiographic finding of a focal mediastinal contour abnormality suggests a primary mediastinal lesion, such as a thymoma, teratoma, bronchogenic cyst, or a vascular lesion (e.g., varices, aneurysm). Detection of diffuse mediastinal enlargement on chest radiography suggests lymphadenopathy, including primary and secondary malignant tumors.
3. **A.** It is important to consider vascular lesions (e.g., aneurysm, pseudoaneurysm, varices) in the differential diagnostic consideration of a detected mediastinal abnormality since 10% of mediastinal abnormalities are vascular lesions.
4. **C.** Thymomas and mature teratomas are both anterior mediastinal masses. Thymomas typically occur in patients over the age of 40 years, while mature teratomas characteristically affect patients under the age of 40.

Differential Diagnosis

Lymphadenopathy (neoplastic or non-neoplastic), Pseudoaneurysm, Extramedullary hematopoiesis.

Discussion

Posteroanterior (PA) and lateral views of the chest show a mediastinal mass projecting into the left hemithorax with well-defined borders and a lobulated contour on the PA view (Fig. 10.1). On the lateral radiograph, the mass appears to involve and middle and posterior mediastinal compartments.

Radiographic analysis is often the first step in evaluation of thoracic disorders affecting the mediastinum; and it requires a familiarity with normal mediastinal anatomy including contours, lines, stripes, and interfaces. Localization to a mediastinal compartment helps narrow the differential diagnostic possibilities.

Abnormal mediastinal contours detected on chest radiography may be manifestations of a variety of primary benign and malignant neoplasms, metastatic lymphadenopathy or coalescent lymph node masses, thyroid and thymic enlargement, vascular malformations, and aneurysms, or represent normal variants of anatomy (e.g., hiatal hernia). A focal contour abnormality suggests a primary mediastinal lesion, whereas diffuse mediastinal enlargement is more suggestive of lymphadenopathy, including primary and secondary malignant tumors. Detection of calcification suggests the possibility of granulomatous lymphadenopathy, teratoma, goiter, neurogenic tumor, or aneurysm.

Further evaluation by contrast-enhanced computed tomography (CT) allows visualization of vascular lesions and optimizes characterization of soft tissue elements and areas of necrosis. Approximately 10% of mediastinal abnormalities represent vascular lesions with characteristic contrast-enhanced CT findings of a vascular pattern of enhancement and demonstration of continuity with a vessel lumen (e.g., aneurysm, pseudoaneurysm, paraesophageal varices).

REFERENCES
Agarwal PP, Chughtai A, Matzinger FRK, Kazerooni EA. Multidetector CT of thoracic aortic aneurysms. *Radiographics*. 2009;29(2):537–552.
Carter BW, Tomiyama N, Bhora FY, et al. A modern definition of mediastinal compartments. *J Thorac Oncol*. 2014;9:S97–S101.
Thoracic Radiology: The Requisites, 3rd ed, 97–136.

CASE 11

Lung Contusion and Laceration

1. **C.** In the setting of recent blunt trauma to the thorax, pulmonary contusion is the most likely cause of the ground-glass opacity and peripheral consolidation in the left upper lobe. Note the displaced rib fracture near the involved lung. Atelectasis and aspiration may also occur in conjunction with blunt trauma to the thorax.

2. **C.** Abnormal lucency within an area of posttraumatic contusion often represents an associated area of pneumatocele formation related to shearing forces that disrupt the affected lung during the traumatic event. Other considerations would include underlying bronchiectasis or bullous emphysema, and less likely a cystic neoplasm.

3. **D.** Lung contusions typically begin to improve within 48 hours of injury. If consolidation and ground-glass worsen beyond that time frame, then aspiration, other pneumonia, and acute respiratory distress syndrome should be considered.

4. **D.** DIP typically manifests on CT as ground-glass opacity that is often basilar and peripheral in its pattern of distribution. Small, well-defined cysts do occur but are a less frequent finding. Cysts are a more common finding (70%) in LIP, combined with the more frequent finding of bilateral ground-glass opacity. Pulmonary Langerhans cell histiocytosis typically manifests on CT as irregular nodules and cysts that are variable in their shape.

Comment

Differential Diagnosis

Aspiration, pneumonia, lung cancer (adenocarcinoma).

Discussion

Thoracic trauma may result in two forms of lung parenchymal injury: pulmonary contusion and pulmonary laceration. Pulmonary contusion is the most common form of lung injury and represents hemorrhage into the alveoli.

On radiographs, pulmonary contusion appears as areas of airspace opacification that are usually in close proximity to the site of blunt trauma but may also less commonly be observed in the opposite portion of the lung (*contrecoup* lesion). Thus the identification of consolidation adjacent to sites of rib fractures or bullet fragments should suggest the diagnosis. The consolidation from contusion typically appears on radiographs within 6 hours of the time of injury, and it usually improves within 24 to 72 hours. The consolidation usually completely resolves within 1 week of onset.

CT may detect pulmonary contusion immediately after injury, before abnormalities are visible radiographically. On CT, areas of contusion may sometimes demonstrate characteristic subpleural sparing of the peripheral 1 to 2 mm of the lungs. *Pulmonary laceration* refers to a tear in the lung parenchyma. Such injuries may initially be masked by surrounding contusion. On radiographs of patients with pulmonary laceration injury, you may observe an ovoid cystic lucency that represents a posttraumatic pneumatocele. Such cysts are typically small (5 mm to 1 cm), but larger cysts can be seen in some cases. If the cyst fills with blood, a spherical hematoma is observed.

In some cases, the cyst may contain air and blood, with a resultant air-fluid level.

REFERENCES
Kaewlai R, Avery LL, Asrani AV, Novellline RA. Multidetector CT of blunt thoracic trauma. *Radiographics*. 2008;28:1555–1570.
Thoracic Radiology: The Requisites, 3rd ed, 279–288.

CASE 12

Malpositioned Catheter

1. **B.** Posteroanterior (PA) chest radiograph shows the distal aspect of a port catheter looped along the right superior aspect of the mediastinum. Lateral chest radiograph shows that the catheter extends posteriorly from the expected location of the superior vena cava. This is the location of the azygos vein which drains into the SVC at this level. The central portions of the brachiocephalic veins are more superiorly located within the thorax, just below the thoracic inlet. The great cardiac vein is part of the heart and is not a position to which central venous catheters typically extend.

2. **D.** The ideal location for a central venous line is at the superior cavoatrial junction. High volume can be injected at this site without potential for vascular injury present in cases of smaller caliber veins (brachiocephalic vein, subclavian vein) while avoiding complications of more distal line placement. Lines in the azygos vein should typically be removed given the higher risk of vascular rupture.

3. **A.** The most common complication of lines terminating in the right atrium is cardiac arrhythmia, which usually resolves by repositioning the line. Cardiac thrombus formation, rupture, or tamponade are potential complications of line placement in the right atrium but are exceedingly rare.

4. **C.** The clinical scenario describes arterial placement of a central line, likely in a subclavian artery. Given arterial placement and inability to apply direct pressure to a subclavian artery given the overlying clavicle, vascular surgery consult is mandatory in this setting. The line should not be removed. Moreover, use of the malpositioned line for chemotherapy or vigorous flushing of the line should be avoided.

Comment

Optimal Location of Central Venous Catheter

The ideal termination of a central venous catheter depends on its purpose. In most cases, a superior cavoatrial junction location is optimal. This allows for high flow infusion with minimal complication risk. The superior cavoatrial junction is not directly visible on chest radiography. The junction of the superior vena cava and the superior margin of the right heart is a good approximation of the superior cavoatrial junction as are the junction of the bronchus intermedius and right superior border of the heart or a point 3 to 4 cm below the carina. The azygos vein drains into the SVC above the right mainstem bronchus through the arch of the azygos vein. On PA radiographs, the arch is imaged en face. Therefore central venous lines which extend into the azygos arch will be most readily visible on the lateral radiograph, which more definitively shows the posterior course of the line (Fig. 12.1 and 12.2).

Azygos Line Placement

Inadvertent insertion of a catheter into the azygos vein is a relatively uncommon complication of central venous catheter placement, with an estimated frequency of approximately 1%. Detection of a malpositioned catheter at this site is important because there is a relatively high frequency of associated venous perforation.

Interestingly, azygos vein cannulation occurs most commonly following left-sided catheter insertion. This association is thought to occur secondary to anterocaudal arching of the left brachiocephalic vein, which may preferentially promote entry of a catheter into the azygos vein rather than the superior vena cava. In contrast, catheters placed from the right side of the thorax have a more direct course to the superior vena cava via the right brachiocephalic vein.

REFERENCES

Piciucchi S, Barone D, Sanna S, et al. The azygos vein pathway: an overview from anatomical variations to pathological changes. *Insights Imaging.* 2014;5(5):619–628.

Thoracic Radiology: The Requisites, 3rd ed, 210–225.

CASE 13

Paraspinal Hematoma

1. **B and C.** Anteroposterior (AP) supine chest radiograph demonstrates bilateral widening of the paraspinal lines along the T12 vertebral body. Combined with history, this is highly suggestive of acute fracture at this vertebral level. Conceivably, a focal metastatic lesion in the lower thoracic spine with associated soft tissue component could also demonstrate these imaging manifestations; however, no bony destruction is evident. Achalasia results in diffuse esophageal dilation and may lead to obliteration of the azygoesophageal recess or to displacement of the azygoesophageal line to the right. In this case the paraspinal lines are displaced. A descending thoracic aortic aneurysm, if focal, would preferentially widen the left mediastinal contour.

2. **B.** The thoracoabdominal sign is a useful sign in identifying posterior mediastinal lesions on frontal chest radiography. Air in the lungs is the contrast which allows for delineation of mediastinal contours on radiography. Therefore any area of the mediastinum which does not contact lung cannot be anatomically defined. The thoracoabdominal sign states that any mediastinal lesion which is well-defined below the level of the anterior diaphragm on frontal radiograph must be posterior in location because the posterior mediastinum abuts air-filled lung at that level. In this case, the abnormal bilateral convex margins of the paraspinal at the T12 vertebral body is confirmatory.

3. **C.** CT is the gold-standard imaging modality for detection of acute fractures suspected on radiography. MRI is useful in the setting of blunt trauma in suspected ligamentous or other soft tissue injury because it provides higher soft tissue contrast than CT. Sensitivity of the standard radiograph in the detection of vertebral fractures has been reported to be in the range of only 30%. Axial CT image shows acute fracture of the T12 vertebral body with adjacent paraspinal hematoma.

4. **D.** Although more x-rays are absorbed at lower energy (tube potential), more x-ray photons are created using higher tube potential. The former plays a larger role in radiography while the latter plays a larger role in CT.

Comment

Thoracic spine fracture is an infrequent but serious complication of blunt trauma. Unfortunately, the portable trauma chest radiograph is not very reliable in detecting spinal fractures. Moreover, thoracolumbar spine radiographs have been shown to have a sensitivity of only 32% for detecting acute spinal fractures. Radiographic findings associated with spinal fracture include those related to mediastinal hemorrhage (such as widening of the paraspinal lines, mediastinal widening, and left apical cap) and vertebral abnormalities. The latter are more specific for spinal injury and include loss of height of the vertebral body and obscuration of the pedicle(s).

When you identify a mediastinal hematoma that is confined to the posterior mediastinum, you should diligently search for evidence of a vertebral body fracture. If a spinal fracture is not evident on chest radiography, you should proceed to CT. Multidetector CT (MDCT) has been shown to have a much higher sensitivity than radiographs for detecting fractures and its sensitivity can be further enhanced by coronal and sagittal reformations.

The technique for a posteroanterior (PA) chest radiograph differs from that of an AP thoracic spinal radiography. To ensure adequate soft tissue penetration and optimal lung evaluation, PA chest radiographs are performed with higher tube potential (kV) than AP thoracic spinal radiographs. The higher tube potential results in faster acquisition, which has the advantage of less motion artifact, as well as decreased radiation dose. However, contrast resolution is decreased. This is not an issue for visualization of lung abnormalities, which display high tissue contrast with the air containing lung, but visualization of mediastinal and spinal abnormalities can be limited.

REFERENCES

Ritenour ER. Why does patient dose increase with tube energy in CT when it does the opposite in radiography? *AJR Am J Roentgenol.* 2015 Jul;205(1):W1.

Thoracic Radiology: The Requisites, 3rd ed, 19–60, 279–288.

CASE 14

Miliary Tuberculosis

1. **C and D.** Magnified view of the upper left hemothorax on posteroanterior (PA) radiograph shows diffuse, small pulmonary nodules consistent with a miliary pattern. The diffuse pattern of the small nodules on imaging is most consistent with miliary infection (most commonly tuberculosis) or miliary metastases. Emphysema manifests as focal areas of destroyed lung rather than nodular disease. Nodular pulmonary edema would also be highly unusual.

2. **B.** The diffuse pattern of nodular lung disease presented in this case is termed "random" in the subclassification of diffuse nodular lung disease. Nodules are present throughout the lungs without preference for any portion of the secondary pulmonary lobule. Centrilobular and perilymphatic patterns are the two other subclassifications of diffuse nodular lung disease which favor specific portions of the secondary pulmonary lobule. The tree-in-bud pattern is a subset of the centrilobular category.

3. **A.** The tree-in-bud pattern almost always represents small airway fluid or impaction with mucus or infected material and almost always signifies aspiration or pneumonia in clinical practice. It would be very unusual for pulmonary edema, hemorrhage, or metastases to present in this manner.

4. **B.** A random pattern of diffuse nodular lung disease indicates hematogenous spread of disease because of the relatively uniform distribution of blood supply to the lung parenchyma without respect to the secondary pulmonary lobule. Lymphatic spread leads to perilymphatic nodularity while aerogenous spread most commonly presents with tree-in-bud or centrilobular nodularity.

Comment

Differential Diagnosis

The differential diagnosis for diffuse nodular lung disease is broad. However, if the pattern of diffuse nodular lung disease can be subcategorized into centrilobular, perilymphatic, or random patterns, the differential diagnosis can be more focused. In combination with clinical history, a single, specific diagnosis may be achieved. The differential diagnosis for random diffuse nodular lung disease mainly consists of two entities: hematogenous infection or hematogenous metastases. Though the imaging pattern of both hematogenous infection and metastases are similar, these two entities can often be differentiated based on critical presentation.

The most common causes of the perilymphatic diffuse nodular pattern are sarcoidosis, lymphangitic spread of tumor, and lymphoma; less-common entities include silicosis and coworkers pneumoconiosis. Centrilobular diffuse nodular disease is most often from airway-related conditions including pneumonia, aspiration, pneumoconiosis, hypersensitivity pneumonitis, and respiratory bronchiolitis.

Imaging Findings

On CT, the random and perilymphatic nodular patterns both demonstrate nodules in the subpleural lung and fissures and centrally along the bronchovascular bundles (Fig. S14.2). Centrilobular nodules, by definition, spare the subpleural lung and fissures. The random pattern of diffuse nodular lung disease does not respect the underlying anatomy of secondary pulmonary lobule. In contradistinction, nodularity in perilymphatic diffuse nodular disease tends to cluster along the septal portions of the secondary pulmonary lobule (including the subpleural lung and fissures) and the bronchovascular tree because lymphatics are most concentrated in these areas.

REFERENCES
Boitsios G, Bankier AA, Eisenberg RL. Diffuse pulmonary nodules. *AJR Am J Roentgenol.* 2010 May;194(5):W354–W366.
Thoracic Radiology: The Requisites, 3rd ed, 323–334.

CASE 15

Neurofibromatosis

1. **B and C**. There are multiple nodular opacities on chest radiograph that demonstrate some borders that are well-defined and some borders that are poorly defined, which is highly suggestive of a non-pulmonary process. Therefore A and D (pulmonary conditions) should not be included on the differential diagnosis.
2. **A**. The imaging description above—some borders which are well-defined and some borders which are poorly defined—is the definition of the radiographic incomplete border sign. The hilar overlay and cervicothoracic signs are helpful in determining the location of mediastinal masses on radiography. The Monod sign presents as a thin crescent of gas around a mycetoma within a pre-existing cavitary or cystic space.
3. **C**. Acoustic neuromas are common findings in neurofibromatosis 2. The other findings (Café-au-lait spots, scoliosis, and optic gliomas) are commonly found in Neurofibromatosis 1.
4. **C**. The description of the imaging findings is highly suggestive of bilateral nipple shadows. Definite diagnosis of this normal finding requires repeat frontal radiograph after placement of nipple markers.

Comment

Differential Diagnosis

The incomplete border sign is inconsistent with pulmonary lesions unless there is associated extension into the pleura, mediastinum, or extra-pulmonary structures. Any nonpulmonary lesion, whether cutaneous, chest wall, pleural, or mediastinal can lead to the incomplete border sign. In clinical practice, the most common cause of the incomplete border sign are nipple shadows.

Imaging Findings

Focused view of the left hemithorax from a PA chest radiograph shows multiple nodular opacities overlying the left lung (Fig. 15.1A). Magnified image of the mid left lung zone shows that many of these lesions have margins that are both well-defined and ill-defined, consistent with the incomplete border sign (Fig. 15.1B).

The incomplete border sign is defined as a focal lesion with indistinct margins along a portion of its borders. This sign arises from the unique shape of many extrapulmonary lesions. In chest radiography, the well-defined borders of focal pulmonary nodules or masses arise from the contrast of the lesion with surrounding air in the lungs and the generally round or oval shape of the lesion. Therefore wherever x-ray photons are tangent to the margins of the pulmonary lesion, there will be sufficient contrast to show sharp margins. In contrast, extrapulmonary lesions are seldom round or oval; more often, these lesions conform to the curved shape of the chest wall, have tapered margins, and/or are pedunculated; moreover, they are not completely surrounded by air. Therefore x-ray photons are seldom completely tangent to the margins of the lesion where the lesion contacts air.

REFERENCES
Hsu CC, Henry TS, Chung JH, Little BP. The incomplete border sign. *J Thorac Imaging.* 2014 Jul;29(4):W48.
Thoracic Radiology: The Requisites, 3rd ed, 97–136.

CASE 16

Left Lower Lobe Atelectasis

1. **B**. The imaging findings are essentially diagnostic of left lower lobe collapse. There is a wedge-shaped opacity in the left retrocardiac region with subtle findings of left lung volume loss: leftward mediastinal shift, downward displacement of the left hilum, and superior displacement of the left hemidiaphragm. Pneumonia would not lead to volume loss. Pleural fluid would not commonly take this shape and would lead to contralateral shift of away from rather than towards the involved hemithorax.
2. **C**. In adults in the outpatient setting, the most common cause of lobar atelectasis is an endobronchial lesion, most often lung cancer. Carcinoid tumor also commonly affects the airways but is statistically less common than lung cancer. Hypoventilation does not cause lobar atelectasis; subsegmental atelectasis, typically in the dependent and inferior aspects of the lungs, is more common in this setting.
3. **A**. In children, the most common cause of lobar collapse is aspiration of a foreign body.
4. **D**. The flat waist sign represents loss of the normal "moguls" of the aortic arch and pulmonary artery along the left superior aspect of the mediastinum, which is causes by leftward deviation and rotation of the mediastinum from severe left lower lobe collapse. The cervicothoracic sign is a sign of mediastinal location of an abnormality on frontal chest radiograph. The S sign of Golden and the luftsichel sign are signs of lobar collapse, classically in the right upper lobe and left upper lobe, respectively.

Comment

Differential Diagnosis

The differential diagnosis for this case is very limited. The imaging findings are essentially pathognomonic for left lower lobe collapse. In the presented clinical setting, this is most often secondary to resorptive atelectasis from an underlying malignant endobronchial lesion, most commonly lung cancer (classically, squamous cell carcinoma or small cell, which are more central and tend to cause lobar atelectasis).

Imaging Findings

The chest radiograph and computed tomography (CT) image reveal the classic features of complete left lower lobe atelectasis. On chest radiographs, complete left lower lobe atelectasis appears as a triangular opacity behind the heart. The displaced major fissure is seen as an interface between the opacified atelectatic lobe and the hyperexpanded left upper lobe. Note the presence of several secondary signs of atelectasis in this case, including inferomedial displacement of the left hilum, slight leftward shift of the mediastinum, and compensatory hyperinflation of the left upper lobe.

Two well-known signs associated with left lower lobe atelectasis are the ivory heart sign and the flat waist sign. In the ivory heart sign, the lung vessels of the left lower lobe normally seen behind the left aspect of the heart on a frontal chest radiograph are no longer visible. The left lower lobe has collapsed medially and inferiorly, leading to complete opacification of the left retrocardiac area. In the flat waist sign, the normal "moguls" of the aortic arch and pulmonary artery along the left superior aspect of the mediastinum "flatten" from leftward deviation and rotation of the mediastinum as a result of left lower lobe atelectasis.

REFERENCES
Woodring JH, Reed JC. Radiographic manifestations of lobar atelectasis. *J Thorac Imaging*. 1996 Spring;11(2):109–144.
Thoracic Radiology: The Requisites, 3rd ed, 19–60.

CASE 17
Pulmonary Hypertension

1. **A.** The pulmonary arteries are enlarged with peripheral pruning of pulmonary arteries. The findings are essentially diagnostic of pulmonary hypertension. Differentiation of idiopathic vs. pulmonary hypertension due to known causes is usually not possible on radiography.
2. **C.** All of the listed options are known causes of pulmonary hypertension except for "C." Although medications can lead to pulmonary hypertension, calcium channel blockers are an accepted treatment for pulmonary hypertension and not a cause of this condition.
3. **C.** A cutoff of 3 cm is a commonly accepted measurement for a normal main pulmonary arterial size on CT. The larger the pulmonary artery, the more likely the patient has pulmonary hypertension.
4. **A.** Portopulmonary hypertension is pulmonary hypertension secondary to portal hypertension. The pathogenesis of pulmonary hypertension secondary to portal hypertension is complex but is likely multifactorial including a hyperdynamic circulatory state, high cardiac output, and portosystemic shunting of vasoactive compounds. The other listed conditions are not known causes of pulmonary hypertension.

Comment

Differential Diagnosis

Enlarged central main pulmonary arteries are highly suggestive of pulmonary hypertension (PH). In cases of pulmonic stenosis, there may be isolated central left pulmonary arterial and main pulmonary arterial dilation from chronic flow effects of the post-stenotic jet. However, this condition is very uncommon relative to PH. PH can be idiopathic (no known cause) or more commonly results from other causes or disease states. Although the list of causes of PH is quite extensive, most cases in adults are a result of chronic left-sided heart disease or chronic lung disease; other notable causes include left-to-right shunts, chronic thromboembolic disease, and collagen vascular disease.

Imaging Findings

Regardless of the cause of PH, the characteristic findings on chest radiographs are similar. There is usually marked enlargement of the main and hilar pulmonary arteries, which rapidly taper as they course distally. The degree of pulmonary artery enlargement varies considerably, and significant PH can be present in the setting of a normal chest radiograph. CT is more accurate than chest radiography for detecting pulmonary artery enlargement. Some causes of pulmonary hypertension may be detected on chest CT (e.g., chronic thromboembolic disease, chronic lung disease [emphysema, pulmonary fibrosis, sarcoidosis], left-to-right shunts, and rarely post-capillary conditions).

REFERENCES
Barbosa Jr EJ, Gupta NK, Torigian DA, Gefter WB. Current role of imaging in the diagnosis and management of pulmonary hypertension. *AJR Am J Roentgenol*. 2012 Jun;198(6):1320–1331.
Thoracic Radiology: The Requisites, 3rd ed, 238–258.

CASE 18
Lung Abscess

1. **A, B, C, and D.** All the listed choices can be included in differential diagnosis for a cavitary lung lesion. Small vessel vasculitis (e.g., granulomatosis with polyangiitis [formerly known as *Wegener granulomatosis*]), necrobiotic nodules in rheumatoid arthritis, metastases, and pulmonary abscess may all cause cavitary nodules or masses.
2. **C.** Classically, the most common primary tumors to cause cavitary metastases are squamous cell carcinoma (usually head and neck cancer), sarcomas, and transitional cell cancer. Recent evidence shows that adenocarcinomas also commonly cavitate. Pulmonary metastases from metastatic melanoma may cavitate; however, this is not as common as in the other primary tumors listed.
3. **C.** Lung abscesses most commonly develop from aspiration pneumonia. Though trauma could lead to focal pneumatoceles, which could become infected, this is uncommon compared with aspiration-related lung abscesses. Focal air-trapping is not a major contributor to lung abscess formation. Bland pulmonary emboli may cause pulmonary infarction, which only rarely cavitate unless infected (septic infarcts resulting from septic emboli, which are usually multiple).
4. **A.** The anterior segment of the right upper lobe is almost never the most nondependent bronchopulmonary segment in the supine, decubitus, or upright positions. Therefore this segment is least affected by pulmonary abscesses.

Comment

Differential Diagnosis

Sagittal computed tomography (CT) image shows a focal cavitary lesion with surrounding consolidation in the posterior segment of the right upper lobe (Fig. 18.1). The differential diagnosis for cavitary lung lesions can be recalled using the classic mnemonic NICE: **N**eoplasm (squamous cell primary tumor or metastases), **i**nfection (pulmonary abscess), **c**ollagen vascular disease and vasculitis (rheumatoid arthritis, granulomatosis with polyangiitis), and **e**mboli (septic emboli). In this case, the patient had other findings suggestive of aspiration. Axial CT image in the same patient as in Fig. 18.1 shows centrilobular ground-glass nodules throughout the left lower lobe (consistent with aspiration) and a air-fluid level in a dilated esophagus consistent with esophageal dysmotility. Esophageal pathology predisposes patients to aspiration. Therefore the most likely diagnosis was that of pulmonary abscess, which most commonly develops from aspiration pneumonia.

Discussion

Aspiration pneumonia is most often polymicrobial with both anaerobic and aerobic microbial agents originating in the mouth. Presentation is usually indolent unlike the more acute presentation of *Streptococcus* pneumonia. Sputum is classically foul-smelling because of the presence of large numbers or anaerobic bacteria. Aspiration most commonly affects the dependent portions of the lungs and preferentially involves the right lung as opposed to the left lung because of the relatively obtuse angle of the right mainstem bronchus with the trachea. Associated empyema is quite common, occurring in 30% to 50% of cases. Bronchopleural or alveolopleural fistula should be suspected in the case of associated pneumothorax or hydropneumothorax. Even with appropriate medical therapy, it may take months for a lung abscess to heal completely. In a minority of patients (10%–20%), percutaneous drainage or surgical intervention may be necessary.

REFERENCES
Franquet T, Giménez A, Rosón N, Torrubia S, Sabaté JM, Pérez C. Aspiration diseases: findings, pitfalls, and differential diagnosis. *Radiographics*. 2000 May–Jun;20(3):673–685.
Thoracic Radiology: The Requisites, 3rd ed, 289–309.

CASE 19

Pneumomediastinum

1. **A, B, and D**. The chest radiograph demonstrates classic findings of pneumomediastinum (see figure captions below). The most common cause of pneumomediastinum is the Macklin effect—alveolar rupture with dissection of gas along the axial interstitium into the mediastinum—which is usually due to asthma. Rupture of the trachea and esophagus are other causes of pneumomediastinum. Blebs are associated with spontaneous pneumothorax.
2. **B**. Pneumomediastinum represents extension of gas along tissue planes and interfaces of the mediastinum. Mediastinal gas does not rapidly shift with patient position as in the other listed conditions and can help in the differentiation of this condition from other causes of ectopic gas.
3. **C**. Typically, the pericardium surrounds the heart and then extends along the proximal margins of the great vessels for a variable distance. Although nearly the entire aorta and the caudal half of the superior vena cava (SVC) can be encompassed by pericardium, the pericardium does not extend above the level of the aortic arch or above the azygous portion of the SVC.
4. **B**. The continuous diaphragm sign represents gas lucency outlining the superior surface of the diaphragm, demarcating it from the inferior margin of the heart. This sign can be seen in either pneumomediastinum or pneumopericardium. However, it is more common in pneumomediastinum. A pneumopericardium is often associated with some degree of pericardial effusion which usually prevents gas accumulation in an inferior position adjacent to the diaphragm. Theoretically, the

ring around the artery sign could be seen in the setting of a pneumopericardium because the pericardium encompasses the proximal right pulmonary artery extending to the level of the truncus anterior. However, in clinical practice, this sign is highly diagnostic of a pneumomediastinum. A large amount of gas must surround the extra-pericardial portion of right pulmonary artery to be clearly visible on lateral radiography.

Comment

Differential Diagnosis

The causes of pneumomediastinum can be categorized into four main groups: conditions that increase alveolar pressure, conditions that disrupt alveolar walls, rupture of gas containing organs (tracheal or esophageal rupture), and extension of gas from other sites. The most common cause is asthma, which leads to elevated alveolar pressure, rupture, and central extension of gas into the mediastinum via the axial interstitium. Other causes of elevated alveolar pressure (central large airway obstruction, mechanical ventilation, blunt trauma) and damage to alveolar walls (pulmonary fibrosis, emphysema, pneumonia, diffuse alveolar damage) can also lead to pneumomediastinum. Extension of gas from the neck or abdomen (whether iatrogenic, traumatic, or infectious) can also extend into the mediastinum although ectopic gas is more concentrated in the area of origin. Except in newborns or young infants, air in the mediastinum will always eventually dissect into the neck, a finding that is useful for determining the location of the ectopic gas.

Discussion

Pneumomediastinum is most often asymptomatic; however, some patients may complain of chest pain or discomfort. Usually, pneumomediastinum, in and of itself, is harmless. The underlying cause of pneumomediastinum, on the other hand, must be addressed. Rarely, pneumomediastinum may lead to tension phenomenon and impair venous return to the heart, though this is much more common in the setting of tension pneumothorax. Pneumomediastinum may rupture into the pleural space and directly cause pneumothorax. Conversely, pneumothorax does not extend into the mediastinum to cause pneumomediastinum.

In addition to typical findings of pneumomediastinum (lucent streaks or punctate foci of gas which outline mediastinal structures), there are multiple signs which, if present, can help facilitate diagnosis. The ring around the artery sign represents gas around the main right pulmonary artery and is visible on lateral radiograph. The Naclerio V sign represents mediastinal gas along the lateral aspect of the inferior thoracic aorta combined with gas between the parietal pleura and left hemidiaphragm. Continuous diaphragm sign can be seen in pneumomediastinum or pneumopericardium and represents ectopic gas superior to the diaphragm but inferior to the heart.

REFERENCES
Bejvan SM, Godwin JD. Pneumomediastinum: old signs and new signs. *AJR Am J Roentgenol*. 1996 May;166(5):1041–1048.
Thoracic Radiology: The Requisites, 3rd ed, 97–136.

CASE 20

Subpulmonic Pleural Effusion

1. **B**. The chest radiograph demonstrates typical findings of a subpulmonic pleural effusion: apparent elevation of the right hemidiaphragm, lateral peaking of superior margin of the right pseudo-hemidiaphragm, and subtle blunting of the

right lateral costophrenic angle. A liver mass and diaphragmatic paralysis would cause elevation of the diaphragm but not cause a lateral peak or blunting of the costophrenic angle. Diaphragmatic eventration usually leads to focal elevation of the diaphragm as opposed to the more diffuse right-sided process in the current case.

2. **D.** Lateral decubitus radiographs are by far the most sensitive means to detect pleural effusion, followed by the lateral radiograph, the PA radiograph, and—finally—the AP (supine) radiograph.

3. **A.** Though all the listed disease processes can cause transudative pleural effusions, congestive heart failure is the most common cause.

4. **A.** Though all the listed disease processes can cause exudative pleural effusions, pneumonia (parapneumonic pleural effusion) is the most common cause.

Comment

On an upright chest radiograph, a pleural effusion is usually manifested by the presence of a meniscus sign, which refers to a blunted appearance of the costophrenic angle, with a concave upward slope. In general, it requires approximately 200 mL of fluid to blunt the lateral costophrenic angle but only approximately 75 ml of fluid to blunt the posterior costophrenic angle. A lateral decubitus view can demonstrate as little as 5 mL of fluid.

In some patients, a large amount of free-flowing pleural fluid may collect in the subpulmonic space before spilling into the costophrenic angle. For unknown reasons, this occurs more often in the right hemithorax. In such cases, one may observe a characteristic appearance on the frontal chest radiograph, including an apparent elevation of the hemidiaphragm, flattening of the diaphragm contour medially, displacement of the peak of the diaphragm laterally, opacification of the lung posterior to the diaphragm on PA view, and greater than 2 cm distance between the inferior left lung margin and the gastric bubble. A suspected subpulmonic effusion can be confirmed by obtaining a lateral decubitus radiograph

REFERENCES
Hansell DM, et al. Imaging of Diseases of the Chest, 5th ed. 2009.
Thoracic Radiology: The Requisites, 3rd ed, 159–192.

CASE 21

Pneumothorax on Supine Radiograph

1. **A.** The chest radiograph demonstrates classic findings of a left-sided pneumothorax on supine radiograph: increased lucency of the left hemidiaphragm, deep left lateral sulcus relative to the normal right sulcus, mass-like configuration of the left pericardial fat pad, and partial visualization of the lateral aspect of the anterior costophrenic sulcus (arrow on appended image).

2. **D.** Lateral decubitus radiograph is by the most sensitive means to detect pneumothorax on radiography. The side of concern should be positioned superiorly (therefore, in this case of suspected left pneumothorax, the patient would be imaged with a right lateral decubitus radiograph).

3. **A.** Primary, spontaneous pneumothorax (not precipitated by trauma and in those without underlying lung disease) is the most common cause of pneumothorax in young individuals. This type of pneumothorax is caused by rupture of small subpleural blebs and classically occurs in tall, slender, young men who smoke. A change in atmospheric pressure has been implicated as a precipitating factor. It has been rarely described in the young individuals listening to loud music.

4. **B.** The deep sulcus sign is high suggestive of a pneumothorax on a supine radiograph. Air within the pleural space rises to the most nondependent of the thorax (in the supine position, the anteromedial, subpulmonic, and lateral basilar space). The ring around the artery sign is a finding in pneumomediastinum. The Westermark sign is a rare finding of pulmonary embolism on radiography, which manifests as localized hypovascularity distal to a focus of pulmonary embolism. The air crescent sign is classically associated with invasive fungal pneumonias. It appears as a superior crescent of air in a cavity filled with solid tissue.

Comment

A pneumothorax is usually readily identifiable on an upright chest radiograph as an apicolateral white line (the visceral pleural line) with an absence of vessels beyond it. However, in the supine position, the apicolateral portion of the lung is no longer the most nondependent portion. Rather, air collects preferentially in the anteromedial and subpulmonic portions of the chest. AP supine chest radiograph demonstrates classic findings of a left-sided pneumothorax on supine radiograph: increased lucency of the left hemidiaphragm, deep left lateral sulcus relative to the normal right sulcus, mass-like configuration of the left pericardial fat pad, and partial visualization of the lateral aspect of the anterior costophrenic sulcus (arrow). Only when a large volume of air is present in the pleural space will you visualize an apicolateral pleural line on a supine radiograph. Thus, although highly specific for pneumothorax, this is not a highly sensitive sign on supine radiographs.

Unfortunately, even with high levels of clinical suspicion, the majority of pneumothoraces are subtle or invisible on supine radiography. Because many patients with pneumothoraces are too ill to undergo upright radiographs, recognition of the appearance of pneumothoraces on supine radiograph is essential. Common manifestations of a pneumothorax on supine radiography include the following:

1. Relative hyperlucency of the ipsilateral hemidiaphragm or whole hemithorax
2. Increased sharpness of the ipsilateral mediastinal and/or cardiac borders or hemidiaphragm
3. Deep lateral sulcus (aka the "deep sulcus sign")
4. Visualization of two apparent ipsilateral hemidiaphragms, and delineation of the edge of the anterior costophrenic sulcus caused by the lucency of the basilar pneumothorax

If pneumothorax is suspected, further evaluation with upright PA radiograph, lateral decubitus radiograph (with suspected side of pneumothorax positioned superiorly), or computed tomography (CT) may be mandatory. In the critically ill patient in whom these imaging choices are not possible, a bedside cross table lateral will demonstrate the anterior location of a pneumothorax.

REFERENCES
Tocino IM, Miller MH, Fairfax WR. Distribution of pneumothorax in the supine and semirecumbent critically ill adult. *AJR Am J Roentgenol*. 1985 May;144(5):901–905.
Thoracic Radiology: The Requisites, 3rd ed, 159–192.

CASE 22

Loculated Pleural Fluid in the Major Fissure (Pseudotumor)

1. **D.** The lesion in question is not in the lung. The presence of incomplete borders on the PA view and the tapered margins of the opacity superiorly and inferiorly on lateral view are diagnostic of an extrapulmonary lesion within the right

major fissure. This is the classic appearance for loculated pleural fluid in a fissure.

2. **D.** A pseudotumor, phantom tumor, or vanishing tumor are common names given to loculated pleural fluid in a fissure because it may simulate a large pulmonary mass. As pleural fluid eventually resolves, the apparent pulmonary mass disappears.

3. **C.** Metastatic disease is the most common cause of neoplastic disease involving the pleural. Adenocarcinoma is the most common cell type. The most common sites of the primary tumors are lung and breast cancer. Lymphoma may also involve the pleural space. The most common primary malignancy of the pleura is mesothelioma secondary to asbestos exposure.

4. **C.** The inferior accessory fissure in the most common accessory fissure in the lungs and is present in up to half of the population. This fissure separates the medial basal segment from the other basal lower lobe segments. The next most common accessory fissure in the superior accessory fissure which demarcates the superior lower lobe segment from the basal segments and is present in up to 20% to30% of the population. The left minor fissure is present in up to 20% of the population while the azygous fissure is present in 1% to 2% of the population.

Comment

The chest radiograph in this case demonstrates the characteristic appearance of a loculated pleural fluid collection within the major fissure. When fluid is loculated within the major fissure, it may appear on the PA projection as either a discrete, masslike opacity with incomplete borders (as demonstrated in the first figure) or as a hazy, veil-like opacity. On the lateral radiograph, such a loculated fluid collection appears as a well-marginated, elliptical opacity coursing along the obliquely oriented axis of the major fissure (as demonstrated in the second figure). The rapid onset and resolution of such fluid collections distinguishes loculated fluid from a solid pleural mass. When the diagnosis is in doubt, a decubitus view may be helpful because it will demonstrate shift of the free fluid. Computed tomography (CT) can readily differentiate pleural fluid collections from solid masses and may be useful in selected problem cases in which there is a lack of shift on decubitus radiographs due to loculation.

Such loculation occurs most commonly in patients with heart failure. Loculated fluid is seen more often in the right pleural space than in the left, and the minor fissure is more commonly involved than the major fissure. Because of the transient nature of loculated fluid collections, they have been referred to as "vanishing tumors," "phantom tumors," and "pseudotumors." Such terms should be avoided in radiology reports to avoid possible confusion.

REFERENCES
Walker CM, Takasugi JE, Chung JH, Reddy GP, Done SL, Pipavath SN, Schmidt RA, Godwin 2nd JD. Tumorlike conditions of the pleura. *Radiographics.* 2012, Jul–Aug;32(4):971–985.
Thoracic Radiology: The Requisites, 3rd ed, 159–192.

CASE 23

Esophageal Cancer

1. **A, B, and C.** The azygoesophageal recess is an interface that extends from the horizontal aspect of the azygous vein superiorly and terminates inferiorly at the esophageal hiatus. This interface is demarcated by air in the right lower lobe abutting the mediastinal contours adjacent to the esophagus. The superior aspect of the recess is contiguous with the subcarinal space. In this case, there is focal convexity along the superior aspect of the azygoesophageal recess. Esophageal

cancer, lung cancer, and a foregut cyst (usually a bronchogenic cyst) could all cause this imaging findings. Thymomas develop in the anterior mediastinum and, therefore, would not lead to abnormality in the azygoesophageal recess.

2. **C.** Because of the typically avid FDG uptake within a primary esophageal cancer, FDG-PET imaging is not dependable for detection of regional lymph nodes adjacent to the primary tumor. Furthermore, FDG-PET lacks the spatial and contrast resolution necessary for accurate T staging in esophageal cancer; endoscopic ultrasound is the best imaging tool for T staging. FDG-PET can detect distant occult metastatic foci, however, and may also be a useful biomarker in treatment response.

3. **A.** There are many causes of an abnormal azygoesophageal recess. In about 80% of posteroanterior (PA) chest radiographs, the azygoesophageal recess is visible as a straight or concave interface posterior to the right heart border. The most common cause of abnormality in the superior aspect of the azygoesophageal recess is lymphadenopathy. The most common cause of pathology in the inferior azygoesophageal recess is a hiatal hernia, which can often be diagnosed definitively by identifying a gas/fluid level in the hernia either on PA or lateral radiographs. Left atrial dilation may also lead to an abnormality in the azygoesophageal recess more superiorly in the subcarinal area. It may be associated with splaying of the carina.

4. **C.** The most common risk factor for AC is gastroesophageal reflux disease. Unlike SCC, AC is more common in the lower third of the esophagus Fig. 23.3. SCC is more common than AC worldwide. AC also has a better prognosis than SCC.

Comment

The azygoesophageal recess normally presents as a smooth interface posterior to the heart and projected over the spine close to the midline on the frontal chest radiograph. It is intimately associated with the azygous vein and the esophagus, from which it derives its name. Normally, the azygoesophageal recess has slightly concave margin without focal convexity or nodularity. In children, the superior aspect of the recess may have mild convexity until early adolescence because of the course of the azygous vein. Frontal scout image from chest computed tomography (CT) shows loss of the normal contour of the azygoesophageal recess superiorly. The azygoesophageal recess is well defined more inferiorly (see arrow in annotated image). Focal convexity in this region on chest radiography requires further assessment with CT or comparison to remote chest imaging to determine the presence of a pathologic process such as a mass or adenopathy. However, many cases are due to the mild rightward course of the esophagus in 20% of young adults.

The differential diagnosis of an abnormality of the azygoesophageal recess is broad. Superiorly, lymphadenopathy (whether malignant or benign) in the subcarinal space is most common. Slightly more inferiorly in the azygoesophageal recess, mild left atrial enlargement may also disrupt the recess. As left atrial dilation worsens, other signs of left atrial enlargement should become apparent including widening of the carinal angle, posterior displacement of the left lower lobe bronchus, and convexity along the posterior margin of the heart border on lateral radiograph. Hiatal hernias are the most common cause of focal convexity in the lower azygoesophageal recess. However, care must be taken not to assume that all lesions in this area as benign, because esophageal cancer may lead to a focal abnormality in the azygoesophageal recess at any level. Gastroesophageal varices may mimic hiatal hernias on radiography though hernias will often have a diagnostic internal gas/fluid level. Bronchogenic cysts are incidentally detected lesions with no serious clinical ramifications; they are usually found inferior to the level of the carina and often cause focal convexity of the azygoesophageal recess. Esophageal duplication cysts arise more inferiorly just above the diaphragm and often on the right side. They also may cause a convexity in the azygoesophageal recess.

REFERENCES
Ravenel JG, Erasmus JJ. Azygoesophageal recess. *J Thorac Imaging.* 2002 Jul;17(3):219–226.
Thoracic Radiology: The Requisites, 3rd ed, 19–60, 97–136.

CASE 24

Benign Calcified Granuloma

1. **A and C.** The radiograph shows the typical appearance of a calcified granuloma, most commonly from previous tuberculosis or histoplasmosis. The "classic" pattern of calcification in pulmonary hamartomas is one with a coarse "popcorn" appearance. However, CT is superior to radiography for showing the true pattern of calcification. Lung adenocarcinoma can present as a solitary nodule. Most are not calcified, and when calcium is present, it is typically faint, eccentric, or stippled. The calcified nodule on the radiograph has sharp margins and is surrounded by aerated lung, indicating that it is pulmonary in location and not a pleural plaque.

2. **C.** A stippled pattern of calcification cannot be considered benign and may be seen in neoplasms such as pulmonary carcinoid. A diffuse pattern of calcification is considered benign. The one exception occurs when the patient has a history of a matrix-forming tumor such as osteosarcoma. A central pattern of calcification is considered benign. A laminar or concentric pattern of calcification can be considered benign and may be encountered in nodules from previous histoplasmosis or tuberculosis.

3. **D.** The presence of macroscopic fat in a solitary lung nodule on CT is diagnostic of a pulmonary hamartoma. Thin section CT is often required to appreciate the small foci of fat. Eccentric calcification is not a reliable indicator of benignity. A small percentage of lung carcinomas can contain calcification, although it is usually scattered throughout the lesion; alternatively, a lung carcinoma can engulf a calcified granuloma, resulting in an eccentric calcification. Although smooth margins suggest a less-aggressive lesion, they are not reliable enough to indicate benignity. For example, some pulmonary carcinoids have smooth margins. A mixed solid and ground-glass attenuation nodule is highly suggestive of low-grade lung adenocarcinoma and should be resected or biopsied because of the high likelihood of malignancy.

4. **B.** A lung nodule with spiculated margins has the highest likelihood ratio (5.54) of being malignant. Larger nodules are more likely to be malignant than smaller nodules. The likelihood ratio of a nodule >3 cm being malignant is 5.23. A lung nodule doubling time between 30 and 400 days has a likelihood ratio of 3.40 of being malignant. Nodules that double in volume in less than 30 days are most likely benign, typically infectious. Lung cancers occur more commonly in the upper lobes than the lower lobes, with slight right upper lobe predominance. The likelihood ratio of an upper lobe nodule being malignant is 1.22.

Comment

Differential Diagnosis

The chest radiograph demonstrates a densely calcified nodule in the left lower lung, recognized benign pattern. These calcified nodules are typically the result of remote granulomatous infection such as tuberculosis or histoplasmosis.

Solitary Pulmonary Nodule

There are two accepted radiographic criteria for a benign solitary pulmonary nodule: lack of growth over at least 2 years and identification of a benign calcification pattern within a smoothly marginated pulmonary nodule.

Roughly half of all resected solitary pulmonary nodules prove to be benign. Clinical indicators that suggest a benign diagnosis include age younger than 35 years and history of exposure to tuberculosis or residence in areas with endemic tuberculosis or fungal infections. Such indicators are, unfortunately, insufficiently specific to be helpful in most individual cases.

For patients with nodules that do not meet the accepted radiographic criteria for benignancy, noncontrast CT with thin-section imaging is usually the preferred method for further evaluation. CT is more sensitive than conventional radiographs for detecting calcium and fat within a nodule. In certain cases, CT imaging allows a confident diagnosis of a specific benign entity such as granuloma, hamartoma, arteriovenous malformation, pulmonary infarction, mucoid impaction, and pulmonary sequestration.

When CT is nondiagnostic, the method of further evaluation depends on patient characteristics and nodule morphology. Noninvasive imaging modalities include contrast-enhanced CT to assess for abnormal nodule enhancement and fluorodeoxyglucose (FDG)-positron emission tomography (PET)/CT imaging, which relies on abnormal glucose analogue (FDG) uptake to distinguish benign from malignant nodules. However, false positive and false negative examinations can occur with FDG-PET/CT because of increased metabolic activity in inflammatory nodules and low metabolic activity in low-grade malignancies.

REFERENCES
Erasmus JJ, Connoly JE, McAdams HP, Roggli VL. Solitary pulmonary nodules: part I. Morphologic evaluation for differentiation of benign and malignant lesions. *Radiographics.* 2000;20:43–58.
Erasmus JJ, McAdams HP, Connoly JE. Solitary pulmonary nodules: part II. Evaluation of the indeterminate nodule. *Radiographics.* 2000;20:59–66.
Thoracic Radiology: The Requisites, 3rd ed, 428–440.

CASE 25

Radiation Pneumonitis

1. **C and D.** The sharp and relatively straight lateral and superior margins, nonanatomic distribution on the lateral view, and distortion and volume loss are highly suggestive of radiation induced injury because the inflammation occurs only within the radiation port. Infection can cause perihilar dense consolidation as well, although margins are typically less well defined except when consolidation abuts a pulmonary fissure. Sarcoidosis can cause perihilar and central opacities, which occasionally appear consolidative, but it is nearly always bilateral and typically symmetric. Idiopathic pulmonary fibrosis is characterized by peripheral and basal predominant interstitial fibrosis. In this patient, there is consolidation, which is limited to the central portion of the right lung.

2. **C.** Radiation pneumonitis is usually apparent on the chest radiograph by 6 to 8 weeks following completion of therapy. On occasion, radiation pneumonitis can have a rapid or delayed onset. However, this is not the usual time course. Numerous factors such as radiation dose, concomitant chemotherapy, and host factors contribute to radiation induced lung injury. Computed tomography (CT) can show show abnormalities before they become apparent on chest radiography.

3. **A.** Although different tumor types can alter the radiation treatment plan for a patient, the tumor histology itself does not directly contribute to the patient's risk for developing

radiation-induced lung injury. Some chemotherapeutic agents such as gemcitabine can predispose a patient to developing radiation-induced lung disease. Higher radiation doses increase the risk of lung injury. Larger tumors require targeting therapy to a larger volume of tissue, thus increasing a patient's risk of developing radiation-induced lung disease.

4. **D**. Radiation fibrosis usually develops 6 to 12 months after the completion of therapy. Radiation pneumonitis is not a prerequisite for developing radiation fibrosis, and patients with radiation pneumonitis might not develop fibrosis. Patients who have radiation pneumonitis and are symptomatic can have a normal radiograph, while some patients with abnormal radiographs are asymptomatic. Radiation fibrosis usually stabilizes 12 to 24 months after completion of therapy, depending on the technique(s) used. A progressing abnormality on the chest radiograph after this time should raise suspicion for recurrent neoplasm or another process.

Comment

Differential Diagnosis

Posteroanterior (PA) and lateral radiographs show dense perihilar consolidation in the right lung with associated volume loss. Note the sharp lateral and superior margins on the PA radiograph and the nonanatomic distribution on the lateral view where consolidation crosses the pulmonary fissures. This nonanatomic distribution of dense consolidation with volume loss is typical of radiation induced injury. Infection and aspiration could have a similar appearance, although the margins typically are less well defined. Adenocarcinoma could be considered with chronic consolidation.

Discussion

The chest radiograph (Figure 1) shows dense right lung consolidation with sharp lateral and superior margins with a nonanatomic distribution, spanning the right lung in the sagittal plane. The geographic margins and geometric shape correspond to the field of irradiation.

Radiation pneumonitis and fibrosis can occur in patients who have received definitive radiation therapy for lung cancer. Radiation pneumonitis is generally observed on chest radiographs within 6 to 8 weeks following completion of treatment, but CT might detect subtle abnormalities earlier than radiography (within a few weeks after completion of treatment). Such opacities are characteristically sharply demarcated and are not limited by anatomic boundaries such as fissures. Fibrosis usually develops within 6 to 12 months following radiation therapy. With time, radiation fibrosis can ensue. The parenchymal opacities generally become more linear in configuration and are usually accompanied by volume loss and traction bronchiectasis.

Several methods have been developed to deliver an adequate dose of radiation to tumors while limiting the amount of exposure to normal lung parenchyma. These techniques include limited radiation portals, tangential beams, conformed therapy, intensity-modulated radiation therapy. These methods can result in variable patterns of radiation-induced lung injury and stereotactic body radiation therapy (SBRT). Knowledge of the temporal relationship and type of therapy can help to distinguish radiation changes from infection and malignancy. Fluorodeoxyglucose positron emission tomography (FDG PET)/CT can be helpful for distinguishing radiation-induced lung disease from malignancy when performed at least 6 to 12 months after completion of radiation therapy.

Radiation pneumonitis can be treated expectantly, or patients may be given corticosteroids. Severe pneumonitis can require supplementary oxygen or mechanical ventilation.

REFERENCES
Choi YW, Munden RF, Erasmus JJ, et al. Effects of radiation therapy on the lung: radiologic appearances and differential diagnosis. *Radiographics*. 2004;24:985–997.
Thoracic Radiology: The Requisites, 3rd ed, 405–427.

CASE 26

Acute Respiratory Distress Syndrome With Barotrauma

1. **A, B, and D**. ARDS is a form of acute hypoxic respiratory failure with myriad causes including infection, trauma, inhalational injury, drug toxicity, aspiration, and collagen-vascular disease. The chest radiograph is always abnormal and usually shows extensive lung opacification with air bronchograms. Sarcoidosis most commonly presents as symmetric mediastinal and hilar lymphadenopathy with or without lung involvement, which includes bilateral perilymphatic nodules and less commonly large opacities.

2. **A and D**. The chest radiograph (Fig. 26.1) shows a lucent gas collection in the right hemithorax separating the visceral and parietal pleura laterally. There is also a pneumomediastinum. There is air streaking into the next superimposed on the spinous processes of the upper vertebral bodies. The computed tomography (CT) (Supplemental Fig. 26.1) shows air in the anterior mediastinum. Pneumomediastinum typically consists of streaks of air in the mediastinum on the frontal radiograph, with gas sometimes outlining structures such as the aorta. Subcutaneous gas is often a secondary sign of pneumomediastinum. Pneumopericardium is much less common than pneumomediastinum except for patients who had recent heart surgery. Pneumopericardium usually surrounds one or both ventricles as a thin band of gas. No ectopic subdiaphragmatic gas is evident on this chest radiograph.

3. **B**. With evolution of ARDS, organization and healing, often with fibrosis, ensue. The lungs become stiff, and barotrauma can result from higher pressure ventilation, which is required to maintain oxygenation. Pneumothorax or pneumomediastinum can develop. Central venous catheter placement can also cause pneumothorax, although increased used of ultrasound guidance has reduced this complication. Pulmonary laceration can cause pneumothorax, but there are not other signs of traumatic injury to the chest in this patient.

4. **D**. Pleural effusion is not a requirement for the diagnosis of ARDS. By definition, $Pao_2/Fio_2 \leq 300$ is required for ARDS, and the severity is assessed by the degree of impaired oxygenation. Bilateral lung opacity on chest radiography is a criterion for the diagnosis of ARDS. Hypoxemic respiratory failure must develop within one week of an insult.

Comment

Differential Diagnosis

The AP portable radiograph shows support tubes in expected locations, diffuse lung opacity, and small right pneumothorax as well as pneumomediastinum. The differential diagnosis of diffuse lung opacity in an acutely hypoxemic patient is usually limited to cardiogenic or non-cardiogenic edema, diffuse alveolar hemorrhage, or infection; and distinction among these causes is often difficult on imaging alone.

Discussion

ARDS is a severe form of acute lung injury that is thought to encompass a variety of distinct disorders that share common pathophysiologic and clinical features. The definition of ARDS was updated in 2012 (the Berlin Definition) to better reflect understanding of ARDS and pitfalls in diagnosis.

A variety of pulmonary and extrapulmonary conditions, can precipitate ARDS including infection, trauma, inhalational injury, drug toxicity, aspiration, and collagen-vascular disease. The clinical definition of ARDS includes $Pao_2/Fio_2 \leq 300$, bilateral lung opacity on the chest radiograph, acute onset, and exclusion of hydrostatic lung edema.

Because of decreased lung compliance and the need for prolonged mechanical ventilation, patients with ARDS can develop barotrauma, including subcutaneous emphysema, pneumothorax, pneumomediastinum, and pulmonary interstitial emphysema.

Treatment of ARDS includes ventilatory support and treatment of the underlying cause. The mortality rate is high, approximately 50%. Survivors can have residual pulmonary deficits.

REFERENCES

ARDS Definition Task Force. Acute respiratory distress syndrome: the Berlin Definition. *JAMA*. 2012 Jun 20;307(23):2526–2533.

Thoracic Radiology: The Requisites, 3rd ed, 226–237.

CASE 27
Cavity From Postprimary Tuberculosis

1. **A, B, and D**. Lung cancer can cavitate, usually as the result of necrosis. Granulomatosis with polyangiitis (formerly Wegener's granulomatosis) can present as a solitary cavitary mass lesion with an irregular, thickened wall, although multiple lesions are more common. Postprimary tuberculosis (reactivation or reinfection) often manifests as cavitary disease. However, the status of the patient's immune system determines the presentation of tuberculosis, whether it is primary infection, reactivation, or reinfection. Cavities can form in sarcoidosis but are typically the sequelae of fibrosis and bronchiectasis. Unilateral upper lobe disease in sarcoidosis would be highly unusual.

2. **C**. Squamous cell carcinomas have the highest association with cavitation, especially when they are large. Adenocarcinomas, small cell lung carcinomas, and large cell carcinomas can cavitate, albeit less frequently than with squamous cell carcinomas.

3. **A**. Wall thickness is not specific for the nature of a cavitary mass lesion, but wall thickness <4 mm is usually associated with a benign lesion. Fluid levels more commonly occur in benign cavitary lesions. However, hemorrhage or necrosis within a neoplasm can produce an intracavitary fluid level. Cavitation in a pre-existing area of lung consolidation is most suggestive of a lung abscess.

4. **C**. In a patient with a cavitary lesion in the apical and posterior segments of the upper lobes or in the superior segment of the lower lobes, respiratory isolation is critical until active tuberculosis is excluded, because spread of mycobacteria into the tracheobronchial tree can result in transmission of the infection to others. Bronchoscopy with bronchoalveolar lavage may be useful in establishing a diagnosis, but respiratory isolation and sputum analysis should be performed first. Transthoracic needle biopsy can help establish the diagnosis, especially if the cavitary lesion is malignant. However, fine needle aspiration typically cannot establish a specific benign diagnosis. However, core needle biopsies have a higher lead in benign lesions. FDG PET/CT is not the next best step because it cannot distinguish between infection or malignancy in this case. First, the patient must be isolated until active tuberculosis has been excluded. Second, a cavitary lesion as such will likely be FDG avid. FDG PET/CT would be more suitable once a diagnosis of lung cancer is made.

Comment
Differential Diagnosis

The posteroanterior (PA) chest radiograph (Fig. 27.1) shows a cavity in the right upper lobe with surrounding nodules, confirmed on CT (Fig. 27.2). There are a variety of causes of cavities in the lung, including infection (pyogenic and granulomatous), neoplasm (usually squamous cell), vasculitides (especially granulomatosis with polyangiitis), and rarely, infarction. The most common causes of a solitary cavity are infections and neoplasms.

Discussion

Certain features can help determine the likely cause of a cavity, but they are not specific enough to allow one to establish a definitive diagnosis in most cases. Features to consider include wall thickness, presence or absence of a fluid level, location, and presence of adjacent lung parenchymal abnormalities. Regarding wall thickness, very thin walled (<4 mm) cavities are often benign. In contrast, neoplasms typically demonstrate very thick walls. There is considerable overlap in this feature, however, and it should not be used as a sole criterion. Regarding the presence of a fluid level, it is most often associated with benign lesions; however, fluid levels are occasionally observed in cavitary neoplasms that have been complicated by secondary infection or hemorrhage. Regarding the location of a cavity, cavities resulting from hematogenous dissemination of disease often occur in the lower lobes, reflecting the gravitational distribution of blood flow. Cavities associated with postprimary tuberculosis are most often located in the apical and posterior segments of the upper lobes and the superior segments of the lower lobes. Primary lung cancer is most common in the upper lobes, slightly more on the right, but any lobe may be affected. Regarding the presence of adjacent lung abnormalities, the development of a cavity within a preexisting area of consolidation is typical of a lung abscess.

Respiratory isolation is a critical step in managing patients with known or suspected tuberculosis because spread of mycobacteria throughout the tracheobronchial tree can result in transmission to close contacts. Treatment for tuberculosis includes multiple antibiotics, depending on the susceptibility profile for the isolated organism. If tuberculosis is confidently excluded, biopsy (transthoracic, bronchoscopic, or thoracoscopic) may be warranted to establish the diagnosis. With transthoracic needle biopsy, the needle should pass tangential to the cavity wall to optimize sampling of cells.

REFERENCES

Reed JC. Solitary localized lucent defect. In: *Chest Radiology: Plain Film Patterns and Differential Diagnoses*. 5th ed. Philadelphia: Mosby–Year Book; 2003:406–426.

Jeong YJ, Lee KS. Pulmonary tuberculosis: up-to-date imaging and management. *AJR Am J Roentgenol*. 2008;191:834–844.

Thoracic Radiology: The Requisites, 3rd ed, pp. 323–334.

CASE 28
Mycetoma

1. **C**. A mycetoma (aspergilloma) is the most likely cause of intracavitary mass in this patient. One characteristic of mycetomas is that they change position in the cavity, resting dependently, as the patient changes position (as demonstrated on the computed tomography [CT] scan). Lung carcinoma can cavitate and contain intracavitary fluid and debris. The wall of the cavity is often thick and irregular. Squamous cell carcinomas are most often associated with cavitation, although any cell type can cavitate. The large opacities of

progressive massive fibrosis associated with silicosis or coal workers' pneumoconiosis can cavitate secondary to necrosis. However, the large opacities are typically bilateral, and small pneumoconiotic nodules should also be present. Pulmonary Langerhans cell histiocytosis is associated with multiple bilateral lung cysts and nodules. A solitary cavitary lesion is not a feature of this disease.

2. **A**. *Aspergillus* is the most common cause of mycetoma, which forms in a pre-existing cavity, cyst, bulla, or bronchiectasis. *Blastomyces* can cause cavitary lung disease. However, mycetoma is not a manifestation of this endemic fungus. *Candida* usually affects the lungs of immunocompromised patients and causes disseminated infection. Mycetoma is not a manifestation of this opportunistic fungus. *Coccidioides* is found in the deserts of the American Southwest and can cause pneumonia and cavitary lung lesions. However, mycetoma is not a manifestation of this infection.

3. **B**. Hemoptysis is a common and potentially life-threatening complication of mycetoma. The wall of the cavity containing the mycetoma is very friable and hyperemic, and bleeding can be extensive. A mycetoma is a saprophytic form of fungal infection that occurs in a pre-existing cavity, cyst, bulla, or bronchiectasis. *Aspergillus* is ubiquitous in the environment and affects susceptible hosts. It is not spread directly from one person to another. A mycetoma can become invasive if host immune function declines but this rarely occurs. However, most patients with mycetomas have structural lung disease without or with mild immune suppression, such as some patients with sarcoidosis. Development of lung carcinoma is not associated with the presence of a mycetoma. However, patients who smoke cigarettes are at greater risk of developing lung carcinoma.

4. **C**. Bronchial artery embolization is the preferred treatment for patients with mycetoma and acute severe hemoptysis. Antifungal therapy is typically not effective and would not be appropriate in the setting of acute hemoptysis. Pneumonectomy or lobectomy may be performed, but elective resection is preferred. Surgical resection is often difficult due to accompanying pleural fibrosis. Poor lung function in diseases such as end stage sarcoidosis may preclude surgical resection. Radiation therapy is not appropriate treatment for mycetoma.

Comment

Differential Diagnosis

Posteroanterior (PA) and lateral radiographs (Figs. 28.1 and 28.2) show left apical thickening, a left apical cavity, and an intracavitary left upper lobe mass layering dependently. Sagittal reformatted CT image (Fig. 28.3) confirms the intracavitary mass, which layers posteriorly with the patient supine. The imaging findings are characteristic of a mycetoma (aspergilloma), the most common radiographic form of aspergillosis. The unilateral apical scarring and cavitary disease favor infection, particularly mycobacterial, as the underlying etiology.

Discussion

Aspergilloma refers to a saprophytic infection that occurs within a pre-existing cyst, cavity, bulla, or area of bronchiectasis. Pathologically, the fungus ball represents a combination of *Aspergillus* hyphae, mucus, and cellular debris.

Patients at risk for aspergilloma formation include those with cystic fibrosis (CF), sarcoidosis, tuberculosis (TB), and emphysema. The infection is typically clinically silent for many years. Presenting symptoms can include cough, weight loss, and recurrent hemoptysis. Although hemoptysis is usually minimal,

a minority of patients present with massive, life-threatening hemoptysis. Severe hemoptysis requires therapeutic intervention such as bronchial artery embolization.

Characteristic imaging findings include a round, dependent opacity located within a cavity or thin-walled cyst. The dependent opacity is often heterogeneous owing to the presence of multiple linear collections of air, resulting in a sponge-like appearance. It occurs most commonly in the upper lobes and is often accompanied by pleural thickening. In most cases, the fungus ball demonstrates mobility with changes in patient position. An aspergilloma is often surrounded by a crescent of air, referred to as the Monod sign. In a minority of cases, however, the fungus ball completely fills the cavity, with no visible air between the cavity and the ball.

Bronchial artery embolization and surgical resection are the most common therapeutic options. Other reported treatments include direct instillation of amphotericin B via a percutaneous catheter into the cavity, although this approach is no longer used. Systemic antifungal therapy is usually of no benefit.

REFERENCES

Franquet T, Müller NL, Giménez A, et al. Spectrum of pulmonary aspergillosis: histologic, clinical, and radiologic findings. *Radiographics*. 2001;21:825–837.

Nitschke A, Sachs P, Suby-Long T, Restauri N. Monod sign. *J Thorac Imaging*. 2013;28(6):W120.

Thoracic Radiology: The Requisites, 3rd ed, 289–309.

CASE 29

Pericardial Cyst

1. **A, B, and D**. Pericardial cyst is a very common cause of a right cardiophrenic angle mass. They typically have smooth margins, as in this example. Lymphoma involving the anterior diaphragmatic lymph nodes can result in pericardiophrenic angle mass. However, lymphoma limited to this location is atypical. Nevertheless, this location is a common site of recurrence of Hodgkin lymphoma treated with mantle external beam radiation therapy because it is outside the typical treatment field. Herniation of intra-abdominal contents through the foramen of Morgagni can occur in the right pericardiophrenic space. Paraganglioma should not be included because anterior mediastinal neoplasms of neural origin are very uncommon; the majority occur in the posterior mediastinum or in the aortopulmonary window.

2. **A**. The CT scan shows a homogeneous water attenuation mass in the right pericardiophrenic space with smooth margins, consistent with a pericardial cyst. There are no imaging features to suggest lymphoma, paraganglioma (which are typically hypervascular), or Morgagni hernia (which typically contains bowel or omental fat).

3. **C**. Most pericardial cysts attach to the parietal pericardium. Pericardial cysts in the pericardiophrenic space occur much more commonly on the right, 2 to 3 times more so than on the left. Most pericardial cysts do not communicate with the pericardium. Those that do are referred to as *pericardial diverticula*. Pericardial cysts are often incidental findings. A small number of patients have chest pain, but a causal relationship usually cannot be confirmed.

4. **D**. Pericardial cysts show no enhancement on postcontrast T1-weighted images. Most pericardial cysts have intermediate to low signal intensity on T1-weighted images. Occasionally, pericardial cysts contain proteinaceous material, which can result in high T1-signal intensity. Pericardial cysts have homogeneous high T2-signal intensity.

Comment

Differential Diagnosis

The posteroanterior (PA) chest radiograph shows a smoothly marginated, homogeneous mass in the right pericardiophrenic space (Fig. 29.1). Most causes of a right cardiophrenic angle mass are benign and include pericardial cyst, Morgagni hernia, lipoma, and thymolipoma. CT image (Fig. 29.2) shows the mass to abut the pericardium and to have homogeneous water attenuation.

Pericardiophrenic Mass

Although the various causes of a right cardiophrenic angle mass might appear similar radiographically, the CT appearances differ depending on the contents of the lesion. The presence of fluid attenuation within a cardiophrenic angle mass is consistent with a pericardial cyst, the diagnosis in this case (see Fig. 29.2). Such cysts are attached to the parietal pericardium, but they typically do not communicate with the pericardial space.

The presence of fat attenuation within a cardiophrenic angle mass can be seen in lipoma, thymolipoma, and Morgagni foramen hernia. Lipomas typically have homogeneous fat attenuation. Thymolipomas, on the other hand, contain a variable mixture of fat and soft tissue elements. Herniated omental fat can be recognized by identifying omental vessels, which appear as serpentine, tubular soft tissue structures. In many cases, colon liver, or both also accompany herniated omental fat. Occasionally, herniated bowel is visible radiographically, precluding the need for CT in most cases.

A soft tissue attenuation cardiophrenic angle mass suggests enlarged pericardiophrenic lymph nodes. Such lymph nodes are a common site of recurrent Hodgkin lymphoma treated with mantle radiation because this region is usually outside of the radiation treatment field. Occasionally, metastases from abdominal tumors may involve these nodes.

Imaging Findings

Pericardial cysts can occur anywhere in the mediastinum in the vicinity of the pericardium. However, most of them occur in the right pericardiophrenic space. Their margins can vary with patient position on imaging studies. On CT, pericardial cysts have homogeneous, water attenuation and do not enhance following IV contrast administration. Mass effect on adjacent structures is typically absent. Pericardial cysts show no enhancement on postcontrast T1-weighted magnetic resonance imaging (MRI), and most have intermediate to low signal intensity on T1-weighted images. Occasionally, pericardial cysts contain proteinaceous material, which can result in high T1-signal intensity. Pericardial cysts have homogeneous high T2-signal intensity.

REFERENCES
Rajiah P, Kanne JP, Kalahasti V, Schoenhagen P. Computed tomography of cardiac and pericardiac masses. *J Cardiovasc Comput Tomogr.* 2011 Jan–Feb;5(1):16–29.
Thoracic Radiology: The Requisites, 3rd ed, 97–136.

CASE 30

Right Lower Lobe Pneumonia

1. **B**. Community-acquired pneumonia is one of the most common causes of lobar consolidation. Lung consolidation is a rare manifestation of acute pulmonary histoplasmosis. Lung nodules and lymphadenopathy are much more typical. The chest radiographs show consolidation in the right lower lobe confined by the major fissure and the hemidiaphragm, indicating an intrapulmonary location of the abnormality. Pulmonary septic emboli result is infected infarcts which contain microabscesses. They often seen in association with bacterial endocarditis or infected central venous catheters.

2. **A**. Air bronchograms refer to air-filled bronchi, which are visible because they are surrounded by consolidated lung. Pneumonia and compressive (relaxation) atelectasis are most associated with air bronchograms. *Pseudocavitation* is a term used to describe small bubble lucencies within a lung nodule and is usually associated with lung adenocarcinoma. Pulmonary interstitial emphysema refers to ectopic air tracking in the pulmonary interstitium and is usually associated with alveolar rupture. The black bronchus sign is the dark black appearance of the bronchi seen in areas of diffuse ground-glass opacity on computed tomography (CT). It is not a sign on chest radiographs.

3. **D**. *Streptococcus pneumoniae* (pneumococcus) is the most common cause of community-acquired pneumonia and most commonly manifests as lobar consolidation. *Aspergillus* species. Can cause lung consolidation. They occur almost exclusively as opportunistic infections in immunocompromised patients. Early in its course, *Legionella pneumophila* can cause lobar consolidation, but it typically progresses to multilobar consolidation with involvement of both lungs. *Staphylococcus aureus* usually causes bronchopneumonia or septic emboli with infarction. Lobar consolidation is not a typical appearance for this organism. Nevertheless, imaging findings in pulmonary infections are very nonspecific and usually cannot be associated with a specific causal organism.

4. **C**. The *silhouette sign* refers to loss of the normal lung–tissue interface when the normally aerated lung becomes consolidated. In this patient, the interface between the consolidated right lower lobe and the hemidiaphragm is lost. The *sail sign* refers to the sail-like appearance of the normal thymus in young children. It should not be mistaken for a mediastinal mass. The *spine sign* refers to increased opacity projected over the spine on the lateral view secondary to lower lobe consolidation. Normally, the vertebral bodies become more lucent on the lateral view from apex to base. The *continuous hemidiaphragm sign* refers to sharp band of lucency outlining the medial portion of the hemidiaphragm by ectopic gas, indicating pneumomediastinum or pneumopericardium if above the diaphragm and pneumoperitoneum above the diaphragm.

Comment

Differential Diagnosis

PA and lateral chest radiographs (Figs.30.1 and 30.2) show confluent opacity in the right lower lobe obscuring underlying vessels without volume loss, compatible with consolidation in the acute setting. Pulmonary hemorrhage and asymmetric edema can have this appearance. In the chronic setting, one should consider lung adenocarcinoma.

Lobar Consolidation

Consolidation is defined in the Fleischner glossary of terms as an exudate or other product of disease that replaces alveolar air rending the lung solid. It is usually produced by infection. Once a pattern of lung consolidation has been identified, it is important to determine the distribution and chronicity of the process and correlate the imaging findings with the clinical presentation of the patient.

In this patient there is a striking lobar distribution of consolidation, a pattern that is most associated with infection. The most common organism to produce a lobar pneumonia is *S. pneumoniae.* Other organisms such as *Klebsiella pneumoniae, Legionella pneumophila*, and *Mycoplasma pneumoniae* can also produce a lobar consolidation pattern.

Regarding the chronicity of a consolidative pattern, this factor is best determined by comparing the current study with earlier chest radiographs or CT scans. The presence of chronic consolidation is associated with a limited differential diagnosis that includes neoplasms such as primary lung adenocarcinoma and lymphoma and rarely lipoid pneumonia. Chronic lobar consolidation may suggest an unusual organism unresponsive to commonly used antibiotics or the presence of endobronchial obstruction most commonly due to lung cancer. In the latter situation there is almost always evidence of some volume loss (atelectasis) of the lobe involved.

Patients with community-acquired pneumonia are treated with antibiotics. CT is generally reserved for patients with suspected complications such as empyema, those not responding to therapy, and patients with recurrent pneumonia.

Imaging Findings

Consolidation is the most common radiographic manifestation of pulmonary infection. Single or multiple lobes can be involved. Other findings may include tree-in-bud nodules, pleural effusion, and lymphadenopathy. CT scans are typically reserved for the identification of complications of pneumonia such as empyema. As a rule, imaging alone cannot reliably determine the causative organism.

REFERENCES
Gharib AM, Stern EJ. Radiology of pneumonia. *Med Clin North Am.* 2001;85:1461–1491.
Thoracic Radiology: The Requisites, 3rd ed, 289–309.

CASE 31

Empyema

1. **B and C.** Noncontrast CT shows a large, complex right pleural collection containing pockets of gas. The presence of pleural thickening posteriorly could be the result of tumor deposits along the pleural space. Chylothorax is typically indistinguishable from a simple pleural effusion and would not contain gas. Hemothorax can lead to a complex pleural collection, but gas would not be expected to be present in the absence of instrumentation or superinfection. In addition, there would be high attenuation areas within the collection.
2. **C.** In the absence of instrumentation, gas in the pleural space typically indicates infection. Empyemas are loculated, so they will not layer dependently with changes in patient position. Although many empyemas have a lenticular configuration, this finding is not specific to empyema and can be seen with other loculated pleural collections. Any large pleural collection can cause compressive atelectasis of the adjacent lung.
3. **D.** Bronchopleural fistula is the most likely cause of an air fluid level within a pleural collection. Thin-section CT may show a direct communication between the lung and pleura. Gas-forming organisms can result in empyema, but this is quite uncommon. They usually cause numerous tiny pockets of loculated gas rather than discrete air fluid levels. Pulmonary gangrene, an uncommon but life-threatening complication of surgery or pneumonia, is not a common cause of a pleural air fluid level, but it is associated with multiple cavities in the affected lung parenchyma. Pleurocutaneous fistulas (empyema necessitans) usually occur with long-standing empyemas, or empyemas due to infection with tuberculous organisms or actinomycetes. They can present acutely following tube thoracostomy.

4. **A.** Bacteria are the most common cause of empyema, particularly *Staphylococcus aureus* and *Streptococcus spp.* Fungi can occasionally cause empyema, most often in immunocompromised patients. Amoebic infection, paragonimiasis, and cystic echinococcal infection are common parasitic causes of pleural infection. Viruses are typically not directly associated with empyema, but bacterial superinfection of the pleural space following a viral lung infection (especially influenza) can occur.

Comment

Differential Diagnosis

Unenhanced chest CT shows a large, complex collection in the right pleural space containing gas and liquid. This most likely is empyema, although the soft tissue thickening posteriorly should raise the question of underlying malignancy.

Discussion

CT is the preferred imaging study to demonstrate the features and extent of a pleural empyema, including smooth thickening and enhancement of visceral and parietal pleura surrounding the abnormal fluid collection (split pleura sign), a finding that suggests empyema but is not specific. This sign can be seen with any cause of pleural inflammation. Additional CT features of empyema include a lenticular-shaped fluid collection, typically forming obtuse margins at its interface with pleural surface, and compression of adjacent lung parenchyma. CT can also show increased extrapleural fat with stranding between the empyema space and the chest wall, particularly if the empyema is chronic. The fat might have increased attenuation because of surrounding edema.

REFERENCES
Kuhlman JE, Singha NK. Complex disease of the pleural space: radiographic and CT evaluation. *Radiographics.* 1997;17:63–79.
Thoracic Radiology: The Requisites, 3rd ed, 159–192.

CASE 32

Neurogenic Tumor (Schwannoma)

1. **A, C.** Postanterior (PA) and lateral radiographs (see Fig. 32.1 and Fig. 32.2) show a smoothly marginated right paraspinal mass. The mass preserves the right paratracheal stripe and subtly obliterates the right paraspinal line on the frontal radiograph and overlies the spine on the lateral projection. Note the incomplete, well-circumscribed margins (incomplete border sign) on the lateral view. The CT image (see Fig. 32.3) confirms the paraspinal location and shows expansion of and extension into the adjacent spinal neuroforamen. Neurogenic tumors are the most common cause of a posterior mediastinal mass. Thymomas almost always occur in the anterior mediastinum. Germ cell tumors primarily occur in the anterior mediastinum. Splaying of the ribs and loss of the left paraspinal line indicate a posterior mediastinal location.
2. **C.** The mass obliterates the right paraspinal line on the frontal radiograph and overlies the spine on the lateral projection. Note the incomplete, well-circumscribed margins (incomplete border sign) on the lateral view. The PA and lateral radiographs clearly show that this mass is neither in the anterior nor the middle mediastinal compartments. An inferior mediastinal compartment has not been described.
3. **B.** MRI of the thoracic spine is the test of choice in this patient because most posterior mediastinal masses are of neural origin. CT can show the extent of the mass and precisely localize it, but MRI is superior in showing intraspinal

extension and any possible associated spinal cord abnormality. FDG-PET/CT will not fully delineate the extent of the lesion and does not provide a diagnosis. Low-grade tumors may have little metabolic activity on FDG-PET. Neurogenic tumors are typically surgical lesions; therefore a biopsy will not significantly alter patient management.

4. **D**. Calcification is uncommon in neurogenic tumors but occurs more often in sympathetic chain tumors than peripheral nerve tumors. Approximately 70% of posterior mediastinal neurogenic tumors are benign. Rib spreading and erosions are common with neurogenic tumors, but rib destruction implies malignancy. Peripheral nerve tumors widen the neural foramen; sympathetic chain tumors more often result in anterolateral vertebral body erosion.

Comment

Differential diagnosis

The majority of paraspinal masses are of neural origin, most commonly schwannoma and neurofibroma. Ganglioneuromas can also occur in this location, but they tend to be more vertically oriented, spanning multiple vertebral bodies. Other possible causes of a paraspinal mass include lymphoma, sarcoma, metastasis, infection (especially tuberculosis), hematoma, and extramedullary hematopoiesis.

Discussion

Neurogenic tumors are the most common cause of a posterior mediastinal mass. Such lesions can be classified into three groups: those arising from peripheral nerves (schwannoma, neurofibroma), those arising from the sympathetic chain (ganglioneuroma, ganglioneuroblastoma, and neuroblastoma), and those arising from the paraganglia (pheochromocytoma, chemodectoma). Most lesions (roughly 70%) are benign.

Neurogenic tumors typically affect patients during the first 4 decades of life. Most lesions are detected incidentally in asymptomatic patients. Symptomatic lesions typically produce neurologic symptoms, such as radicular pain and neuresthesias. Intravertebral extension can result in symptoms of cord compression. Interestingly, tumors arising from peripheral nerves, such as schwannoma, tend to differ in shape from those arising from the sympathetic chain, such as ganglioneuroma. The former lesions are generally round, and the latter are usually fusiform, with a vertical orientation.

Rib abnormalities, such as rib spreading and rib erosion, are commonly associated with neurogenic tumors and do not imply malignancy. In contrast, bone destruction is usually associated with malignancy. Vertebral body abnormalities are often present. Such abnormalities are best demonstrated on CT examinations. Tumors arising from peripheral nerves are often associated with widening of the neural foramen. In contrast, lesions arising from the sympathetic chain more often result in anterolateral vertebral body erosion.

On cross-sectional imaging, benign neurogenic tumors are usually homogeneous in appearance and have well-defined margins. Malignant lesions are more likely to be heterogeneous and to demonstrate irregular margins. Foci of calcification are present in a minority of cases. Such calcifications are more often identified on CT than on chest radiographs. Calcification is more commonly observed in tumors arising from the sympathetic chain than in those arising from the peripheral nerves.

When a neurogenic tumor is suspected on chest radiographs, MRI is generally the preferred cross-sectional imaging test for further evaluation because of its superb ability to demonstrate intraspinal extension of tumor or the presence of an associated spinal cord abnormality. Surgical resection of neurogenic tumors is the mainstay treatment. Chemotherapy and radiation therapy may be used in conjunction with surgery in patients with malignant tumors.

REFERENCES
Duwe BV, Sterman DH, Musani AI. Tumors of the mediastinum. *Chest.* 2006;128:2893–2909.
Thoracic Radiology: The Requisites, 3rd ed., pp. 97–136.

CASE 33
Hemothorax

1. **A**. A homogenously high attenuation pleural collection or a pleural collection with high attenuation foci is consistent with a hemothorax. Empyemas are typically loculated and associated with pleural thickening. Their attenuation is usually lower. Chylothoraces have water attenuation on CT. Solitary fibrous tumors of the pleura present as pleural masses of varying sizes with varying degrees of heterogeneity.

2. **A**. A rapidly enlarging pleural collection should suggest a hemothorax in the correct clinical setting (e.g., trauma, surgery, line placement, anticoagulation). A slowly enlarging pleural collection is most likely an effusion or empyema and not a hemothorax. Although hemothoraces can become loculated, such an appearance is not specific for hemothorax and can occur with effusions and empyema. Acute and subacute hemothoraces have high attenuation and are usually heterogeneous. Over time, the attenuation of a hemothorax can diminish, but it typically remains greater than that of water.

3. **D**. The hematocrit sign describes differing layers of pleural blood products produced by differing degrees of coagulation. The split pleura sign describes fluid separating the two layers of enhancing pleura and can be seen with empyema and other causes of pleural inflammation. The collar sign and dependent viscera sign are both associated with diaphragmatic injury. The former describes narrowing of abdominal viscera as they pass through a diaphragmatic defect, and the latter describes a herniated abdominal viscus layering along the posterior chest wall.

4. **B**. Evacuation of a hemothorax is essential to avoid complications such as compressive atelectasis, fibrothorax, and empyema. Tube thoracostomy is appropriate for stable patients. Patients with severe bleeding may require thoracotomy or embolization. Talc pleurodesis is no appropriate for a traumatic hemothorax.

Comment
Differential Diagnosis

The differential diagnosis for a pleural collection includes pleural effusion (transudative or exudative), empyema, chylothorax, hemothorax, and pleural tumor. The presence of high attenuation dependent material suggests hemothorax (Fig. 33.1). Enhancing pleural tumor deposits could potentially be confused with blood products. However, such deposits are usually nodular and associated with diffuse pleural thickening as well as fluid.

Hemothorax

A collection of blood in the pleural space is called a hemothorax and occurs in up to 50% of patients sustaining blunt chest trauma. Hemothorax can also develop as a complication of surgery or other pleural instrumentation, anticoagulation therapy, and tumor. Catmenial hemothorax is a rare condition characterized by recurrent bleeding into the pleural space during menses because of ectopic endometrial tissue. Most hemothoraces require drainage, usually with a thoracostomy tube. Undrained hemothoraces can result in fibrothorax or empyema.

Imaging Findings

Hemothorax is indistinguishable from other pleural collections on chest radiography but is easily identified as high attenuation (35-70 HU) pleural fluid on CT. Because the attenuation of blood products varies with acuity and the presence of clot, a hemothorax may have a heterogeneous or layering appearance.

REFERENCES
Palas J, Matos AP, Mascarenhas V, Herédia V, Ramalho M. Multidetector computer tomography: evaluation of blunt chest trauma in adults. *Radiol Res Pract. 2014.* 2014:864369. https://doi.org/10.1155/2014/864369. Epub 2014 Sep 8.
Thoracic Radiology: The Requisites, 3rd ed, 279–288.

CASE 34
Rib Notching

1. **C.** Neurofibromatosis type 1 (NF-1) can cause rib notching secondary to neural tumor formation along the intercostal nerves. Furthermore, NF-1 can cause apparent lung nodules from chest wall lesions as well as mediastinal masses from neural tumors. Metastases can cause multiple pulmonary nodules, but metastatic tumor is not considered a cause of multifocal rib notching. Takayasu arteritis can cause central systemic arterial stenosis and occlusion and rarely may produce rib notching if there is stenosis of the subclavian artery but it does not produce chest wall or pulmonary nodules. Rib erosions, multiple thoracic nodules and masses are not typical of tuberous sclerosis complex.
2. **A.** Vertebra plana is not a typical manifestation of NF-1, which does not involve the marrow space of vertebral bodies. Neural foraminal widening is a common manifestation of NF-1 and usually results from dumbbell-shaped neural tumors. NF-1 can cause rib erosions from neural tumor formation in the intercostal nerves, and scoliosis is common in patients with NF-1.
3. **B.** Metastases are the most common causes of rib destruction in an adult. Primary osseous sarcomas of the ribs are rare. Multiple myeloma commonly causes rib destruction but is far less common than metastases. Metabolic bone disease usually causes rib demineralization, and insufficiency fractures can occur. However, rib destruction is not a typical feature.
4. **D.** Aortic coarctation can cause rib notching from enlarged intercostal arterial collateral vessels. Right aortic arch, cervical aortic arch, and aberrant subclavian artery do not cause rib notching.

Comment
Differential Diagnosis

Rib notching is most frequently caused by enlarged collateral vessels, for example in coarctation of the aorta where collateral blood flow occurs through dilated intercostal arteries. Other causes include arterial venous malformations of the chest wall and superior vena caval obstruction. The second most common cause of rib notching is growth of an intercostal neurogenic tumors, particularly neurofibromas, as in this case. Frank destructive changes in a rib should prompt suspicion for malignancy, typically caused by a metastatic lesion.

Neurofibromatosis Type 1 (NF-1)

Neurofibromatosis type 1 (von Recklinghausen disease) is the most common neurocutaneous disorder (phakomatosis), with an incidence of 1:2000 to 1:3000. Although caused by an autosomal dominant mutation of the *NF1* gene, which encodes for the tumor suppressor protein neurofibromin, approximately half of cases result from a spontaneous mutation. Common clinical manifestations include cutaneous neurofibromas and "café au lait" spots, which are large patches of increased skin pigmentation. Other outward manifestations include short stature, scoliosis, macrocephaly, and Lisch nodules (benign growths on the iris that typically do not affect vision). Other clinical findings include hypertension and vision impairment, the latter resulting from optic gliomas.

Imaging Findings

Thoracic manifestations of NF-1 include cutaneous, paraspinal, mediastinal, and intercostal neurofibromas. Cutaneous neurofibromas can mimic lung nodules on chest radiography. Scoliosis is also common in patients with NF-1. Pulmonary manifestations include fibrosis and cysts. Numerous pulmonary nodules should raise the suspicion of metastases from malignant degeneration of a neurofibroma. In this case, biapical paraspinal masses and nodular soft tissue opacities associated with several lower ribs bilaterally are characteristic findings in neurofibromatosis.

REFERENCES
Rossi SE, Erasmus JJ, McAdams HP, Donnelly LF. Thoracic manifestations of neurofibromatosis-I. *AJR Am J Roentgenol.* 1999 Dec;173(6):1631–1638.
Boone ML, Swenson BE, Felson B. Rib notching: its many causes. *Am J Roentgenol Radium Ther Nucl Med.* 1964;91:1075–1088.
Thoracic Radiology: The Requisites, 3rd ed, 159–192.

Fair Game

CASE 35

Left Upper Lobe Atelectasis (Lung Cancer)

1. **C.**
2. **C.**
3. **B.**
4. **B.**

Comment

Posteroanterior chest radiograph (Fig. 35.1) shows a veil-like opacity throughout the left hemithorax with leftward shift of mediastinal structures, hyperexpansion of the right lung, and elevation of the left hemidiaphragm. Note the vertically oriented crescentic shaped lucency to the left of the aortic arch, representing the superior segment of the left lower lobe manifesting as the luftsichel sign. Coronal contrast-enhanced computed tomography (CT) (Fig. 35.2) shows the collapsed left upper lobe. Note the superiorly displaced left major fissure along its inferior border.

Differential Diagnosis

Pneumonia, lobectomy, lung cancer, pleural effusion or tumor, mediastinal mass or widening.

Discussion

Atelectasis refers to variable causes of incomplete expansion of alveoli, each with unique imaging manifestations. Lobar atelectasis refers to incomplete expansion of an entire lobe or lobes of a lung, most commonly from obstruction of the supplying lobar bronchus and resorption of air distal to the obstruction. Causes may be from within the bronchus lumen (mucus plugs, foreign bodies, malpositioned support devices, broncholith, endobronchial tumors) or extrinsic compression of the bronchi (lymphadenopathy, masses, vasculature.) In a review by Naidich and colleagues, endobronchial lesions were responsible for 40% of cases lobar atelectasis, 95% of which were a result of endobronchial tumors (lung cancer, bronchial carcinoids, endobronchial metastases, and lymphoma). The remaining cases were from benign etiologies (mucus plug and bronchial stenosis). Thus, lobar atelectasis patterns should prompt further investigation into the cause of the obstructive atelectasis (CT, bronchoscopy).

Direct imaging signs of atelectasis include displacement of fissures and crowding of bronchovascular structures. Indirect signs include increased lung opacity, mediastinal shift toward the affected lung with compensatory hyperinflation of adjacent lobes, displacement of hilar structures, and elevation of the ipsilateral hemidiaphragm. Upper lobe volume loss may result in tethering of the inferior accessory fissure (if present), manifesting the *juxtaphrenic peak sign*, another indirect sign of atelectasis. Specific signs of left upper lobe atelectasis include opacification and volume loss in the left hemithorax, obscuration of the upper mediastinum/aortic arch (i.e., silhouette sign), and an elevated left hilum. Crescentic lucency lateral to the aortic arch (i.e., luftsichel sign) may be seen, representing compensated hyperinflation of the superior segment of the left lower lobe as it reorients to fill the void created between the atelectatic left upper lobe and aortic arch.

In the revised 2017 8th edition of the *TNM Staging System for Lung Cancer*, complete and partial lung atelectasis and pneumonitis extending to the hilum have been combined under the T2 classification. The previous 7th edition separated partial and complete lung atelectasis/pneumonitis into T2 and T3 lesions, respectively. Re-examination of a large database informed the change, as partial atelectasis/pneumonitis was associated with similar 5-year survival of other T2 descriptors. However, patients with complete lung atelectasis/pneumonitis had a better 5-year prognosis than those with other T3 descriptors when staged clinically (60%–67% for T2 versus 52% for T3) and pathologically (65%–74% for T2 versus 57% for T3).

REFERENCES

Parker MS, Chasen MH, Paul N. Radiologic signs in thoracic imaging: case-based review and self-assessment module. *AJR.* 2009;192:S34–S48.

Naidich DP, McCauley DI, Khouri NF, et al. Computed tomography of lobar collapse: endobronchial obstruction. *J Comput Assist Tomogr.* 1983;7(5):745–757.

Detterbeck FC, Boffa DJ, Kim AW, Tanoue LT. The eighth edition lung cancer stage classification. *Chest.* 2017;151(1):193–203.

Goldstraw P, Chansky K, Crowley J, et al. The IASLC lung cancer staging project: proposals for revision of the TNM stage groupings in the forthcoming (8th) edition of the TNM Classification for. *Lung Cancer. J Thoracic Oncol.* 2015;1:39–51.

Thoracic Radiology: The Requisites, 3rd ed, 47–60, 450–459.

CASE 36

Interstitial Pulmonary Edema

1. **A**
2. **A**
3. **B**
4. **E**

Comment

Anteroposterior chest radiograph (Fig. 36.1) shows diffuse smooth interstitial thickening and perihilar haziness. Note the enlarged cardiac silhouette and sequela of prior coronary artery bypass surgery. Axial contrast-enhanced chest computed tomography (CT) (lung windows) (Fig. 36.2) shows smooth interlobular septal thickening and smooth bronchial wall thickening and mosaic attenuation. The normal polyhedral shape of the secondary pulmonary lobule is preserved.

Differential Diagnosis

Pneumonia, hemorrhage, lymphangitic carcinomatosis, pulmonary alveolar proteinosis, acute eosinophilic pneumonia, Erdheim-Chester disease, lymphangiectasia.

Discussion

Pulmonary edema refers to abnormal accumulation of fluid in compartments outside of the lung vasculature (i.e., the lung interstitium or alveolar space). This redistribution of fluid occurs by several mechanisms including (1) increased hydrostatic gradient across the microvasculature (left heart failure or fluid overload), (2) decreased intravascular oncotic pressure (hypoalbuminemia, hepatic and renal failure), or (3) increased capillary and/or alveolar endothelial permeability (transfusion-associated lung injury, opiate overdose, high-altitude edema, and acute respiratory distress syndrome, among others).

There are physiologic alterations which have been described in cardiogenic edema as left heart pressures elevate and are transferred to the pulmonary veins (pulmonary venous hypertension) and capillary beds. Cephalization of pulmonary veins refers to increase in caliber of upper lobe vessels relative to the lower lobes, which occurs early as pulmonary capillary wedge pressures (PCWP) reach 12 to 25 mmHg. Progressive elevations of PCWP (20–30 mmHg) will cause transudation of fluid into the interstitium, producing radiographic findings such as interlobular septal thickening and subpleural edema with fluid outlining the secondary pulmonary lobules and interlobar fissures, respectively. Alveoli will begin to fill with fluid at PCWP above 25 to 30 mmHg, producing radiographic findings of increased lung density and consolidations, most prominent in the central, perihilar regions (so-called *perihilar haze*). Although theoretical, this sequence is not necessarily predictable.

Septal lines produced from fluid within deep lung septae are referred to as Kerley A lines, which extend from the hilum and cross normal vascular markings toward the lung periphery and are about 5 to 10 cm in length. Kerley B lines are shorter (<2 cm) present at the periphery of the lung extending perpendicular to the pleural surface. Fluid accumulation in the axial interstitium will manifest as peribronchial thickening or "cuffing." Additional radiographic findings of cardiogenic pulmonary edema include widened vascular pedicle, measured on upright frontal chest radiographs from the right lateral margin of the superior vena cava interface as it crosses the right mainstem bronchus and left lateral margin of the proximal left subclavian artery. Although variable, abnormal vascular pedicle widths are greater than 5.8 cm and indicate elevated central venous pressure and intravascular blood volumes. Cardiomegaly and pleural effusions may also be seen. As cardiogenic edema is treated, clinical improvement may precede the radiographic clearing of the above findings.

REFERENCES
Gluecker T, et al. Clinical and radiologic features of pulmonary edema. *Radiographics*. 1999;19(6):150–153, discussion 1532–33.
Thoracic Radiology: The Requisites, 3rd ed, 229–233.

CASE 37

Thyroid Goiter

1. **D**
2. **B**
3. **A**
4. **G**

Comment

Differential Diagnosis

Thymic lesion (hyperplasia, thymolipoma, thymic cyst, thymic epithelial neoplasm, thymic neuroendocrine tumor), Lymphadenopathy (lymphoma, metastases, Castleman disease), Germ cell neoplasms, Lymphangioma, Congenital cysts, Tortuous or aneurysmal neck vessels, Mediastinal hematoma.

Discussion

A goiter refers to an enlarged thyroid gland. Goiters may be primary (rare, ectopic rests of thyroid tissue from embryologic migrational anomalies, with blood supply derived from intrathoracic vessels) or secondary (downward extension of thyroid tissue maintaining vascular connection to the cervical thyroid), the latter being far more common. Although most are confined to the thyroid bed (cervical goiter), intrathoracic extension intrathoracic extension occurs in 3% to 35% of cases. Of intrathoracic goiters, most (75% to 90%) involve the prevascular mediastinal

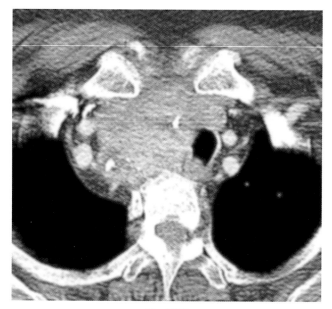

Fig. 37.3

compartment (retrosternal) with fewer (10% to 25%) extending into the visceral mediastinal compartment (retrotracheal or retroesophageal). Factors associated with increased likelihood of thyroid goiter include a deficiency in dietary iodine, advancing age, female sex, low thyroid-stimulating hormone (TSH) levels, smoking, high body mass index (BMI), and the existence of thyroid nodules.

Radiographic features include tracheal deviation beginning at the level of the larynx and occasionally extending below the thoracic inlet (Fig. 37.1). The mass typically creates well-defined convex upper mediastinal contours and thickening of the paratracheal stripes, which become faded and obscured above the clavicles, indicating continuity with the soft tissues of the neck (*cervicothoracic sign*). Prevascular goiters often fill the retrosternal space (Fig. 37.2) while visceral goiters will fill the retrotracheal (Raider's) triangle on lateral radiographs. Coarse calcification may be detected with radiography. Computed tomography (CT) features include a high-attenuation (70–80 HU) mass resulting from intrinsic iodine content (Fig. 37.3). Heterogeneity in the attenuation may be from cystic and nodular changes. Calcifications are often coarse and irregular. CT with contrast material will show enhancement of the thyroid parenchyma. Enhancing lymph nodes to the same degree of the thyroid should raise suspicion for metastatic thyroid carcinoma. If the tissue origin is in question, nuclear medicine scintigraphy with iodine radionuclides may be considered.

Cross-sectional imaging is often necessary for presurgical planning of substernal goiters as ultrasound evaluation of the mediastinal component is limited. Although most prevascular goiters may be resected via transcervical thyroidectomy, several features of the mass may predict the need for extended surgery (e.g., sternotomy or thoracotomy). These include less-pliable thyroid tissue, visceral or paravertebral mediastinal extension, aortic arch or subcarinal extension, dumbbell "conical" configuration with a waste at the thoracic inlet, or if the intrathoracic component of the mass is larger than the inlet.

REFERENCES
Brichkov I, et al. Simultaneous unilateral anterior thoracoscopy with transcervical thyroidectomy for resection of large mediastinal goiter. *J Thorac Dis*. 2017;9(8):2484–2490.

Buckley JA, Stark P. Intrathoracic mediastinal thyroid goiter: imaging manifestations. *AJR Am J Roentgenol.* 1999;173:471–475.
Riffat F, et al. Radiologically predicting when a sternotomy may be required in the management of retrosternal goiters. *Ann Otol Rhinol, & Larngol.* 2013;122(1):15–19.
Thoracic Radiology: The Requisites, 3rd ed, 110–112.

CASE 38

Community Acquired Pneumonia

1. **A**
2. **A and D**
3. **D**

Comment

Differential Diagnosis

Aspiration, atelectasis, pulmonary edema, hemorrhage, pulmonary infarction, organizing pneumonia, eosinophilic pneumonia, lung cancer.

Discussion

Pneumonia refers to an infection of the lungs with typical and atypical bacteria, viruses, fungi, or parasites, and continues to be a significant source of morbidity and mortality, especially among the aging population. Lower respiratory infections were responsible for 3.2 million of the 56.4 million deaths worldwide. Classification of pneumonia is according to the setting in which the infection occurred, including community-acquired (CAP), hospital-acquired (HAP), health care–associated (HCAP), and ventilator-associated pneumonia (VAP). The diagnosis of CAP includes the presence of symptoms suggesting a lower respiratory infection (cough, chest pain, dyspnea) with accompanying opacities on imaging, in a patient without hospitalization, intubation, or associations with risk factors related to healthcare (e.g. dialysis, nursing home) for at least 14 days before symptom onset. *Streptococcus pneumoniae* is a gram-positive coccus that is the most common bacterial etiology in CAP. Other common organisms include *Haemophilus influenzae, Staphylococcus aureus,* viruses, and others. In over half of cases, a specific pathogen may not be isolated.

Radiographic features range from normal (no findings) to extensive, multifocal bilateral opacities or increased lung density depending on the causative agent, mechanism and timing of inoculation, and host response. Opacities are typically seen on radiographs within 12 hours of symptom onset. Most CAP manifests via three radiographic and pathologic patterns: (1) focal non-segmental or lobar pneumonia (Figs. 38.1 and 38.2), (2) bronchopneumonia, and (3) focal or diffuse interstitial pneumonia. Bacterial lobar pneumonia results from an inflammatory alveolar exudate which fills terminal airways and adjacent acini via pores of Kohn, resulting in the typical consolidative pattern on radiography. Consolidation is defined as lung opacification which obscures adjacent structures of similar attenuation (*silhouette sign*). Air-filled bronchi coursing within the consolidation may become visible producing the *air-bronchogram sign.* Lack of volume loss in the affected lobe and the presence of air-bronchograms help distinguish pneumonia from obstructive atelectasis. All adults with radiographic evidence of pneumonia should be reimaged in 6 to 8 weeks to ensure complete radiographic resolution after treatment, as an underlying malignancy or structural abnormality may have contributed to the finding.

CT may allow a more specific microbiologic pattern and is typically employed in cases of unresolved pneumonia or suspected complications. Some nodules or consolidations may be marginated by a rim of ground-glass opacity on CT (*halo sign*), which represents perilesional hemorrhage and inflammation, often described in the setting of an immunocompromised patient who is infected with angioinvasive aspergillosis but can be seen in other infections with other organisms and in other conditions (e.g., granulomatosis with polyangiitis.) CT with contrast material also permits assessment of attenuation values within areas of consolidation and can better define areas of necrosis or abscess. Pleural complications include empyema or bronchopleural fistula.

REFERENCES

Kirsch J, et al. ACR Appropriateness Criteria® Acute Respiratory Illness in Immunocompetent Patients. *J Thorac Imaging.* 2011;26:W42–W44.
Walker CW, et al. Imaging pulmonary infection: classic signs and patterns. *AJR Am J Roentgenol.* 2014;202:479–492.
Franquet T. Imaging of community-acquired pneumonia. *J Thorac Imaging.* 2018;33(5):282–294.
Thoracic Radiology: The Requisites, 3rd ed, 289–309.

CASE 39

Pulmonary Langerhans Cell Histiocytosis

1. **C**
2. **D**
3. **B**
4. **C**

Comment

Differential Diagnosis

Centrilobular emphysema, lymphangioleiomyomatosis (LAM), multifocal micronodular pneumocyte hyperplasia (MMPH), desquamative interstitial pneumonia (DIP), lymphocytic interstitial pneumonia (LIP), Birt-Hogg-Dube syndrome, light chain deposition disorder (LCDD), amyloidosis, post-infectious cysts (*Pneumocystis pneumoniae*), cystic pulmonary metastases, tracheobronchial papillomatosis, neurofibromatosis.

Discussion

Pulmonary Langerhans cell histiocytosis (PLCH) is a single-system variant of a diverse group of histiocytoses and is the most common form in adults. The pathophysiology involves infiltration of the terminal and respiratory bronchiolar interstitium by pulmonary Langerhans cells, which are dendritic antigen-presenting cells found normally in tracheobronchial epithelium. The cellular proliferation leads to loose cellular nodule formation and progressive destruction of the terminal airways resulting in progressive dilatation of the small airways (cyst formation). Fibrosis surrounding the destroyed airway produces a stellate scar and parenchymal distortion.

PLCH is characterized by distinct clinical, epidemiologic, and radiologic features which include young and middle-aged adult smokers (90%) who present with nonproductive cough and dyspnea. Treatment is centered around smoking cessation, with over 70% of patients having resolution of symptoms. Patients with progressive disease may be treated with corticosteroids or immunomodulating therapies (cyclophosphamide, methotrexate). Lung transplantation may be considered for those with progressive, end-stage disease. However, PLCH may recur in the transplanted lungs in up to 20% of cases.

Imaging features suggestive of PLCH include an upper lung zone-predominant reticulonodular pattern and occasional cysts, with notable sparing of the bases and costophrenic sulci (Fig. 39.1). CT findings including upper lung zone predominant thin-walled, often bizarre-shaped cysts, admixed with 1–10 mm centrilobular nodules, with or without cavitation (Fig. 39.2). Cavitary nodules on CT may exhibit mildly thickened walls, manifesting the "Cheerio sign." Occasionally, coalescent cysts can evolve into larger cavities, predisposing to recurrent pneumothorax (15%–25%). There is a strong association with secondary pulmonary hypertension.

REFERENCES

Raoof S, Bondalapati P, Vydyula R, et al. Cystic lung diseases: algorithmic approach. *Chest.* 2016;150(4):945–965.

Roden AC, Yi ES. Pulmonary Langerhans cell histiocytosis: an update from the pathologists' perspective. *Arch Pathol Lab Med.* 2016;140:230–240.

Thoracic Radiology: The Requisites, 3rd ed, 368–369, 368b, 369f.

CASE 40

Lymphangitic Carcinomatosis

1. **A**
2. **E**
3. **E**
4. **C**

Comment

Differential Diagnosis

Pulmonary edema, atypical infection, drug toxicity, idiopathic pulmonary fibrosis, lymphoma, leukemia, sarcoidosis, silicosis, asbestosis, alveolar proteinosis, diffuse pulmonary lymphangiomatosis, Erdheim-Chester disease, IgG4-related disease.

Discussion

Pulmonary lymphangitic carcinomatosis (PLC) refers to infiltration of the pulmonary lymphatic system by neoplastic cells. It is usually a result of hematogenous embolization of neoplastic cells into pulmonary capillaries with secondary invasion of the lymphatics and interstitium. In about 25% of cases, it may occur via retrograde extension of tumor into lymphatics adjacent to involved mediastinal or hilar lymph nodes or a central lung cancer. The most common malignancies associated with PLC include lung and breast cancers, as well as carcinomas of the stomach, pancreas, colon, prostate, cervix, and thyroid. Adenocarcinomas are primarily implicated in PLC.

The pulmonary lymphatics are located within the lung interstitium, which is divided into three anatomic compartments: axial (central/bronchoarterial), peripheral (interlobular septal/subpleural/fissural), and parenchymal (intralobular/interalveolar). Lymphangitic carcinomatosis leads to thickening of the interstitial compartments due to cellular infiltration, desmoplastic reaction, and lymphatic obstruction. The axial interstitium was more commonly and more severely affected than axial and peripheral (diffuse) or only peripheral compartments. Patients with involvement of the peripheral interstitium also suffered more frequent and more severe symptoms of dyspnea and cough, and adverse alterations in pulmonary function testing (marked decrease in vital capacity and widening of alveolar-arterial oxygen gradients.) In general, the presence of PLC is a poor prognostic sign (average survival 142 days), particularly in patients with more diffuse or peripheral interstitial involvement.

Chest radiographs are normal in 25% to 50% of cases of PLC, but when identifiable, abnormalities include interlobular septal thickening (Kerley's lines) with or without hilar lymphadenopathy. A primary lung tumor surrounded by septal thickening may be seen. HRCT more readily depicts the anatomy of the secondary pulmonary lobule and lymphatic-containing structures. PLC manifests with nodular (beaded) septal thickening of peripheral interlobular septa and central bronchovascular structures (Fig. 40.1). An important distinction of PLC from other causes of septal thickening (i.e., pulmonary fibrosis, sarcoidosis) is the preservation of lung architecture. Ancillary findings might include metastatic pulmonary nodules, mediastinal or hilar lymphadenopathy, or pleural effusion. Alterations in pulmonary perfusion may be seen on ventilation-perfusion scintigraphy, as a consequence of tumor microemboli. Fluorodeoxyglucose positron emission tomography (FDG PET) CT has been shown to have utility in identification of PLC, with FDG avidity significantly increased (average standard uptake value 1.37 ± 0.29) in PLC lung relative to spared lung and background uptake in the mediastinal blood pool, with a sensitivity of 86% and a specificity of 100%. However, FDG PET/CT may miss cases of PLC which surround focally avid primary tumor may mask detection.

REFERENCES

Johkoh T, et al. CT findings in lymphangitic carcinomatosis of the lung: correlation with histologic findings and pulmonary function tests. *AJR Am J Roentgenol.* 1992;158(6):1217–1222.

Prakash P, et al. FDG PET/CT in assessment of pulmonary lymphangitic carcinomatosis. *AJR Am J Roentgenol.* 2010;194(1):231–236.

Thoracic Radiology: The Requisites, 3rd ed, 336–339, 344–346, 416–418.

CASE 41

Rounded Atelectasis

1. **E**
2. **B**
3. **B**
4. **E**

Comment

Differential Diagnosis

Pneumonia, lung cancer, pulmonary infarct, localized fibrous tumor of the pleura.

Discussion

Atelectasis refers to variable causes of incomplete expansion of alveoli, each with unique imaging manifestations. Rounded atelectasis refers to a unique form of peripheral focal atelectasis that is nearly always associated with a pleural abnormality. The most common association is with that of asbestos-related pleural disease. However, it may occur as a sequela of any cause of pleural thickening including empyema, effusion (hepatic hydrothorax, congestive heart failure, uremia, and end-stage renal disease), or post-surgical (especially coronary artery bypass grafting [CABG]). Rounded atelectasis develops secondary to tethering of the lung by an area of pleural thickening or fluid, which then creates an invagination of the adjacent pleura along the margin of involved lung tissue. The lung further contracts over time and creates a progressive infolding of the lung which lies in contact with the abnormal pleural surface.

Radiographic features include a subpleural round or lentiform, marginated mass-like opacity forming acute angles with the adjacent lung and often adjacent to pleural thickening or calcifications. Tethering and swirling of bronchovascular structures may also be evident (Fig. 41.1). Signs of volume loss are minimally present on chest radiography. CT is superior to radiography in demonstrating the four characteristic features of rounded atelectasis, including a focal subpleural parenchymal mass, adjacent pleural abnormality, volume loss, and comet tail sign (Fig. 41.2). Azour and colleagues conducted a review of CT features present in 189 cases of rounded atelectasis. The right lower lobe was involved more than half of the time and affected the posterior pleural surfaces in 73% of cases. Rounded atelectasis occurred with equal frequency in the setting of asbestos exposure and hepatic hydrothorax (26%), followed by post-infectious pleuritis (22%) and congestive heart failure (12%). Pleural abnormalities included pleural thickening (88%), pleural fluid (60%), and/or pleural calcification (40%). When CT features are equivocal, additional evaluation with positron emission tomography (PET)/CT may be necessary to exclude malignancy, particularly in the setting of asbestos exposure and smoking. PET imaging typically shows none to low-level fluorodeoxyglucose (FDG) avidity (average standard uptake value 2.2, range 0s–7.8).

Serial CT examinations tend to show stability or slight decrease in size of the atelectatic parenchyma. Recognition of typical CT features of rounded atelectasis may prevent unnecessary follow-up examinations or diagnostic interventions.

REFERENCES

Azour L, Billah T, Salvatore MM, et al. Causative factors, imaging findings, and CT course of round atelectasis. *Clinical Imaging.* 2018;50:250–257.

Riley JY, Naidoo P. Imaging assessment of rounded atelectasis: A pictoral essay. *J Med Imaging Radiat Oncol.* 2018;62(2):211–216.

Thoracic Radiology: The Requisites, 3rd ed, 47, 50f, 385, 424.

CASE 42

Sarcoidosis (Stage IV)

1. **E**
2. **E**
3. **A**
4. **B**

Comment

Differential Diagnosis

Pneumoconiosis (silicosis, coal workers pneumoconiosis, berylliosis), tuberculosis, pulmonary Langerhans cell histiocytosis, chronic hypersensitivity pneumonitis, ankylosing spondylitis, pleuroparenchymal fibroelastosis (PPFE), radiation fibrosis, lung cancer.

Discussion

Sarcoidosis is an idiopathic multisystem disorder characterized by non-caseating granulomas, with lung and mediastinal involvement in over 90% of cases. The diagnosis of sarcoidosis is achieved through exclusion of other entities which share clinical and radiopathologic similarities. The disorder tends to affect younger adults (age <40), with women affected nearly twice as often as males. There is also a higher prevalence of sarcoidosis in the African Americans than other ethnic and racial groups. The diagnosis is often found incidentally, as over 50% of patients are asymptomatic, and when symptoms occur, are more commonly systemic rather than respiratory. Interestingly, there is an inverse relationship between smoking and sarcoidosis.

The most common imaging feature of sarcoidosis is bilateral mediastinal or hilar lymphadenopathy, with or without pulmonary abnormalities. Parenchymal involvement manifests as a reticulonodular pattern of perilymphatic nodules in an upper lung zone distribution. Up to 20% of patients with parenchymal disease will progress to irreversible fibrosis (Stage IV), portending a poor prognosis.

Imaging features of Stage IV sarcoidosis include upper lung zone architectural distortion, volume loss with upward hilar traction, traction bronchiectasis, and peribronchovascular reticulation (Figs. 42.1, 42.2 and 42.3). Fibrosis tends to be more pronounced in the apical and posterior portions of the upper lobes, causing characteristic posterior displacement of fissures. Occasionally, large fibrotic masses may develop mimicking progressive massive fibrosis. Apical bullous change may lead to mycetoma formation. Pulmonary hypertension is a frequent complication of the disease. Furthermore, patients with sarcoidosis are at increased risk for lung cancer.

REFERENCES

Askling J, et al. Increased risk for cancer following sarcoidosis. *Am J Respir Crit Care Med.* 1999;160:1668–1672.

Little BP. Sarcoidosis: overview of pulmonary manifestations and imaging. *Semin Roentgenol.* 2015;50(1):52–64.

Thoracic Radiology: The Requisites, 3rd ed, 365–366.

CASE 43

Emphysema (Centrilobular)

1. **B**
2. **C**
3. **B**
4. **B**

Comment

Differential Diagnosis

Cystic lung disease (pulmonary Langerhans cell histiocytosis, lymphangioleiomyomatosis, lymphoid interstitial pneumonia, desquamative interstitial pneumonia, Birt-Hogg-Dube, light chain deposition disease), HIV-associated cystic lung disease, *Pneumocystis* pneumonia, pneumatocele, cystic metastases, constrictive bronchiolitis, pneumothorax, asthma.

Discussion

Emphysema refers to irreversible destruction of the walls of alveoli, leading to enlargement of the terminal airspaces. Smoking is the most common cause of emphysema. Patients may present with chronic dyspnea and obstructive symptoms. Pulmonary function tests (PFT) quantify the degree of obstruction and parenchymal damage with diminution of forced expiratory volume in one second (FEV1) and its ratio to the forced vital capacity. Lung volumes may increase from airway obstruction and hyperinflation, resulting in increased total lung capacity, functional residual capacity, and residual volume. Measures of vital capacity and diffusing capacity for carbon monoxide (DLCO) decrease as alveolar surface area is reduced. Up to 30% of the lung may need to be destroyed before abnormalities are detected with PFT.

Distribution of emphysema on an anatomical basis includes *centrilobular*, *paraseptal*, *panlobular*, and *paracicatricial* categories. *Centrilobular emphysema* refers to a pattern of lung destruction predominantly affecting the respiratory bronchioles located centrally in the secondary pulmonary lobule. *Paraseptal emphysema* refers to destruction of the alveolar ducts and sacs in the periphery of the secondary pulmonary lobule, manifesting with subpleural lung and along the fissures. Thin walls may be evident and represent interlobular septa outlining the periphery of the secondary pulmonary lobule. Confluent areas of paraseptal emphysema are termed bullae when enlarged airspaces reach greater than 1 cm. When the entire lobule is involved it is described as *panlobular*. This pattern results in loss of respiratory tissues leaving behind only supporting elements such as vessels, conducting airways, and septae. Panlobular emphysema may occur in smokers, elderly, or distal to areas of bronchiolar obstruction. However, it has a strong association with alpha-1-antitrypsin deficiency, and this etiology should be raised when panlobular emphysema is recognized. Alpha-1-antitrypsin normally serves as an inhibitor of neutrophil elastase, which contributes to alveolar destruction triggered by smoking. Individuals with deficiency in the enzyme suffer unregulated and accelerated alveolar destruction. Unlike typical smoking-related emphysema, panlobular emphysema tends to be more prominent in the lung bases. *Paracicatricial* emphysema refers to irregular patterns of localized emphysema occurring adjacent to areas of fibrosis and may not necessarily be associated with smoking and airflow obstruction.

Computed tomography (CT) is more sensitive and specific than radiography for detection of the various forms of emphysema, manifesting as small foci of low attenuation relative normal parenchyma without discernable walls, usually concentrated in the upper lung zones (Fig. 43.1 and Fig. 43.2). Features which distinguish emphysema from other causes of lucent spaces in the lung (i.e., cystic lung disease) include invisible walls and the presence of a central dot within the lucent areas, representing the centrilobular arteriole and bronchiole. Whereas, lung cysts tend to displace the centrilobular arteriole and bronchiole to the edge of the cystic space. Bullous change occurring along the lung periphery predispose patients to secondary spontaneous pneumothoraces. In addition, giant bullae may compress adjacent lung and lead to impaired ventilation or may become chronically infected particularly with *Aspergillus* species.

REFERENCES
Edwards RM, et al. Imaging of small airways and emphysema. *Clin Chest Med*. 2015;36:335–347.
Thoracic Radiology: The Requisites, 3rd ed, 392–399.

CASE 44

Anterior Mediastinal Mass

1. **A**
2. **A**
3. **D**
4. **A**

Comment

Differential Diagnosis

Other thymic epithelial neoplasm (thymic carcinoma, thymic neuroendocrine tumor), thymic cyst, thymic hyperplasia, thymolipoma, lymphoma, lymphangioma, metastases, thyroid goiter, germ cell tumor, parathyroid mass, mediastinal lipomatosis

Discussion

The mediastinum is bounded laterally by the mediastinal pleura of both lungs, anteriorly by the sternum, posteriorly by the spine, superiorly by the thoracic inlet, and inferiorly by the diaphragm. Mediastinal compartments have been historically classified according to semi-anatomic divisions based on lateral chest radiographs. Modern approaches to characterization of mediastinal lesions require cross sectional imaging with computed tomography (CT) and magnetic resonance imaging (MRI). The International Thymic Malignancy Interest Group (ITMIG) improved upon earlier designations and created a new definition and standard consensus for compartmentalization of the mediastinum, which includes the prevascular, visceral, and paravertebral compartments.

Compartment	Prevascular	Visceral	Paravertebral
Boundaries	Anterior: sternum Posterior: anterior aspect of pericardium	Anterior: posterior boundary of the prevascular mediastinum Posterior: vertical line extending 1 cm behind the anterior cortex of each thoracic vertebral body	Anterior: posterior boundary of visceral mediastinum Posterolateral: vertical line in posterior chest wall at the lateral margin of the thoracic spine transverse processes

All three compartments are bound superiorly by the thoracic inlet, laterally by the parietal mediastinal pleura, and inferiorly by the diaphragm.

Thymoma is the most common subclass of thymic epithelial neoplasms, comprised of epithelial cells and lymphocytes in varying proportions and morphologies, which determines their prognosis. Most are contained by a fibrous capsule (non-invasive thymoma, Stage I). More aggressive lesions invade through their capsule and into adjacent structures (Stage II and III, respectively). Metastases are rare and usually involve local structures such as the pleura or pericardium (Stage IVA). The stage of disease determines treatment approach and prognosis. Non-invasive thymoma is treated with surgical resection alone while Stage II disease is treated with surgical resection with or without postoperative radiation. Stage III and IVA disease are treated with neoadjuvant chemotherapy and surgery, whereas Stage IVB disease (distant metastases) is treated with palliative chemotherapy.

Thymomas are usually discovered as incidental findings in patients 40 years of age. Occasionally, patients may present with paraneoplastic sequelae, most commonly myasthenia gravis (1/3 of patients with thymoma). Others include pure red blood cell aplasia and hypogammaglobulinemia, as well as associations with autoimmune disorders such as systemic lupus erythematosus, rheumatoid arthritis, and inflammatory bowel disease.

Small lesions may escape detection by radiography or may present as a prevascular mediastinal mass (Fig. 44.1 and 44.2). Subtle thickening of the anterior junction line may be the only radiographic feature. On CT, thymomas typically manifest as round or ovoid homogenous tumors (Fig. 44.3). When necrosis or hemorrhage is present, they may become more heterogeneous. Calcification has also been described. Lymphadenopathy is not a typical feature, as advanced thymoma typically exhibits local invasion as opposed to lymphatic dissemination. Larger lesions exert mass effect on adjacent structures. Invasive thymomas exhibit intrinsic heterogeneity and irregular borders and will violate mediastinal fat planes between adjacent structures. "Drop metastases" are typical of these tumors manifesting as pleural or pericardial nodules or effusions. MRI features include intermediate and hyperintense signal on T1 and T2 weighted images, respectively. Chemical shift ratio greater than 0.9 between in- and opposed-phase T1-weighted images indicates the presence of intravoxel fat, which is typical of thymic hyperplasia but not of thymoma which would have a chemical shift ratio of 0.7 or less. Differentiation of thymoma from hyperattenuating thymic cysts and cystic thymoma is readily accomplished with MRI. Dynamic contrast enhanced MRI might also differentiate low-risk thymomas from high-risk thymomas, thymic carcinoma, and lymphoma. fluorodeoxyglucose (FDG)-positron emission tomography (PET) /CT has limited utility in evaluation of thymoma, as normal or hyperplastic tissue can show FDG avidity.

REFERENCES
Carter BW, et al. ITMIG classification of mediastinal compartments and multidisciplinary approach to mediastinal masses. *RadioGraphics*. 2017;37:413–436.
Thoracic Radiology: The Requisites, 3rd ed, 103–115.

CASE 45

Subcarinal Lymph Node Enlargement Secondary to Metastatic Disease

1. **D**
2. **D**
3. **C**
4. **E**

Comment

Differential Diagnosis

Lymphadenopathy (infection, metastases, lymphoma, sarcoidosis, Castleman disease), foregut duplication cysts, hiatal hernia, aortic aneurysm, esophageal mass, mediastinal hemorrhage, tracheal neoplasm.

Discussion

Accurate staging of lung cancer facilitates tailoring of evidence-based treatment strategies as well as prognostic information for patients. The staging process allows determination of the extent of intra- and extrathoracic tumor involvement. The American Joint Committee on Cancer (AJCC) and Union for International Cancer Control (UICC) work jointly to unify lung cancer staging classifications. Lymph node metastases are an important component of the TNM staging system and accurate description of regional or nonregional lymph node involvement is essential. The International Association for the Study of Lung Cancer (IASLC) established a standardized map of the intrathoracic lymph nodes, which should be used along with the current 8th edition TNM classification for malignant lung tumors.

Regional lymph nodes are named by structures which are in close anatomic relationships. The IASLC lymph node map describes 14 stations grouped into 7 zones. Most lung cancers first drain to intrapulmonary lymph nodes of the involved lobe, then sequentially to ipsilateral interlobar, hilar, and paratracheal nodal stations. However, lymphatics from all lung segments may have direct drainage to paratracheal or subcarinal stations. Such communications allow metastases to "skip" nodal stations and explain the importance of subcarinal lymphadenopathy in the TNM staging paradigm. The subcarinal zone is defined anatomically by the carina superiorly and inferiorly by the upper border of the left lower lobe bronchus and lower border of the bronchus intermedius.

Subcarinal zone lymph nodes are considered pathologically enlarged at 1.2 cm short axis diameter and designated as N2 disease in the current TNM staging system for lung cancer. This is an important designation for determining prognosis and treatment strategy. Patients with subcarinal lymphadenopathy are considered as having either Stage IIIA or IIIB disease (depending on the size of the primary tumor) with 5-year survival of 36% and 26%, respectively. Patients with Stage IIIA disease may be considered for surgical resection in addition to chemoradiation, which is not the case for patients with Stage IIIB disease.

Staging may involve a combination of non-invasive imaging (computed tomography [CT] and positron emission tomography [PET]/CT) and more invasive bronchoscopic and surgical procedures. Endobronchial and endoscopic options include bronchoscopy, endobronchial ultrasound, and esophageal endoscopic ultrasound. Surgical options include mediastinoscopy, anterior mediastinotomy (Chamberlin procedure), and video-assisted thorascopic surgery (VATS). Of these, bronchoscopy, endoscopy, and mediastinoscopy allow access to the subcarinal space, with mediastinoscopy considered the gold standard.

REFERENCES

Goldstraw P, et al. The IASLC Lung Cancer Staging Project: Proposals for revision of the TNM stage grouping in the forthcoming (Eight) edition of the TNM Classification for Lung Cancer. *J Thoracic Oncol.* 2015;1:39–51.

El-Sherief AH, et al. International Association for the Study of Lung Cancer (IASLC) Lymph Node Map: Radiologic Review with CT Illustration. *RadioGraphics.* 2014;34:1680–1691.

Lanuti M, et al. Mediastinoscopy and other thoracic staging procedures. *Mastery of Cardiothoracic Surgery.* Philadelphia: Lippincott Williams & Wilkins; 2014:14–27.

Thoracic Radiology: The Requisites, 3rd ed, 450–459.

CASE 46

Silicosis

1. **B**
2. **D**
3. **D**
4. **C**

Comment

Differential Diagnosis

Other pneumoconiosis (coal workers pneumoconiosis, talcosis, berylliosis, etc), sarcoidosis, tuberculosis & other military infections, pulmonary Langerhans cell histiocytosis, hypersensitivity pneumonitis, metastases, lung cancer (in progressive massive fibrosis).

Discussion

Silicosis represents one of several lung disorders which share a common etiology related to inhalation of aerosolized particulates and deposition in the pulmonary parenchyma (pneumoconioses). Silicon dioxide is an abundant component of Earth's crust, found in many rocks. Exposure to silica dust may occur more frequently in the setting of certain occupations such as mining, quarrying, ceramics, sandblasting, and others. Larger (>5 μm) inhaled particles are readily cleared through the central airways and mucociliary transport. However, smaller particles may remain in the lung, become ingested by pulmonary macrophages, and carried into the lymphatics for clearance. Prolonged exposure to silica dust may overwhelm the lymphatic clearance mechanisms and result in silicosis.

Three subtypes of silicosis have been described and include acute, classic, and accelerated forms. Acute silicosis (silicoproteinosis) occurs from a very large exposure to silica dust over a short period of time leading to acute onset of symptoms including dyspnea, cough, fever, and weight loss. The disease can progress rapidly and result in respiratory failure. Classic silicosis has an indolent course, occurring 10 to 20 years after low-level exposures. Patients are typically asymptomatic. Accelerated silicosis exists as a spectrum of disease between acute and classic forms, with radiographic manifestations occurring 4 to 8 years after exposure to large amounts of silica. Complications of silicosis include a higher risk for infection with tuberculosis and development of lung cancer.

In 2011, the International Labor Organization updated its guidelines for objective classification of pneumoconiosis, including digital radiography as the standard for assessing disease extent in comparison to reference standards. Classic silicosis manifests in two forms radiographically: simple and complicated. Simple classic silicosis most commonly manifests on radiographs as multiple bilateral nodules (3–5 μm) distributed mostly in the upper lung zones. Lymphadenopathy is a common secondary finding and may be calcified in up to 20% of cases, with eggshell pattern in 5-10%, a highly suggestive feature of silicosis. High resolution computed tomography (CT) findings are more sensitive and specific than radiography for early detection and characterization of the disease, showing a perilymphatic pattern of well-defined nodules in the upper lobes (typically posterior), as well as hilar and mediastinal lymphadenopathy. Complicated silicosis (also called progressive massive fibrosis) is defined as formation of conglomerate nodules measuring over 1 cm on imaging. These are also typically distributed in the posterior bilateral upper lobes, are often bilateral, may have associated paracicatricial emphysema near the lesion. Progressive massive fibrosis especially when cavitary can mimic lung cancer and may even exhibit avidity on fluorodeoxyglucose (FDG)-positron emission tomography (PET) imaging.

REFERENCES

Cox CW, Rose CS, Lynch DA. State of the art: imaging of occupational lung disease. *Radiology.* 2014;270(3):681–696.

International Labor Office. Guidelines for the Use of ILO International Classifications of Radiographs of Pneumoconioses Revised Edition. 2011 Geneva: International Labor Office.

Thoracic Radiology: The Requisites, 3rd ed, 377–390.

CASE 47

Connective Tissue Disease-Associated Interstitial Lung Disease (Systemic Sclerosis [Scleroderma] With Nonspecific Interstitial Pneumonia [NSIP] Pattern)

1. **B**
2. **B**
3. **D**
4. **C**

Comment

Differential Diagnosis

Idiopathic NSIP, drug-induced NSIP, usual interstitial pneumonia (UIP), interstitial pneumonia with autoimmune features (IPAF), hypersensitivity pneumonitis, desquamative interstitial pneumonia (DIP), airway-centered interstitial fibrosis (ACIF), organizing pneumonia, dependent atelectasis, edema, infection, hemorrhage, aspiration.

Discussion

Systemic sclerosis (scleroderma) is a multisystem autoimmune disorder characterized by inflammation, excess collagen production, and vasculopathy. The lung is the second most site of involvement, typically manifesting as interstitial lung disease and pulmonary hypertension. The disease tends to affect women of childbearing age and is associated with a poor prognosis (30% 10-year mortality), especially if diagnosed at an older age. Pulmonary disease may lead to the initial diagnosis of an underlying connective tissue disorders (CTD). However, most CTDs are diagnosed clinically including investigation for unique patterns of elevated serum antibodies for each. Serologic markers for systemic sclerosis include anti-centromere antibody and anti-Scl-70, with the latter being associated with greater likelihood of pulmonary fibrosis and an overall poorer prognosis. Unlike for desquamative interstitial pneumonia, there is no strong association with smoking in NSIP. Other associated findings include a high incidence of esophageal dysmotility (75%) which may be considered when esophageal dilation, gas–fluid level, and open esophageal sphincter are present on CT. Pulmonary arterial enlargement may be seen, implicating pulmonary hypertension in up to 41% of patients.

The most common histologic pattern of systemic sclerosis is that of NSIP, followed by UIP. Histologically, NSIP is classified as one of two subtypes—cellular or fibrotic—depending on the degree of fibrosis present. Unlike for UIP, histological changes in NSIP are both spatially and temporally homogenous ranging from inflammatory infiltrate within alveolar septae (cellular) to intramural collagen deposition (fibrotic). Unlike for UIP, alveolar septal architecture is preserved, and areas of organization or fibroblastic foci are minimal to absent.

Radiographic features consist of lower lung zone predominant reticulation or patchy mid-to-lower lung zone hazy opacities. Classic CT findings (Fig. 47.1) include symmetric, subpleural, basilar-predominant ground-glass opacities (especially in the cellular form) with varying degrees of reticulation and traction bronchiectasis/bronchiolectasis (typically associated with the fibrotic form). Axial distribution may be central, peripheral, or diffuse. Subpleural sparing, wherein the lung immediately adjacent to the visceral pleura appears relatively unaffected, is highly suggestive of NSIP. Although uncommon, honeycombing is usually mild and associated with the fibrotic form.

REFERENCES

Kim EA, et al. Interstitial lung disease associated with collagen vascular diseases: radiologic and histopathologic findings. *RadioGraphics.* 2002;22:S151–S165.

Capobianco J, et al. Thoracic manifestations of collagen vascular diseases. *RadioGraphics.* 2012;32:33–50.

Thoracic Radiology: The Requisites, 3rd ed, 355–357, 361–363.

CASE 48

Ranke Complex

1. **D**
2. **B**
3. **A**
4. **G**

Comment

Differential Diagnosis

Healed granulomatous disease (tuberculosis, fungi, etc), healed varicella infection, hamartoma, pneumoconiosis (silicosis, coal workers pneumoconiosis), carcinoid tumor, calcified or ossified metastases (mucinous tumors, sarcomas, medullary thyroid carcinoma), metastatic pulmonary calcification, pulmonary ossification, alveolar microlithiasis.

Discussion

Tuberculosis refers to infection with mycobacterial species, which include most commonly *Mycobacterium tuberculosis*, or other atypical organisms such as *Mycobacterium bovis*, *Mycobacterium microti*, and *Mycobacterium kansasii*. In humans, thoracic infections with these species are divided broadly into tuberculous (TB) or nontuberculous (NTM) infection.

When persons with active infection cough, sneeze, or speak, airborne mycobacteria are transferred via 1 to 5 μm droplets to the terminal airspaces and become ingested by alveolar macrophages. In most cases, the host immune system can adequately control the infection, preventing replication and spread of the organisms, and the host will remain asymptomatic and noncontagious, harboring the infection at a subclinical level (*latent TB*). In 5% of infected hosts, the initial infection is controlled, but dormant mycobacteria become active, or the host may become infected with a different strain at a later time (*postprimary, reactivation TB*). In the remainder of infected individuals, the immune system fails to control the initial infection in the first 1 to 2 years, giving rise to *primary TB*.

Imaging plays a critical role in the diagnosis and management of patients with TB, with variable manifestations depending on the integrity of the host immune response (as opposed to the long-held classic teachings relating imaging patterns to the temporal relationship to infection). Parenchymal consolidation and necrotic hilar and mediastinal lymphadenopathy are hallmarks of primary TB. In patients with primary TB and an adequate host immune response, the parenchymal consolidation may resolve leaving a residual scar or often calcified nodule (*Ghon focus*). At the same time, lymphadenopathy may regress leaving behind residual calcified lymph nodes in the drainage pathway of the parenchymal infection. The combination of the Ghon focus and calcified ipsilateral lymph nodes is referred to as *Ranke complex*, signifying healed primary TB (*inactive TB*).

Testing for latent TB with tuberculin skin test or interferon-γ release assays is advised for asymptomatic persons at high risk of exposure or reactivation and persons with incidental imaging findings suggestive of inactive TB. In the tuberculin skin test (purified protein derivative, PPD), a protein derived from *M tuberculosis* is injected intradermally to elicit a localized delayed cell-mediated hypersensitivity response to the bacterial proteins, which would indicate prior infection, but false positive and false negative tests can occur. All individuals with positive screening tests will undergo chest radiography (single PA view) to look for imaging features of active TB (consolidation, centrilobular tree-in-bud nodules, cavitation, lymphadenopathy, pleural effusion) which would prompt treatment or previous TB (fibronodular scarring, peribronchial fibrosis, bronchiectasis, apical volume loss, Ghon focus or Ranke complex).

REFERENCES
Jeong YJ, Lee KS. Pulmonary tuberculosis: up-to-date imaging and management. *AJR Am J Roentgenol.* 2008;191(3):834–844.
Nachiappan AC, et al. Pulmonary tuberculosis: role of radiology in diagnosis and management. *RadioGraphics.* 2017;37:52–72.
Rozenshtein A, et al. Radiographic appearance of pulmonary tuberculosis: dogma disproved. *AJR Am J Roentgenol.* 2015;204:974–978.
Thoracic Radiology: The Requisites, 3rd ed, 323–333.

CASE 49

Bronchiectasis

1. **A.** The case demonstrates primarily lower lung zone predominant cylindrical, varicoid, and cystic bronchiectasis. None of the other options are included on these images.
2. **B.** Bronchiectasis is defined by dilatation of the bronchial diameter to 1.5 times that of the accompanying pulmonary artery or arteriole. Bronchomalacia is defined by greater than 70% luminal cross-sectional area collapse on expiration (choice D). Choice E refers to saber sheath configuration of the trachea, typically associated with COPD.
3. **C.** The signet ring sign refers to the CT cross-section appearance in the dilated bronchial wall ("ring") appears to have a "jewel" affixed to it, representing the accompanying pulmonary artery. The three-density sign (formerly "headcheese sign") is used to describe geographic areas of lucent, normal, and ground-glass lung attenuation in the setting of hypersensitivity pneumonitis. The fallen viscera sign is evoked in the setting of traumatic diaphragmatic rupture. The reverse halo sign is a CT pattern commonly associated with organizing pneumonia and sometimes pulmonary infarcts.
4. **G.** All of the listed conditions typically manifest with some pattern of bronchiectasis.

Comment

Differential Diagnosis

Chronic infection/inflammation (bronchitis, aspiration, toxic inhalation, allergic bronchopulmonary aspergillosis, rheumatoid arthritis), congenital causes (cystic fibrosis, primary ciliary dyskinesia, tracheobronchomegaly, Williams-Campbell syndrome, bronchial atresia, immune deficiency, yellow nail syndrome), traction bronchiectasis (interstitial pneumonias, sarcoidosis, radiation fibrosis), bronchial obstruction (tumor, foreign body, extrinsic compression), cystic or cavitary lung disease.

Discussion

There are approximately 23 divisions of the airway beyond the trachea and main bronchi comprised of lobar, segmental, and intrapulmonary bronchiole divisions. Airways may have a purely conductive function or a combined conductive-and-gas-exchange function (respiratory bronchioles). Hyaline cartilage and muscular fibers form the intrapulmonary bronchi while bronchioles are defined by their lack mural cartilage.

Bronchiectasis refers to irreversible dilation of the bronchi, most commonly the medium-sized 4th to 6th divisions. Lack of bronchiolar tapering in the peripheral lung is often the earliest and most sensitive imaging sign. However, direct signs of bronchial dilation include elevated bronchoarterial ratios, wherein a bronchial diameter measures greater than its accompanying pulmonary artery. Bronchoarterial ratios of 1.0 to 1.5 are nonspecific and can be normal findings in elderly subjects and those living at high altitude. However, bronchoarterial >1.5 indicates bronchiectasis, and may also manifest on cross-section as the *signet ring sign* on CT in which the round pulmonary arteriole simulates a "jewel" affixed to a "ring" (the bronchial wall).

Many processes may result in bronchiectasis, most commonly infections and associated inflammation of the airway wall. Respiratory syncytial virus (RSV) is a frequent cause in children, while chronic aspiration is a common cause. Bronchiectatic airways often become chronically colonized with organisms such as *Haemophilus, Pseudomonas,* and other species. In order of severity, bronchiectasis may manifest with cylindrical (tram track, uniformly spaced walls), varicoid (alternating dilation and narrowing), or cystic (rounded, often clustered) patterns. Traction bronchiectasis reflects desmoplastic reaction and retractile tethering of airways by adjacent fibrosis as opposed to intrinsic airway abnormalities.

The distribution of bronchiectasis may suggest a specific underlying cause. For example, central mucus plugging may be seen in cystic fibrosis and allergic bronchopulmonary aspergillosis, often with upper lobe predominance. Tuberculosis also tends to produce upper lobe predominant bronchiectasis. Traction bronchiectasis may occur within areas of prior radiation therapy or in regions affected by diffuse lung diseases such as sarcoidosis, silicosis, or berylliosis. Diffuse bronchiectasis may be caused by congenital bronchial abnormalities, deficiencies of host defense, mucus production, or altered ciliary clearance. Focal bronchiectasis typically occurs from long-standing bronchial obstruction of a lobe or segment, which may be secondary to tumor, foreign body, or other extrinsic compression.

REFERENCES
Milliron B, et al. Bronchiectasis: mechanisms and imaging clues of associated common and uncommon diseases. *RadioGraphics.* 2015;35(4):1011–1030.
Dodd JD, et al. Imaging in cystic fibrosis and non-cystic fibrosis bronchiectasis. *Semin Respir Crit Care Med.* 2015;36(2):194–206.
Thoracic Radiology: The Requisites, 3rd ed, 137–158.

CASE 50

Arteriovenous Malformation

1. **E**
2. **F**
3. **D**

Comment

Differential Diagnosis

Metastasis, septic emboli, solitary pulmonary nodule, pulmonary artery pseudoaneurysm, meandering pulmonary vein, pulmonary varix, anomalous pulmonary venous return.

Discussion

A pulmonary arteriovenous malformation (AVM) is a direct communication between a pulmonary artery and pulmonary vein without an intervening capillary network, resulting in a right-to-left shunt. Arteriovenous malformations may be congenital or acquired, with congenital variants believed to develop from errors in capillary formation. Acquired AVMs are typically encountered in patients with underlying congenital heart disease, chronic liver disease, or certain infections such as tuberculosis or actinomycosis. Pulmonary AVMs may be single or multiple (30%) or may be multisystem. Between 80% and 90% of patients with pulmonary AVMs have the inherited disorder known as hereditary hemorrhagic telangiectasia (Osler-Weber-Rendu disease), characterized by cutaneous and mucosal telangiectasias and occasionally AVMs in other organs. The classic morphology of pulmonary AVMs includes a feeding artery, a vascular nidus, and a draining vein. Lesions are classified as simple (single feeding artery and single draining vein) or complex (two or more feeding arteries or draining veins).

Although most patients with AVMs are asymptomatic, they may develop cyanosis, dyspnea, and digital clubbing in the setting of significant right-to-left shunting. Central nervous system complications such as stroke and brain abscess may occur as a result of paradoxical emboli. Hemoptysis is a less common complaint.

Chest radiographic manifestations of the vascular nidus include single or multiple nodules (Fig. 50.1), typically in the medial or lower thirds of the lung. A feeding artery may be recognized as a dilated vessel extending to the nidus from the hilum; a draining vein may be traced into the left atrium – manifesting as a dilated vessel that is typically larger than the feeding artery.

Multidetector computed tomography (CT) is helpful for the detection of small AVMs and in the delineation of the angioarchitecture before therapeutic embolization via pulmonary angiography (Fig. 50.2). Radiologists should report on the size and number of feeding pulmonary arteries and pulmonary, the size of the vascular nidus, and any draining veins, as well as the presence of other AVMs, as these have implications for the interventionalist who may consider catheter-based treatment. After treatment, patients will undergo life-long imaging follow-up with a 6-month baseline scan to ensure nidus involution and serially in 3 to 5-year intervals.

REFERENCES

Shovlin CL. Pulmonary arteriovenous malformations. *Am J Respir Crit Care Med*. 2014;190(11):1217–1228.

Trerotola SO, Pyeritz RE. PAVM embolization: an update. *AJR Am J Roentgenol*. 2010;195(4):837–845.

Thoracic Radiology: The Requisites, 3rd ed, 193–209.

CASE 51

Aortic Aneurysm

1. **C**
2. **B**
3. **C**

Comment

Differential Diagnosis

Mediastinal mass (e.g., lymphadenopathy, goiter, thymic neoplasm, esophageal mass, etc.), tortuous vasculature, anomalous vessels (e.g., aberrant subclavian artery or double aortic arch).

Discussion

Thoracic aortic aneurysms are considered when there is abnormal dilation of the ascending aortic lumen >5 cm (>50% normal diameter). Measurements may be made on axial computed tomography (CT) images at the level of the right pulmonary artery, or more accurately on double-oblique reformatted images. The ascending thoracic aorta is considered ectatic at diameters between 4 and 5 cm. However, some consider an ascending aorta to be aneurysmal at 4.5 cm. Serial surveillance imaging is employed to assess the rate of dilation because the incidence of rupture correlates with aneurysm size, especially for those >5 cm in diameter. Elective surgical repair has been recommended for ascending aortic aneurysms of 5 to 5.5 cm and for descending thoracic aortic aneurysms 5.5 to 6.5 cm in diameter, with early repair recommended for patients with existing conditions such as Marfan syndrome.

True aneurysms have intact layers of the aortic wall while false (pseudoaneurysms) have some degree of mural disruption and containment of blood only by adventitia. Aneurysms may have fusiform or saccular morphology, with fusiform aneurysms exhibiting long-segment cylindrical dilation, and saccular aneurysms manifesting as focal outpouchings.

Involvement of the ascending aorta and aortic root should raise suspicion of distinct conditions such as connective tissue diseases including Marfan, Ehlers-Danlos, and Loeys-Dietz syndromes, as well as those caused by syphilis or associated with Turner syndrome. Assessment should also be made for a bicuspid aortic valve. Complications of ascending aortic aneurysms include rupture, dissection, aortic insufficiency, and pericardial tamponade. Descending aortic aneurysms may result from atherosclerotic, posttraumatic, and infectious (mycotic) etiologies. Aneurysms may also arise from inflammatory conditions, including large vessel vasculitis (e.g., Takayasu or giant cell arteritis.)

Aortic aneurysm should be considered in the differential diagnosis of a mediastinal mass, as 10% of mediastinal masses

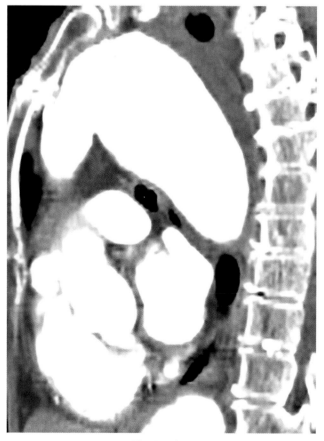

Fig. 51.1C

are of vascular etiology. When normal aortic contours are indistinguishable from a mediastinal mass, the silhouette sign may assist in localizing the lesion to the aorta. Other radiographic clues might include convexity of the right superior mediastinum, the hilum overlay sign, tracheal deviation, and lateralization of the left paraaortic interface. Peripheral calcification may be a clue to the presence of an atherosclerotic aneurysm. Contrast-enhanced CT and magnetic resonance imaging (MRI) play important roles in the diagnosis and surveillance of aortic aneurysms (Fig. 51.1C).

REFERENCES

Meyersohn NM, et al. Role of computed CT in the assessment of the thoracic aorta. *Curr Treat Options Cardio Med.* 2015;17:35.
Thoracic Radiology: The Requisites, 3rd ed, 97–136.

CASE 52

Pulmonary Infarct

1. **E**
2. **B**
3. **C**

Comment

Differential Diagnosis

Tumor thrombus, primary pulmonary artery sarcoma, vasculitis, artifact (respiratory motion, flow, streak), mimics (pulmonary vein, mucoid impaction).

Discussion

Pulmonary embolus (PE) is a common clinical problem requiring prompt diagnosis and management, as untreated PE is associated with up to 30% mortality. Symptoms of acute PE are non-specific and include dyspnea and pleuritic chest pain, as are the clinical signs of tachypnea, tachycardia, and hemoptysis. Clinical decision support and validated clinical scoring systems (Wells, simplified Wells, and modified Geneva scores) can assist the clinician in directing appropriate work-up and management. If PE is suspected in a patient with low pretest probability and a negative D-dimer test, an alternate diagnosis other than PE should be considered. If the D-dimer test is positive, then imaging is the next step in diagnostic workup.

Chest radiographs are often the first imaging performed but may show no abnormality. Signs of PE on radiography include atelectasis, Westermark sign (parenchymal lucency beyond the occluded vessel), Fleischner sign (an enlarged central pulmonary artery), and "knuckle sign" (tapered distal vessels due to central thrombus.) Pulmonary infarction may manifest as peripheral wedge-shaped consolidation in the lower lateral aspect of the involved hemithorax that abuts the pleura (Hampton hump) (Fig 52.1), or as atelectasis, an elevated hemidiaphragm, or pleural effusion. Chest radiography is primarily used to exclude other diagnoses that might mimic a PE, such as pneumothorax, pneumonia, or rib fracture. A recent chest radiograph is required to interpret any subsequent ventilation-perfusion scintigraphy scan.

Ventilation scintigraphy utilizes inhaled radiotracers xenon 133 or technetium-99m (^{99m}Tc) diethylenetriamine-pentaacetic acid which are distributed through the lungs. ^{99m}Tc macroaggregated human albumin is injected intravenously to map the lung perfusion. Diagnosis of PE is made when two or more segmental or larger wedge-shaped perfusion defects are found in areas of normal ventilation (V/Q mismatch).

Computed tomography pulmonary angiography (CTPA) has become the modality of choice for diagnosis of PE with sensitivity and specificity reaching 96% and 100%, respectively. Conversely, in patients with low pre-test probability for PE, CTPA may produce false-positive rates as high as 42%. Findings of PE include complete occlusion or partial filling defects within pulmonary arteries. Occasionally, PE can be detected as a hyperattenuating filling defect on non-contrast computed tomography (CT). Dual-energy CT maps iodine perfusion within normal lung tissue, analogous to scintigraphy, and may allow visualization of perfusion defects distal to small emboli.

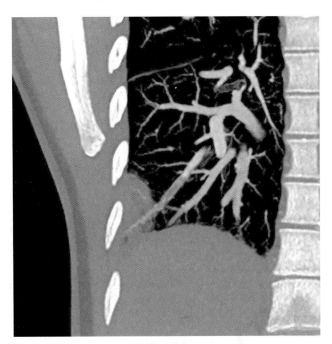

Fig. 52.2

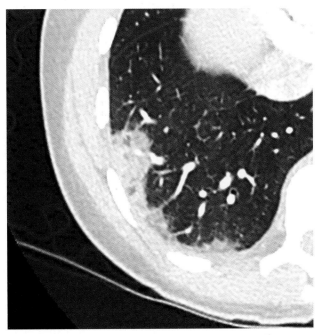

Fig. 52.3

On CT, pulmonary infarcts typically manifest as peripheral, often wedge-shaped consolidation that extends to the pleural surface (Figs. 52.23 and 52.3). Ground-glass opacity and bubble-like lucencies may be seen—representing hemorrhage and infarcted tissue—and become more nodular as they resolve. CTPA may identify patients with hemodynamic compromise who are at increased risk for fatal or nonfatal adverse events. Imaging signs of right heart strain (right ventricle–left ventricle ratio of >1.0), straightening or leftward bowing of the interventricular septum, contrast reflux into the hepatic veins, and dilated main pulmonary artery. CTPA can also detect alternative diagnoses such as pneumonia, pneumothorax, pericarditis, and aortic dissection. Pitfalls in CTPA interpretation include respiratory motion, image noise, flow-related artifact, and streak artifact from concentrated contrast material within the superior vena cava. Mimics of PE include slow flow in vessels (especially within areas of consolidation or atelectasis) and mucus-plugged bronchi.

Treatment includes anticoagulation, inferior vena cava filter, systemic thrombolysis, catheter–directed mechanical or pharmacologic thrombolysis, and surgical embolectomy. Most pulmonary emboli resolve without sequelae. Others may result in incomplete resolution and chronic thromboembolic disease.

REFERENCES
Kirsh J, et al. American College of Radiology Appropriateness Criteria ® Acute Chest Pain—Suspected Pulmonary Embolism. *J Am Coll Radiol.* 2017;14(5):S2–S12.
Kligerman SJ, et al. Radiologist performance in the detection of pulmonary embolism: features that favor correct interpretation and risk factors for errors. *J Thorac Imaging.* 2018;33(6):350–357.
Thoracic Radiology: The Requisites, 3rd ed, 238–258.

CASE 53

Lymphoma

1. **E**
2. **D**
3. **C**

Comment

Differential Diagnosis

Mediastinal Hodgkin lymphoma, thymic epithelial neoplasm, mediastinal germ cell neoplasm, mediastinal goiter, lymph node metastasis.

Discussion

Primary mediastinal lymphoma (PML) arises from the thymus or lymph nodes, typically manifesting as a prevascular or (less commonly) visceral mediastinal mass. Classification of PML is divided into Hodgkin (HL) or non-Hodgkin (NHL). HL is defined by the presence of Reed-Sternberg cells and includes classical HL and nodular lymphocyte predominant subtypes. Subtypes of primary mediastinal NHL include diffuse large B-cell lymphoma, lymphoblastic lymphoma, and primary thymic large B-cell lymphoma. Clinical symptoms are non-specific including cough or tachypnea. Occasionally, mass effect might cause dysphagia or superior vena cava (SVC) syndrome. Fever and weight loss can also be present.

Radiographic features of lymphoma most commonly include mediastinal widening on the frontal projection and retrosternal clear space filling on the lateral projection. A *hilum overlay sign* may be seen as preservation of hilar vasculature interfaces, indicating the mass is not in the same anteroposterior

plane as the hila. There may be tracheal deviation or narrowing from mass effect. CT features typically include a midline mass of homogeneous soft tissue attenuation. Masses tend to be large and are defined as "bulky" if over 10 cm or if greater than one-third of the intrathoracic diameter is occupied, portending poor prognosis. If cystic change and necrosis are present, the mass may appear more heterogeneous. Lymphoma tends to exert significant mass effect on and displace adjacent mediastinal structures. Invasion of adjacent chest wall or lung parenchyma may occur. Midline location of the mass favors lymphoma, while an off-midline location might suggest an alternate diagnosis such as thymoma. Treated lymphoma will decrease in size and attenuation with occasional calcification. Calcifications are rare in untreated lymphoma. Treatment response on MRI may manifest as increased T2 signal in areas of tumor necrosis and eventually, low T2 signal indicating fibrosis. ^{18}FDG-PET-CT plays an important role in staging and restaging of lymphoma, with complete response considered with resolution of FDG activity whether there is decrease in lesion size. Whole-body and PET-MRI may be employed for serial imaging in surveillance for lymphoma with added benefit of no ionizing radiation.

REFERENCES
Barrington SF, et al. Role of imaging in the staging and response assessment of lymphoma: consensus of the International Conference on Malignant Lymphomas Imaging Working Group. *J Clin Oncol.* 2014;32(27):3048–3058.
Shah KJ, et al. Diffuse large B-cell lymphoma in the era of precision oncology: how imaging is helpful. *Korean J Radiol.* 2017;18(1):54–70.
Thoracic Radiology: The Requisites, 3rd ed., p. 113.

CASE 54

Traumatic Aortic Injury (Transection)

1. **A, B, and E**
2. **D**
3. **E**

Comment

Differential Diagnosis

Ductus bump, aortic spindle, bronchial artery infundibulum, aortic pseudoaneurysm, penetrating atherosclerotic ulcer, pseudocoarctation.

Discussion

Prompt exclusion of traumatic aortic injury (TAI) after blunt chest trauma is critical as such injuries have a greater than 70% in-field mortality and up to 50% 24-hour mortality if left untreated. TAI occurs most commonly at sites where the aorta is relatively fixed, namely the root, isthmus, and descending aorta at the level of the diaphragmatic hiatus. Patients who survive long enough to receive hospital care typically have injuries at the aortic isthmus, just distal to the left subclavian artery origin, near the ligamentum arteriosum. Proposed injury mechanisms include (1) rapid differential deceleration of the fixed portions of the aorta relative to other mediastinal structures, (2) shear stress on the wall, (3) osseous pinch secondary to posterior translation of the sternum, and (4) hydrostatic or water-hammer phenomenon caused by sudden increases in intrathoracic pressure resulting in tears. Root injuries are associated with other serious cardiovascular

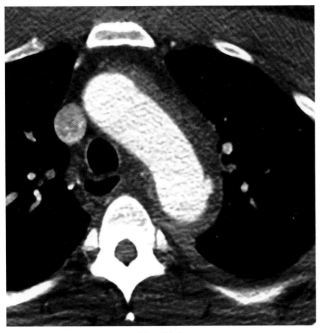

Fig. 54.2

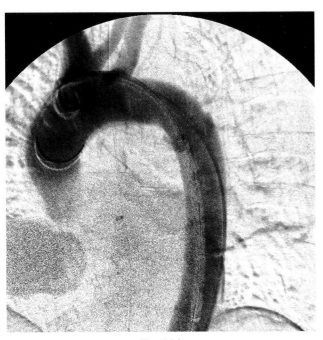

Fig. 54.3

esophagus, or nasogastric tube; and a left apical cap, indicating hemorrhage extending into the apical extrapleural space.

Computed tomography angiography (CTA) is the most appropriate study for evaluation of TAI, yielding rapid, high-resolution depiction of the injury and associated findings with a sensitivity and specificity of more than 90% for detection of TAI. Direct CT signs of TAI include aortic contour abnormality, intimal flap, intraluminal thrombus, pseudoaneurysm, and frank contrast extravasation. Precise CT characterization of the lesion is important for treatment planning (stent versus surgery) and should include information related to the length of defect, aortic diameter above and below, and distance from the great vessel origins. Detection of a periaortic hematoma is an indirect sign of TAI, demonstrating blood in contact with the aorta (Fig. 54.2). Mediastinal blood with a preserved fat plane around the aorta suggests a different source of bleeding – from mediastinal veins or intercostal or internal mammary arteries. Fractures of the first or second ribs should prompt close examination of the aorta and arch vessels to exclude traumatic vascular injury. Treatment of TAI typically includes surgical or endovascular graft repair (Fig. 54.3).

REFERENCES

Steenburg SD, et al. Acute traumatic aortic injury: imaging evaluation and management. *Radiology.* 2008;248:748–762.
Cullen EL, et al. Traumatic aortic injury: CT findings, mimics, and therapeutic options. *Cardiovasc Diagn Ther.* 2014;4(3):238–244.
Thoracic Radiology: The Requisites, 3rd ed, 279–288.

CASE 55

Lipoid Pneumonia

1. **A, B, C, D, E**
2. **C**
3. **D**

Comment

Differential Diagnosis

Lung adenocarcinoma (mucinous), lymphoma, alveolar proteinosis, alveolar sarcoid, chronic eosinophilic pneumonia, organizing pneumonia.

Discussion

Lipoid pneumonia (LP) is an uncommon cause of chronic lung opacification on chest radiography and computed tomography (CT). The etiologies include exogenous and endogenous causes of lipid accumulation in alveoli. Exogenous sources include aspiration of animal fats, mineral oil, or vegetable oils. Endogenous LP results from phagocytosis of lipids by intraalveolar macrophages that occur secondary to secretions that may accumulate beyond a point of endobronchial obstruction, fat storage diseases, or alveolar proteinosis. Exogenous LP may have an acute onset if a large quantity of petroleum-based product is introduced to the lung, resulting in an acute pneumonitis. Chronic LP typically follows from repeated, long-standing aspiration of animal fats or other oils and manifests similarly to acute LP. Predisposing conditions to chronic LP include older age, intellectual developmental disorders, oropharyngeal dysphagia, gastroesophageal reflux, or other factors which may cause aspiration (e.g., Zenker diverticulum). Chronic use of mineral oil laxative is also classically associated.

Radiographic manifestations vary according to the cause, with acute exogenous lipoid pneumonia producing ground-glass and consolidative opacities often in a lobar and basilar distribution. Chronic LP may manifest as a non-resolving consolidation

complications, including coronary arterial injury, hemopericardium, and tamponade.

Supine chest radiography is the first imaging modality used in the trauma setting, mainly to exclude acute life-threatening conditions like tension pneumothorax (Fig. 54.1). Several clues may assist in the diagnosis of TAI on chest radiography. These include widening of the vascular pedicle (>8 cm or 25% of the width of the thorax); loss of normal aortic arch and descending aortic contours; rightward displacement of the trachea, on chest radiography. On CT, LP is characterized by the demonstration of low attenuation within focal or multifocal areas of parenchymal consolidation equal to that of macroscopic fat (-30 HU) (Figs. 55.1 and 55.2). The areas of consolidation are often irregular or spiculated, forming nodular or mass-like opacities that may mimic lung cancer. CT detection of fat attenuation within a nodule or mass must be differentiated from other fat-containing lung lesions (e.g., hamartoma, fat-containing metastases [sarcomas].)

Chronic LP may be associated with architectural distortion or other evidence of fibrosis due to chronic inflammation. Pneumatoceles may develop in areas of previous pneumonitis and become complicated by pneumomediastinum or pneumothorax if they rupture. A "crazy-paving" pattern may also be seen on CT with non-resolving ground-glass opacity with superimposed interlobular septal thickening. Lipoid pneumonia may be avid on fluorodeoxyglucose (FDG)-positron emission tomography (FDG PET) if there is associated inflammation. Chronic airspace opacities must be differentiated from other causes such as pulmonary infection, alveolar proteinosis, lung cancer, and lymphoma.

REFERENCES

Betancourt SL, et al. Lipoid pneumonia: spectrum of clinical and radiologic manifestations. *AJR Am J Roentgenol.* 2010;194:103–109.
Marchiori E, et al. Exogenous lipoid pneumonia. Clinical and radiological manifestations. *Respiratory Medicine.* 2011;105:659–666.
Thoracic Radiology: The Requisites, 3rd ed, 355–376, 405–427.

CASE 56

Kartagener Syndrome (Primary Ciliary Dyskinesia)

1. **B**
2. **A, C, D**
3. **B**

Comment

Differential Diagnosis

Cystic fibrosis, allergic bronchopulmonary aspergillosis, post-infectious bronchiectasis, common variable immune deficiency, human immunodeficiency virus (HIV).

Discussion

Kartagener syndrome is a subset of the primary ciliary dyskinesia (PCD) spectrum of ciliopathies characterized by a classic triad of bronchiectasis, situs inversus, and sinusitis. Patients with PCD inherit a genetic defect that leads to impaired ciliary structure and function in an autosomal recessive pattern. Early symptoms of bronchitis, sinusitis, otitis media, and rhinitis often lead to early childhood presentation, which may be complicated by recurrent pneumonia. Patients may present later in life with reduced fertility because of impaired spermatozoon ciliary function. Bronchiectasis associated with this disorder is typically less severe than that of cystic fibrosis. Imaging features include situs inversus and bronchiectasis, with or without superimposed infection (Fig. 56.1). Bronchiectasis in this condition typically affects the right middle and lower lobes. Centrilobular nodules and tree-in-bud opacities indicate the small airways affected by mucus and infection. Mosaic attenuation and air-trapping may be seen. Maxillofacial computed tomography (CT) will show sequelae of acute and chronic sinusitis including mucosal thickening and mucoperiosteal reaction, with or without superimposed air-fluid levels (Fig. 56.2). Other associated findings include bronchial wall thickening, lung hyperinflation,

and atelectasis. Fifty percent of patients with PCD will have situs abnormalities (heterotaxy or situs inversus) (Fig. 56.3).

REFERENCES

Knowles MR, et al. Primary ciliary dyskinesia. *Clin Chest Med.* 2016;37(3):449–461.
Thoracic Radiology: The Requisites, 3rd ed, 137–158, 103–209.

CASE 57

Invasive Aspergillus

1. **A, B, and C**
2. **C**
3. **C**
4. **D**

Comment

Differential Diagnosis

Other pneumonia (bacterial, mycobacterial, or fungal), granulomatosis with polyangiitis, pulmonary infarction, lung cancer.

Discussion

Invasive pulmonary aspergillosis is the most common fungal infection to affect immunocompromised patients, usually those with severe neutropenia. Populations at risk for this potentially fatal infection include transplant recipients, hematologic malignancies, or those receiving chronic high-dose steroids.

Radiographic manifestations of invasive aspergillus include solitary or multiple ill-defined pulmonary nodules or masses, and confluent consolidation (Fig. 57.1). When *Aspergillus fumigatus* organisms invade pulmonary blood vessels (angioinvasive form), localized small to medium sized pulmonary arteries become occluded leading to peripheral infarction. CT findings of pulmonary infarction include peripheral wedge-shaped subpleural consolidation with surrounding ground-glass opacity (*CT halo sign*) in which the halo represents hemorrhage (Fig. 57.2). This sign is not specific for *Aspergillus* but is highly suggestive in the appropriate clinical setting. Other invasive fungal organisms such as *Mucor* and *Candida* species may also manifest with halos on CT. Early recognition of the halo sign may prompt the addition of anti-fungal treatment, thereby reducing morbidity and mortality. After onset of therapy, areas of consolidation may cavitate and form the *air crescent sign*, indicating recovery of neutrophil function and response to treatment.

REFERENCES

Walsh S, et al. Importance of the reversed halo sign for the diagnosis of angioinvasive pulmonary aspergillosis. *Respir Med.* 2014;108(8):1240.
Prasad A, et al. Pulmonary aspergillosis: what CT can offer before it is too late! *J Clin Diagn Res.* 2016;10(4):TE01–TE05.
Thoracic Radiology: The Requisites, 3rd ed, 155.

CASE 58

Granulomatosis With Polyangiitis

1. **A, B, C, D, and E**
2. **E**
3. **C**
4. **D**

Comment

Differential Diagnosis

Septic emboli, lung abscesses, tuberculosis, tracheobronchial papillomatosis, pulmonary metastases.

Discussion

Antineutrophil cytoplasm antibody (ANCA)-associated vasculitis is the most common of the primary small vessel vasculitides that include granulomatosis with polyangiitis (GPA) (formerly Wegener granulomatosis), eosinophilic granulomatosis with polyangiitis (E-GPA), and microscopic polyangiitis. GPA represents a multisystem necrotizing vasculitis resulting in the classic clinical triad of upper airway disease with lung and renal involvement (glomerulonephritis). The upper respiratory tract is involved in almost all patients and may include symptoms and signs of otitis, sinusitis, rhinorrhea, epistaxis, or airway stenosis. Lungs and kidneys are involved in 90% and 80% of patients, respectively. The presence of cytoplasmic ANCA (cANCA) suggests the diagnosis. Treatment typically includes cyclophosphamide and steroids.

Chest radiographic and CT findings associated with GPA include multiple pulmonary nodules and masses, seen in up to 90% of patients with pulmonary disease (Fig. 58.1). The distribution of nodules and masses is usually bilateral, lower lung zone, and subpleural. Nodules may coalesce into larger masses >10 cm in diameter, with predisposition to cavitation when greater than 2 cm, forming thick-walled irregular cavities and decreasing in size with treatment (Fig. 58.2). On contrast-enhanced CT, most nodules or masses demonstrate central low attenuation, indicating necrosis. Less commonly ground-glass opacity may surround the nodule (*CT halo sign*). Other CT findings include *reverse CT halo* and *feeding vessel* signs, the latter representing an artery, leading into a nodule or mass. Consolidation and ground-glass opacities are the second most common manifestation after nodules and masses, reflecting pneumonitis or alveolar hemorrhage related to vasculitis. Airway abnormalities include tracheal and bronchial wall thickening. Concentric inflammatory wall thickening can result in airway stenosis, with subglottic tracheal involvement being most typical. The differential diagnosis for subpleural nodules and masses of GPA includes septic emboli and abscess, neoplasms (including hematogenous metastases and lymphoma), organizing pneumonia, and Kaposi sarcoma.

REFERENCES

Feragalli B, et al. The lung in systemic vasculitis: radiological patterns and differential diagnosis. *Br J Radiol.* 2016;89(1061):20150992.

Thoracic Radiology: The Requisites, 3rd ed, 238–258.

CASE 59

Lymphangioleiomyomatosis

1. **A-C.** The CT images show diffuse cystic lung disease throughout the lungs. Of the listed choices, the only choice which is not a known cause of diffuse cystic lung disease is Hermansky-Pudlak syndrome, which is an inherited cause of pulmonary fibrosis and oculocutaneous albinism, more common among people from Puerto Rico.
2. **B.** The cysts in Langerhans cell histiocytosis (LCH) are usually upper lung preponderant with sparing of the costophrenic angles. Cysts can have thicker walls than in other cystic lung diseases and may coalesce to form bizarre shapes. The cysts often arise from centrilobular nodules which

produce small airway obstruction. Combined with a history of smoking, these findings are essentially diagnostic of LCH.
3. **A.** Lymphangioleiomyomatosis (LAM) may cause pleural effusions which are chylous (chylothorax) in up to 1/3 of patients. The most common causes of chylothorax are trauma to the thoracic duct and lymphoma. It would be unusual for the other listed conditions to lead to chylothorax.
4. **C.** Hepatocellular carcinoma is not associated with tuberous sclerosis complex (TSC). Common manifestations of TSC include a LAM-like cystic pattern of lung disease, rhabdomyomas in the heart, renal angiomyolipomas, a myriad of skin lesions, brain lesions, sclerotic bone lesions and multinodular multifocal pneumocyte hyperplasia. The latter entity produces multiple small pulmonary nodules.

Comment

LAM is characterized by abnormal proliferation of immature smooth muscle cells. Thin-walled lung cysts in LAM may rupture, leading to spontaneous pneumothoraces. Lymphatic obstruction may result in chylous pleural effusions. Vascular endothelial growth factor-D (VEGF-D) levels are often elevated in LAM but not in other cystic lung diseases and can be used to support the diagnosis and to monitor progression of disease. Recently, sirolimus has been shown to stabilize lung function in LAM. Recent evidence also suggests that sirolimus may be beneficial in the treatment of other manifestations of TSC.

The differential diagnosis for diffuse cystic lung disease is not as broad as in other diffuse lung diseases. Most cases are either due to TSC, LAM, or LCH. In most cases, the CT imaging manifestations of LAM and TSC in the lungs are indistinguishable, although multinodular multifocal pneumocyte hyperplasia (MMPH) occurs almost exclusively in TSC with or without manifestations of LAM. The features of MMPH on CT consist of multiple small nodular lesions usually 5 mm or less in diameter which can be solid or subsolid in attenuation. Obviously, if other non-pulmonary manifestations of TSC are evident, the diagnosis can be made readily. LAM and LCH are usually quite different in their imaging appearance. Cysts in LAM are uniformly thin-walled and evenly spaced throughout the lungs. In LCH, the cysts may be asymmetric or bizarrely shaped because cysts may coalesce over time. Small nodules may be present in LCH which would be very unusual in LAM. In LCH, the diffuse lung disease classically spares the costophrenic angles. Regarding demographics, all LAM patients (and vast majority with TSC) are women, usually of child-bearing age. LCH also tends to affect young adults who are smokers but is not limited to women.

Less common causes of diffuse cystic lung disease include lymphocytic interstitial pneumonitis (LIP), Birt-Hogg-Dube syndrome (BHD), and amyloidosis.

Helpful diagnostic pearls for these conditions:

LIP: Almost always secondary rather than idiopathic. In adults, most often associated with Sjogren syndrome. May also occur in immunodeficiency syndromes.

BHD: Associated with renal tumors (most often chromophobic renal cell carcinoma) and skin lesions (fibrofolliculomas most common). Autosomal dominant inheritance.

Amyloidosis: May occur with LIP and Sjogren syndrome. Produces nodular amyloid foci which may be partially calcified/ossified.

REFERENCES

Seaman DM, Meyer CA, Gilman MD, McCormack FX. Diffuse cystic lung disease at high-resolution CT. *AJR Am J Roentgenol.* 2011;Jun;196(6):1305–1311.

Thoracic Radiology: The Requisites, 3rd ed, 355–376.

CASE 60

Tuberculosis

1. **A-C.** The computed tomography (CT) images show large necrotic lymph nodes in the mediastinum.), Tuberculous lymphadenitis, lymphoma, and metastatic disease (usually from a squamous cell carcinoma primary) are the most common causes for necrotic lymphadenopathy. Sarcoidosis is a very common cause of large bulky lymph nodes in the mediastinum and hilar regions; however, necrosis within lymph nodes would be unusual.

2. **D.** Consolidation is a common finding of tuberculosis in children. Fibrocavitary disease is seen in active tuberculosis and bronchiectasis may occur in active disease or as late consequence of remote tuberculosis. Both are more frequently identified in adults. Ground-glass opacity is not a major finding in most cases of tuberculosis.

3. **A.** Lymphadenopathy in tuberculosis (TB) is common in children and those with human immunodeficiency virus–acquired immunodeficiency syndrome (HIV-AIDS) with CD4 counts below 200/mm^3.

4. **A.** TB pleural effusions are very uncommon in infants and uncommon in children. Up to 15% of adults may have pleural effusions as a manifestation of TB; this may be the sole and initial manifestation of TB in some cases. Therefore, a high level of clinical suspicion is necessary. A pleural biopsy is required for diagnosis.

Comment

The terms primary and post-primary TB continue to be used in the medical literature. It was previously believed that primary and post-primary TB could be differentiated on clinical and imaging grounds. However, DNA fingerprinting evidence has shown that primary and post-primary TB cannot be differentiated reliably on imaging (i.e., time from initial infection to the inception of active disease cannot predict the imaging manifestations of TB).

However, the imaging manifestations of TB in adults, children, and HIV-positive patients differ. Lymph node enlargement is a characteristic feature of TB in children but is much less common in adults. Lymph node enlargement may occur alone or in association with parenchymal consolidation, though isolated consolidation in children is unusual. On contrast-enhanced CT scans of patients with mediastinal and hilar tuberculous lymphadenitis, enlarged nodes often demonstrate a low-attenuation center and peripheral rim enhancement. Histologically, such nodes have been shown to demonstrate central necrosis and a highly vascular, inflammatory capsular reaction. Although low-attenuation nodes are characteristic of TB, they are not specific for this entity. Such nodes may also be encountered in atypical mycobacterial and fungal infections. Neoplastic lymph nodes (e.g., metastatic squamous cell carcinoma and lymphoma) may also demonstrate this appearance.

Regarding TB in HIV-positive patients, the radiographic appearance varies depending on the patient's CD4 count. In patients with CD4 counts above 200/mm³, a post-primary pattern is typically seen. In patients with CD4 counts below 200/mm³, you will usually observe a primary pattern, including low-attenuation lymph nodes and consolidation.

REFERENCES

Jeong YJ, Lee KS. Pulmonary tuberculosis: up-to-date imaging and management. *AJR Am J Roentgenol.* 2008 Sep;191(3):834–844.

Thoracic Radiology: The Requisites, 3rd ed, 323–334

CASE 61

Pneumocystis jirovecii Pneumonia

1. **A, B, C, and D.** The CT images shows diffuse ground-ground glass opacity with superimposed reticulation septal thickening and intralobular lines consistent with a crazy paving pattern. All the answer choices can manifest this pattern on chest CT. Crazy paving on chest CT is classically described in pulmonary alveolar proteinosis; however, given the relative rarity of this condition, other more common disease processes are usually responsible for the pattern in most clinical practices. Another rare cause of the crazy paving pattern is chronic lipoid pneumonia, which occurs in those who are at risk for aspiration or inhalation of lipid-laden substances (mineral oils, oil-based nose drops, lip gloss, etc).

2. **B.** Up to 1/3 of HIV patients with *Pneumocystis jirovecii* pneumonia (PJP) will have associated air cysts; very often there is an upper lung preponderance. The prevalence of cysts in PJP is lower in non-HIV afflicted patients. Interestingly, cysts may resolve with treatment. As in other cystic lung diseases, these patients are at risk for spontaneous pneumothoraces. Significant pleural effusions or lymphadenopathy is unusual in PJP. In the setting of PJP, tree-in-bud nodules on chest CT suggest superimposed infection in the small airways from another microbial agent or from aspiration.

3. **A.** Lymphangioleiomyomatosis (LAM) may cause pleural effusions which are chylous (chylothorax) in up to 1/3 of patients. The most common causes of chylothorax are trauma to the thoracic duct (often post-surgical) and lymphoma. It would be unusual for the other listed conditions to lead to chylothorax.

4. **A.** Trimethoprim-sulfamethoxazole (Bactrim) is first line therapy and prophylaxis for PJP.

Comment

The incidence of PJP has decreased as highly active antiretroviral therapy (HAARTT) and chemoprophylaxis has become standard treatment in HIV-positive patients. However, PJP continues to be the most common opportunistic infection in people with AIDS. In addition to HIV-positive patients, PJP may also affect other immunocompromised individuals (in the setting of stem cell or solid transplant, chemotherapy for malignancy, hematological malignancy, or chronic corticosteroid therapy).

The classic chest radiographic presentation of PJP consists of bilateral perihilar or diffuse symmetric opacities, which may be finely granular, reticular, or ground glass in appearance. Importantly, the chest radiograph may be normal at the time of presentation in a significant minority of cases of PJP. CT, particularly HRCT, is more sensitive than chest radiographs for detecting PJP and thus may be helpful in evaluating symptomatic patients with normal or equivocal radiographic findings. The classic CT finding in PJP is extensive ground-glass attenuation, which corresponds to the presence of intraalveolar exudate, consisting of fluid, organisms, and debris. It is often distributed in a patchy or geographic fashion, with a predilection for the central, perihilar regions of the lungs. Ground-glass attenuation is occasionally accompanied by thickened septal lines, and foci of consolidation may also be evident in severe cases. In up to a third of cases of PJP, ground-glass opacities are accompanied by cystic lung disease. Such cysts have an upper lobe predominance and demonstrate varying sizes and wall thicknesses.

REFERENCES

Kanne JP, Yandow DR, Meyer CA. Pneumocystis jiroveci pneumonia: high-resolution CT findings in patients with and without HIV infection. *AJR Am J Roentgenol.* 2012 Jun;198(6):W555–W561.

Thoracic Radiology: The Requisites, 3rd ed, 310–322.

CASE 62

Metastatic Osteosarcoma

1. **A, B, C, and D**. There are multiple bilateral calcified mediastinal and hilar lymph nodes. All the listed conditions can cause calcified mediastinal and hilar lymph nodes and would be viable diagnostic considerations although silicosis would be unusual in such a young patient.
2. **D**. Lymphoma frequently calcifies after chemotherapy and radiation therapy. Calcification within lymph nodes affected by lymphoma before therapy is highly unusual.
3. **D**. Of the listed conditions, histoplasmosis is the least likely to cause eggshell calcification.
4. **A**. Garland's triad (also known as the *1-2-3 sign* and described on standard radiography) is defined as lymphadenopathy localized to the right paratracheal and bilateral hilar regions. This symmetric pattern of lymphadenopathy is most often associated with sarcoidosis.

Comment

Axial maximum intensity projection image from chest computed tomography (CT) shows multiple hyperdense mediastinal and hilar lymph nodes as well as scattered hyperdense pulmonary nodules within the lungs consistent with ossified metastatic disease in the setting of osteosarcoma.

Calcified lymph nodes are usually benign, and they are often related to granulomatous processes, such as tuberculosis (TB), histoplasmosis, or sarcoidosis. Neoplastic causes of calcified lymph nodes are less common. They include metastases from mucinous adenocarcinomas and lymphoma. Regarding lymphoma, calcification is frequently seen following radiation therapy, but it is rarely encountered in untreated cases.

Ossified lymph nodes are a rare manifestation of metastatic osteosarcoma. Such nodes appear like calcified lymph nodes. In patients with osteosarcoma, the presence of lymph node metastases indicates a poor prognosis. Lymphatic involvement is usually accompanied by metastases within the lung which is the most common site of metastatic disease. Lung metastases frequently demonstrate ossification.

REFERENCES

Seo JB, Im JG, Goo JM, Chung MJ, Kim MY. Atypical pulmonary metastases: spectrum of radiologic findings. *Radiographics*. 2001 Mar–Apr;21(2):403–417.

Thoracic Radiology: The Requisites, 3rd ed, 428–440.

CASE 63

Septic Infarcts

1. **A, B, and C**. The computed tomography (CT) images show bilateral cavitary nodules with peripheral preponderance and pleural effusions. The differential diagnosis for cavitary nodules includes metastatic disease, septic infarcts, multifocal necrotic pneumonia, and small vessel vasculitis. Cavitary nodules are not a feature of adult respiratory distress syndrome; moreover, pleural effusions are also uncommon in acute respiratory distress syndrome (ARDS) unless there is superimposed heart failure.
2. **B**. In a patient with chronic cavitary nodules, subcutaneous nodular lesions, and joint pain, rheumatoid arthritis is the most likely etiology. Although there are many radiologic manifestations of tuberculosis in the thorax, this constellation of findings is not suggestive of that diagnosis. Granulomatosis with polyangiitis (Wegner granulomatosis) is not

typically associated with joint pain or subcutaneous nodules. Invasive aspergillosis is an acute condition in neutropenic patients.
3. **C**. Indwelling central venous catheters, prosthetic devices, tricuspid endocarditis (often from intravenous drug use), skin infection, and periodontal disease are all common causes of septic infarcts/emboli.
4. **A**. Diffuse ground-glass opacity with mild superimposed nodularity are typical findings in fat embolism. Risk factors for fat embolism include pelvic and long bone fractures, hemoglobinopathies, burns, and pancreatitis. Usually, there is a 1- to 2-day delay in the appearance of abnormalities in the lungs because most of the pulmonary inflammatory response follows the breakdown of fat globules into free fatty acids.

Comment

Axial image from chest CT shows bilateral peripheral predominant cavitary nodules with pleural effusions.

Septic infarcts most often originate from right-sided tricuspid endocarditis or from infected thrombi within systemic veins. Other sources include skin infections, periodontal disease, central venous catheters, and pacemaker wires. On chest radiographs and CT scans of patients with septic infarcts, you may observe poorly defined nodular opacities and areas of wedge-shaped parenchymal opacification. Such opacities are usually peripheral in location and abut the pleural surface. They have a predilection for the lower lobes. Cavitation is frequently observed, particularly on CT scans. A characteristic finding on CT is the identification of feeding vessels leading to the nodules (arrows in the second figure) and wedge-shaped parenchymal opacities. Thus, the CT finding of cavitating nodules with feeding vessels is highly suggestive of septic infarcts.

REFERENCES

Khashper A, Discepola F, Kosiuk J, Qanadli SD, Mesurolle B. Nonthrombotic pulmonary embolism. *AJR Am J Roentgenol*. 2012 Feb;198(2):W152–W159.

Thoracic Radiology: The Requisites, 3rd ed, 289–309.

CASE 64

Bronchopleural Fistula

1. **C**. The original chest radiograph shows near complete opacification of the left hemithorax after left pneumonectomy consistent with fluid filling the left pneumonectomy space. The follow-up chest radiograph shows new gas/fluid levels within the upper left hemithorax, essentially diagnostic of a bronchopleural fistula secondary to a bronchial stump dehiscence.
2. **B**. The shorter bronchial stump after right pneumonectomy as well as the more tenuous blood supply of the right main bronchus relative to the left main bronchus renders bronchopleural fistulas following pneumonectomy more common on the right side.
3. **A**. Right middle lobe torsion after right upper lobectomy is the most common type of lobar torsion. This surgical emergency may result in hemorrhagic infarction or necrosis of the involved lobe due to central kinking of vessels and lymphatics.
4. **D**. The next step in management of a suspected bronchopleural fistula would be bronchoscopy to confirm its presence. In addition, nuclear medicine xenon scans could also be pursued to confirm the diagnosis and pinpoint the location of the fistula.

Comment

Bronchopleural fistula is a relatively uncommon but serious complication following pneumonectomy, with a prevalence of up to 5% and a mortality rate of approximately 20%. Major predisposing factors relate to operative causes of bronchial ischemia, such as a long bronchial stump, ligation of the bronchial arteries too proximally, and disruption of bronchial blood supply from extensive lymph node dissection. Additional risk factors include preoperative radiation therapy, steroid therapy, malnutrition, and resection through infected or cancerous tissue.

Following pneumonectomy, the mediastinum is normally shifted toward the side of resection, and the pneumonectomy space gradually fills with fluid over time. Bronchopleural fistula should be considered when any of the following are observed: (1) the pneumonectomy space fails to fill with fluid; (2) there is an abrupt downward shift in the air-fluid level in the pneumonectomy space identified on an upright radiograph; (3) there is a new collection of air in a previously opacified pneumonectomy space; or (4) there is contralateral shift of the mediastinum associated with any of the above findings. The diagnosis can be confirmed with a xenon ventilation study, which will demonstrate xenon activity in the pneumonectomy space or bronchoscopy.

REFERENCES
Chae EJ, Seo JB, Kim SY, Do KH, Heo JN, Lee JS, Song KS, Song JW, Lim TH. Radiographic and CT findings of thoracic complications after pneumonectomy. *Radiographics.* 2006 Sep–Oct;26(5):1449–1468.
Thoracic Radiology: The Requisites, 3rd ed, 259–278.

CASE 65

Superior Sulcus Tumor

1. **B.** Squamous cell carcinoma is the most common cell type of lung cancer to present in the superior sulcus (apex of the lung) with invasion of mediastinal and chest wall structures.
2. **C.** Stage III B or stage IV lung cancer patients are considered inoperable. In the TNM staging system, chest wall invasion is considered T3 disease. T3 disease is not sufficient to establish stage III B status. Therefore N3 disease (contralateral mediastinal/hilar lymphadenopathy or supraclavicular/anterior scalene lymphadenopathy) would be the only setting in which the patient would be nonoperable.
3. **B.** Invasion of the mediastinum, heart, great vessels, trachea, recurrent laryngeal nerve, esophagus, vertebral body, or carina and separate tumor nodule(s) in another ipsilateral pulmonary lobe is considered T4 disease and nonoperable regardless of other N and M findings.
4. **C.** Standard therapy for superior sulcus tumors include chemotherapy and radiotherapy (CRT) with subsequent surgery 3 to 5 weeks after completion of CRT.

Comment

A lung cancer arising at the extreme apex of the lung is referred to as a superior sulcus tumor or Pancoast tumor. Affected patients typically present with symptoms of shoulder pain in 44% to 96%, Horner's syndrome (ptosis, miosis, anhidrosis) in 14% to 50%, and weakness and atrophy of intrinsic muscles of the hand in 8% to 22%.

Chest radiographs show asymmetric opacity in either apex (Figs. 65.1 and 65.2). Chest computed tomography (CT) better characterizes superior sulcus tumors and can delineate infiltration of the adjacent mediastinal fat and other structures Fig. 65.3. Magnetic resonance imaging (MRI) is more accurate than CT for determining the resectability of a superior sulcus tumor owing to its superior ability to evaluate tumor extension into the vertebral body, neural foramina, spinal cord, and brachial plexus. Positron emission tomography (PET)-CT allows for detection of nodal and distant metastases and is thus helpful for staging. Like other non–small cell lung cancers, superior sulcus tumors are staged using the TNM staging system.

Operable candidates are usually treated with preoperative radiation and chemotherapy followed by surgery.

REFERENCES
Bruzzi JF, Komaki R, Walsh GL, et al. Imaging of non–small cell lung cancer of the superior sulcus. Part 1: anatomy, clinical manifestations, and management. *Radiographics.* 2008;28:551–560.
Thoracic Radiology: The Requisites, 3rd ed, 405–427.

CASE 66

Tuberculosis (Post-Primary Type)

1. **A, B, and C.** The computed tomography (CT) images show a large cavitary lesion in the right lung. TB (post-primary pattern), fungal pneumonia, and primary lung cancer are all possible diagnoses. Pulmonary infarcts are usually smaller, involve a peripheral portion of the lung parenchyma abutting the pleural surface, and seldom cavitate unless infected.
2. **D.** Squamous cell carcinoma is the most frequent lung cancer cell type associated with cavitation.
3. **C.** Tree-in-bud opacities were first described in the setting of TB. They indicate endobronchial spread of disease into the small airways (bronchioles). Typically, the bronchioles are not visualized on chest CT unless there is impaction of material (pus, blood, tumor, etc.) within them.
4. **A.** There is a dual arterial blood supply to the lungs comprised of the pulmonary and bronchial arteries. Localized disruption of pulmonary arterial flow occurs with pulmonary embolism. If there is superimposed congestive heart failure, the bronchial arterial supply is also affected. This combination increases the likelihood of development of focal pulmonary infarct within the territory of the embolism.

Comment

The terms "primary" and "post primary" tuberculosis are inaccurate. DNA fingerprinting has demonstrated that in adults, there is no significant difference in the imaging features between recently acquired tuberculosis and remotely acquired tuberculosis. However, knowledge of the patterns associated with the traditional classification is still important. The primary pattern of tuberculosis manifests as consolidation, often in the mid or lower lung zones, with lymphadenopathy. This pattern is more common in children and in human immunodeficiency virus (HIV) positive patients with low CD4 counts. The post primary pattern of tuberculosis is characterized by upper lung opacities often with associated cavitary or fibrocavitary disease.

Chest computed tomography (CT) axial image demonstrates a cavitary lesion with associated focal areas of tree-in-bud opacities in the right lung. The patient had known tuberculosis. Based on imaging findings, this would be most consistent with a post primary pattern of tuberculosis. Tree-in-bud opacities suggest endobronchial spread of disease. Though originally described in the setting of tuberculosis, and thought to be pathognomonic for this condition, we now know that this imaging pattern is quite common in other inflammatory conditions involving the small airways (bronchioles) including aspiration and non-tuberculous mycobacterial pneumonia. Any condition, which leads to impaction of the bronchioles can produce the tree-in-bud pattern. Rarely, the tree-in-bud pattern is due to small metastatic foci within pulmonary arteries, which mirror the branching pattern of the airways with which they are in proximity.

REFERENCE
Jeong YJ, Lee KS. Pulmonary tuberculosis: up-to-date imaging and management. *AJR Am J Roentgenol.* 2008 Sep;191(3):834–844.

CASE 67

Lymphadenopathy From Lung Cancer

1. **A, B, D, and E.** The subaortic (AP window), low paratracheal, para-aortic, and hilar lymph nodes are all FDG avid consistent with nodal metastases in these stations. FDG PET CT image shows that the right upper lobe nodule, the paratracheal, para-aortic, and prevascular lymph nodes are all FDG-avid, consistent with nodal metastases (Figs. 67.1 and 67.2). FDG PET CT image more inferiorly demonstrates a highly FDG-avid right hilar lymph node (Fig. 67.3). Para-aortic and prevascular lymph nodes are not enlarged. No FDG avid high paratracheal lymph nodes are visualized in the provided images. The distinction between high paratracheal and low paratracheal lymph nodes is the top of the aortic arch.
2. **C.** Contralateral mediastinal lymphadenopathy (N3 disease) makes this patient's disease stage III B which is considered unresectable. Isolated T3 or N2 disease is potentially resectable. Obviously, metastatic disease is a contraindication for surgery (M1) but there is no definite evidence of distant metastases in the provided images.
3. **A.** The right upper lobe is most commonly affected by lung cancer. Interestingly, in the setting of pulmonary fibrosis, lung cancer is most often located within the lower lobes.
4. **D.** Spiculated margins have a high association with lung cancer and would produce a true positive result with PET/CT in most cases. Lesions smaller than 1 cm may be difficult to image reliably using PET imaging unless focal metabolic activity is high. Carcinoid tumors often have low FDG avidity because of their slow growth rate. Lung cancers with ground glass attenuation (typically adenocarcinoma) are associated with low FDG activity.

Comment

Lymph node enlargement is a common cause of a mediastinal or hilar mass and should be suspected whenever a spherical or ovoid mass or masses are identified within a known anatomic lymph node location. There are a variety of infectious, inflammatory, and neoplastic causes of thoracic lymph node enlargement. Neoplastic etiologies include primary lung cancer, metastatic disease, and lymphoma.

Both CT and magnetic resonance imaging (MRI) rely on the anatomic features of lymph nodes, most notably lymph node size (short axis larger than 1 cm), to distinguish between malignant and benign lymph nodes. This strategy is limited by a low sensitivity and specificity. Thus, in patients with primary lung cancer, enlarged nodes must be biopsied for staging purposes. FDG-PET imaging, which relies upon metabolic (glucose metabolism) rather than anatomic features, is the most accurate noninvasive imaging test for assessing mediastinal lymph nodes. False negatives are uncommon and usually related to small lymph node size (microscopic metastases.) However false positives are more frequent because of the FDG avidity seen in inflammatory nodes. The accuracy of FDG-PET can be further enhanced by using an integrated PET-CT scanner, which improves visual quality and quantitative accuracy of PET images, while optimizing

anatomic-metabolic correlation. Recent data indicates that diffusion weighted images (DWI) on MRI offer better specificity than PET-CT.

REFERENCES
Kligerman S, Abbott G. A radiologic review of the new TNM classification for lung cancer. *AJR Am J Roentgenol.* 2010;194:562–573.
Thoracic Radiology: The Requisites, 3rd ed, 405–427.

CASE 68

Subsolid Nodule (Adenocarcinoma)

1. **A, B, C. and D**. The magnified CT image in Fig. 68.1 demonstrates a focal ground-glass nodule within the superior segment of the left lower lobe. All of the listed considerations may manifest in this manner. On sagittal or coronal reformats, scar may be distinguished as having a flat or linear configuration.
2. **B.** A mixed ground-glass and solid pulmonary nodule is most concerning for primary lung cancer (most often adenocarcinoma) (Fig. 68.2). Solid nodules with central cavitation may be malignant but are frequently of infectious origin (e.g., septic emboli, fungal pneumonia) or inflammatory (e.g., granulomatosis with polyangiitis, rheumatoid nodules).
3. **D.** Pure ground-glass nodules measuring 6 mm or smaller require no further dedicated CT follow-up per current Fleischner Society guidelines (see Reference).
4. **B.** Centrilobular ground-glass nodules are commonly found in the setting of hypersensitivity pneumonitis, respiratory bronchiolitis, and pulmonary hemorrhage. Metastatic disease presenting with such a CT pattern would be highly unusual.

Comment

On thin-section CT, a malignant solitary pulmonary nodule (SPN) may be of soft tissue (solid), pure ground-glass attenuation, or a combination of both ground-glass and solid components (i.e., part-solid or mixed attenuation). Of those patterns, the part-solid nodule is the most likely to be malignant (Fig. 68.2),

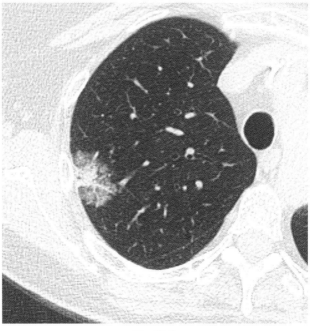

Fig. 68.2

and the soft tissue attenuation nodule is the most likely to be benign.

According to current guidelines, solitary subsolid nodules require no further imaging follow up if they measure less than 6 mm. A ground-glass nodule larger than 6 mm can be reevaluated with CT at 6 to 12 months to confirm persistence. If it persists, annual CT follow-up every 2 years for a minimum of 5 years is then suggested. Part-solid nodules greater than or equal to 6 mm in total dimension are followed by CT at 3 to 6 months to confirm persistence. If unchanged or if the solid component remains <6 mm, annual CT should be performed for 5 years. If the solid component is greater than or equal to 6 mm or increases in size over time, then biopsy or surgical resection is suggested.

Malignant SPNs are also variable in their border characteristics and may manifest as spiculated, ill-defined, or well-defined nodular opacities. Spiculated or irregular margins have a relatively high likelihood of malignancy.

REFERENCES
MacMahon H, Naidich DP, Goo JM, Lee KS, Leung ANC, Mayo JR, Mehta AC, Ohno Y, Powell CA, Prokop M, Rubin GD, Schaefer-Prokop CM, Travis WD, Van Schil PE, Bankier AA. Guidelines for management of incidental pulmonary nodules detected on CT images: from the Fleischner Society 2017. *Radiology*. 2017 Jul;284(1):228–243.
Thoracic Radiology: The Requisites, 3rd ed, 428–440.

CASE 69

Azygos Continuation of the Inferior Vena Cava

1. **A, B, and C.** Postanterior (PA) chest radiograph demonstrates a masslike lesion within the expected location of the azygos vein at the right tracheobronchial angle and lateral displacement of the azygoesophageal interface (arrows). Differential diagnosis includes a very enlarged azygous vein or enlarged lymph nodes. Therefore the differential diagnosis includes lymphoma, azygos continuation of the inferior vena cava, and long-standing superior vena cava obstruction inferior to the level of the azygos vein. Massive azygos vein dilation from partial anomalous pulmonary venous return would be highly unusual.
2. **B.** Azygos continuation of the inferior vena cava. There is massive enlargement of the azygos vein similar in size to the thoracic aorta. No normal intra-abdominal IVC is present. Findings are essentially diagnostic of azygos continuation of the inferior vena cava. Axial and coronal computed tomography (CT) images demonstrate the massively enlarged azygos vein without a normal intra-hepatic IVC. There are multiple spleens (arrows) in the left upper quadrant.
3. **A.** Veins of Sappey. The same phenomenon explains the focal hepatic hot spot sign seen with sulfur colloid nuclear medicine images.
4. **A.** Most patients with polysplenia syndrome have congenital cardiac or vascular abnormalities. Asplenia is associated with more severe and often fatal congenital heart disease, but the prevalence is less than seen in polysplenia syndrome.

Comment

The chest radiograph and CT images demonstrate marked distention of the arch of the azygos vein (Figs. 69.1 and 69.2). The coronal CT image shows dilation of the retrocrural portion of the azygos vein and absence of a definable inferior vena cava. The constellation of findings is diagnostic of azygos continuation of the inferior vena cava, a congenital anomaly that is associated with both the asplenia and the polysplenia syndromes. Note

multiple spleens in the left upper quadrant of the abdomen on the abdominal CT image (Fig. 69.3).

Chest radiographs demonstrate widening of the azygos arch contour and lateral displacement of the azygoesophageal recess below this level. CT can confirm the diagnosis by demonstrating absence of a definable inferior vena cava (Fig. 69.3). CT is also helpful in excluding other causes of azygos vein distention such as obstruction of the vena cava.

Knowledge of this developmental anomaly is important preoperatively for planning cardiopulmonary bypass surgery and may also help to avoid difficulties at cardiac catheterization.

REFERENCES
Kandpal H, Sharma R, Gamangatti S, et al. Imaging the inferior vena cava: a road less traveled. *Radiographics*. 2008;28:669–689.
Thoracic Radiology: The Requisites, 3rd ed, 97–136.

CASE 70

Right Upper Lobe Atelectasis (Lung Cancer)

1. **C.** Posteroanterior (PA) and lateral chest radiographs demonstrate right upper lobe collapse. A mass is present within the central aspect of the right upper lobe which is most likely a primary lung cancer.
2. **D.** Imaging findings are typical of the S sign of Golden in which a central obstructing lesion in the right lung causes a moderate degree of right upper lobe collapse. The peripheral concave interface represents superiorly displaced minor fissure while the central/medial convex interface represents the inferolateral margins of the central mass.
3. **B.** In a young patient, a central calcified nodule with associated postobstructive atelectasis is likely to represent a carcinoid tumor. The other diagnostic considerations are possible but less likely.
4. **B.** T2. Updated criteria for a T2 tumor include the following: greater than 3 cm but less than or equal to 5 cm in size, main bronchus involvement regardless of distance to the carina, invasion of the visceral pleura, and/or any degree of postobstructive atelectasis or pneumonitis of the ipsilateral lobe or lung.

Comment

The most common cause of complete lobar atelectasis is obstruction of a central bronchus. In an adult patient in the outpatient setting, lung cancer is the most likely diagnosis. In intubated patients, mucus plugging is the most common cause of lobar collapse.

The tumor-node-metastases (TNM) system for staging lung cancer was revised in 2017. According to this classification system, a centrally obstructing neoplasm with associated postobstructive atelectasis or obstructive pneumonitis is classified as T2, even if the entire lung is collapsed. The 2017 update made this change to include complete lung atelectasis as a T2 tumor rather than T3 (as in the 2009 revision) based on analysis of a new lung cancer database that demonstrated better survival among patients with complete lung atelectasis than those with other T3 descriptors.

Squamous cell carcinomas typically occur in main, segmental, or subsegmental bronchi and grow endobronchially. In contrast, small cell carcinoma is characterized by a submucosal, peribronchial growth pattern and a discrete endobronchial tumor is seldom identified. Small cell carcinoma typically occurs as a large central mass that may narrow the bronchial lumen by extrinsic compression and is often associated with extensive mediastinal adenopathy. Lung adenocarcinomas are typically peripheral.

REFERENCES
Carter BW, Lichtenberger 3rd JP, Benveniste MK, de Groot PM, Wu CC, Erasmus JJ, Truong MT. Revisions to the TNM staging of

lung cancer: rationale, significance, and clinical application. *Radiographics*. 2018 Mar–Apr;38(2):374–391.
Thoracic Radiology: The Requisites, 3rd ed, 19–60, 450–459.

CASE 71
Traumatic Rupture of the Left Hemidiaphragm

1. **B**. Axial CT image demonstrates colonic bowel adjacent to a left posterior rib (Fig. 71.1). Coronal image demonstrates a focal defect within the left hemidiaphragm (Fig. 71.2, arrows) with extrusion of intra-abdominal contents into the thorax consistent with left hemidiaphragmatic rupture. Findings are diagnostic of left hemidiaphragmatic rupture
2. **D**. In normal patients, the curved nature of the diaphragm prevents the stomach and bowel from abutting the left posterior ribs. The dependent viscera sign (when the stomach or bowel abuts the left posterior ribs or is posterior to the spleen, or on the right side when the liver abuts the right posterior ribs) is a specific sign for diaphragmatic rupture.
3. **D**. The most common location for hemidiaphragmatic rupture is the posterolateral aspect of the left hemidiaphragm. Diaphragmatic rupture is more commonly identified on the left than the right, possibly due to the protective effect of the liver. There is, however, some evidence that some right-sided diaphragmatic injuries may be missed because the liver may prevent extrusion of intra-abdominal contents through a small right hemidiaphragmatic defect.
4. **C**. The presented clinical scenario is suggested of right hemidiaphragmatic dysfunction likely due to iatrogenic right phrenic nerve injury. Functional assessment of the diaphragm is currently performed using fluoroscopy. Functional imaging of the diaphragm could also be the theoretically achieved with MRI or ultrasound although these modalities are not widely used.

Comment

Diaphragmatic rupture is an uncommon but serious complication of blunt and penetrating trauma. The left hemidiaphragm is affected more often than the right side. The left-sided predominance is thought to be secondary to two factors: a protective effect from the liver on the right side and relative weakness of the left hemidiaphragm compared with the right.

Because of the morbidity and mortality from associated gastric and bowel obstruction and strangulation, a prompt diagnosis of diaphragm rupture is important. Unfortunately, however, the diagnosis is often delayed. One should suspect this diagnosis when there is apparent elevation of a hemidiaphragm, changing hemidiaphragm levels on serial radiographs, or an unusual contour of the hemidiaphragm. A more specific finding is the identification of stomach or bowel in the thorax. CT or MRI can confirm the diagnosis. Although the direct multiplanar imaging capability of MRI offered a major advantage, CT now provides high-quality multiplanar reformations that can now be obtained with thin-section multidetector CT (MDCT) scanners. Such CT images have improved sensitivity and specificity in the diagnosis diaphragmatic rupture. CT is the preferred imaging test for suspected diaphragm injury in the acute trauma setting.

REFERENCES
Kaewlai R, Avery LL, Asrani AV, Novelline RA. Multidetector CT of blunt thoracic trauma. *Radiographics*. 2008;28:1555–1570.
Nason LK, Walker CM, McNeeley MF, Burivong W, Fligner CL, Godwin JD. Imaging of the diaphragm: anatomy and function. *Radiographics*. 2012 Mar–Apr;32(2):E51–E70.
Thoracic Radiology: The Requisites, 3rd ed, 159–192.

CASE 72
Persistent Left Superior Vena Cava

1. **A and C**. On axial contrast enhanced chest computed tomography (CT), there is a vascular structure just anterior to the aortic arch. Normally, no large vascular structure is present in this region. The differential diagnosis for this finding includes left superior vena cava and partial anomalous pulmonary venous return, typically of the left upper lobe. Axial image from chest CT shows the left SVC draining into the dilated coronary sinus (arrow).
2. **C**. Up to 90% of left superior vena cavas drain into the coronary sinus, which then drains into the right atrium. Rarely, the left superior vena cava drains into the left atrium directly or by way of an unroofed coronary sinus or left superior pulmonary vein. This creates a right to left shunt.
3. **C**. In a partial anomalous pulmonary venous return involving the right superior pulmonary vein, the anomalous vein most commonly drains into the superior vena cava just above the junction of the superior vena cava and right atrium. There is almost always an associated sinus venosus atrial septal defect high within the atrial septum.
4. **C**. An unroofed coronary sinus represents a direct connection between the coronary sinus and left atrium. Functionally, this creates a connection between the right atrium and left atrium through the coronary sinus and is considered a type of atrial septal defect.

Comment

Left-sided superior vena cavas are quite common and are incidentally discovered in up to 0.5% of the general population. There is a higher prevalence of left-sided superior vena cava in the setting of congenital heart disease (approximately 5%). The left superior vena cava is usually associated with a smaller right superior vena cava. The left superior vena cava most commonly drains into the coronary sinus, and the coronary sinus is often dilated due to increased flow as illustrated in this case.

Most often, the left superior vena cava is invisible or subtle on radiography. There may be focal widening of the left superior aspect of the mediastinum adjacent to the aortic arch. Left-sided central venous catheter placement either via the subclavian or jugular approach will demonstrate the left-sided superior vena cava. The catheter will not across midline into the left innominate vein, but rather extend along the left lateral aspect of the mediastinum adjacent to the aortic arch. On cross-sectional imaging, an anomalous vessel is present along the anterior margin of the aortic arch which connects superiorly to the left-sided jugular and subclavian venous systems.

This anatomic course distinguishes PAPVR from a left sided SVC. The anomalous pulmonary vein arises usually within the left upper lobe and drains superiorly into the left brachiocephalic vein. The left brachiocephalic (innominate) vein is typically absent or atretic in the setting of a left superior vena cava.

REFERENCES
Demos TC, Posniak HV, Pierce KL, Olson MC, Muscato M. Venous anomalies of the thorax. *AJR Am J Roentgenol*. 2004 May;182(5):1139–1150.
Thoracic Radiology: The Requisites, 3rd ed, 19–60.

CASE 73
Aspiration

1. **A, B, C, and D**. All of the listed conditions could cause bronchial wall thickening and tree-in-bud opacities as is present in this case.

2. **C.** Lymphocytic interstitial pneumonitis in adults is almost always related to Sjogren syndrome or an underlying immunodeficiency; there is no association with aspiration. In contrast, chronic aspiration has been associated and may exacerbate usual interstitial pneumonitis. Aspiration may also be the underlying cause of non-cryptogenic organizing pneumonia and diffuse alveolar damage.

3. **A.** Aspiration commonly affects the most dependent portions of the lungs. When a patient is supine, the posterior segments of the upper lobes, superior segments of the lower lobes, and posterior basal segments of the lower lobes are most often affected. When the patient is upright, the basal segments of the lower lobes are most at risk.

4. **A.** Pneumonia and atelectasis are the most common sequelae of foreign body aspiration in adults. In small children air trapping may occur distal to the obstructed bronchus. In the setting of chronic retention of a bronchial foreign body, post obstructive bronchiectasis secondary to chronic post obstructive pneumonia may develop. Pneumothorax related to foreign body aspiration is rare.

Comment

Aspiration is defined as inhalation of solid or liquid materials into the lungs and airways. Even in normal individuals, a small amount of aspiration of nasopharyngeal contents is common. Normal clearance mechanisms and immune defenses prevent development of any significant infection or lung inflammation. There are two main patterns of aspiration, which are commonly encountered in the hospital setting: aspiration pneumonitis and aspiration pneumonia. The latter is the result of superimposed infection. Aspiration of inert fluid or particulate material as well as large foreign bodies may also occur. Predisposing factors for aspiration include alcoholism, decreased level of consciousness, pharyngeal and/or esophageal abnormalities and neuromuscular weakness. Axial chest computed tomography (CT) image demonstrates bilateral lower lobe tree-in-bud nodular opacities, bronchial wall thickening, and endoluminal debris, consistent with aspiration.

Aspiration pneumonitis caused by inhalation of acid gastric contents is associated with diffuse lung injury from chemical pneumonitis. This is known as *Mendelson syndrome*. The severity of lung injury is related to the amount of aspiration and the acidity of aspirated contents. Aspiration pneumonia develops from inhalation of material containing oropharyngeal bacteria (in those with poor oral hygiene) and/or gastric bacteria (especially in the setting of increase in gastric pH) or superinfection of aspiration pneumonitis. Differentiation of aspiration pneumonitis from aspiration pneumonia based on imaging findings may be difficult. The development of focal abscesses and/or parapneumonic effusion would support a diagnosis of infection rather than simple pneumonitis.

REFERENCES
Prather AD, Smith TR, Poletto DM, Tavora F, Chung JH, Nallamshetty L, Hazelton TR, Rojas CA. Aspiration-related lung diseases. *J Thorac Imaging.* 2014 Sep;29(5):304–309.
Thoracic Radiology: The Requisites, 3rd ed, 137–158

CASE 74

Nonspecific Interstitial Pneumonitis (NSIP)

1. **B.** There is basilar predominant pulmonary fibrosis with relative subpleural sparing characterized by ground-glass opacity, reticulation, and traction bronchiectasis essentially diagnostic of NSIP. The subpleural sparing essentially excludes a diagnosis of UIP. AIP is typically not this uniform and symmetric; moreover, this degree of traction bronchiectasis would be unusual. LIP, in the chronic setting, most often presents as a cystic lung disease.

2. **D.** There are 7 findings on computed tomography (CT), which would make a CT fibrotic pulmonary pattern suggestive of a nonidiopathic pulmonary fibrosis pattern:
   a. Upper or mid-lung predominance
   b. Peribronchovascular predominance
   c. Extensive ground-glass abnormality (extent>reticular abnormality)—the answer in this case
   d. Consolidation in bronchopulmonary segment(s)/lobe(s)
   e. Profuse micronodules (bilateral, predominantly upper lobes)
   f. Discrete cysts (multiple, bilateral, away from areas of honeycombing)
   g. Diffuse mosaic attenuation/air-trapping (bilateral, in three or more lobes)

3. **C.** UIP is most commonly basilar and peripheral in distribution. It is characterized by reticular opacities which extend to the pleural surface. Subpleural sparing would be highly unusual in UIP and much more supportive of a NSIP diagnosis. However, a substantial minority of UIP (up to 25%) may not be basilar predominant in zonal distribution.

4. **D.** NSIP is often seen in collagen vascular disease, as a drug reaction or it may be the histologic pattern identified by the pathologist in some patients with hypersensitivity pneumonitis. Idiopathic NSIP is much less common.

Comment

Nonspecific interstitial pneumonitis (NSIP) is classified as one of the idiopathic interstitial pneumonias. Pathologically, it is characterized by temporally and spatially homogeneous interstitial inflammation with or without fibrosis. Traditionally, NSIP has been categorized as either cellular, fibrotic, or mixed cellular and fibrotic. On CT, NSIP is typically basilar predominant but has a variable pattern in the axial plane (peripheral, diffuse, or central). Ground-glass opacity is almost always present with variable degrees of superimposed reticulation and traction bronchiectasis as well as bronchiolectasis. Often the degree of traction bronchiectasis appears to be out of proportion to the degree of concomitant lung disease. A significant degree of subpleural honeycombing is unusual. However, a small minority of cases of NSIP eventually progress to UIP. Therefore a combined NSIP and UIP CT pattern may occasionally be observed. In contrast to UIP, which is most often idiopathic, NSIP is almost always secondary to an underlying condition--most commonly collagen vascular disease, medication/drugs, or hypersensitivity pneumonitis (HP). The esophagus is dilated in this case, consistent with esophageal dysmotility in this patient with underlying history of collagen vascular disease.

The main imaging differential diagnosis for NSIP include UIP and HP. Differentiation of NSIP from UIP and HP may be difficult if not impossible in some cases. The most helpful differentiating findings of NSIP from UIP are substantial ground glass abnormality and subpleural sparing. A substantial degree of ground-glass opacity in UIP without a superimposed condition would be unusual. In addition, subpleural sparing in UIP. UIP classically originates in the subpleural lung and progresses more centrally. In many cases of fibrotic HP, the distribution of lung disease is upper lung predominant, which would be unusual in UIP and rare in NSIP. Also, there is very often substantial air trapping in HP, which would be unusual in isolated UIP or NSIP. In patients with NSIP features of collagen vascular disease may be evident on imaging including esophageal dilation (esophageal dysmotility), pulmonary arterial dilation (pulmonary hypertension), and pleural or pericardial effusion/thickening.

REFERENCES

Koelsch TL, Chung JH, Lynch DA. Radiologic evaluation of idiopathic interstitial pneumonias. *Clin Chest Med.* 2015 Jun;36(2): 269–282.

Thoracic Radiology: The Requisites, 3rd ed, 355–376.

CASE 75

Ascending Aortic Aneurysm

1. **A, B, C, and D**. All of the listed conditions are potential causes for the development of ascending aortic aneurysms.
2. **D**. Typically, thoracic aortic aneurysms are considered for repair when they are larger than 5 to 6 cm or are growing at a rapid rate.
3. **D**. Bicuspid aortic valves are associated with ascending aortic aneurysms, intracranial arterial aneurysms, Turner syndrome, and aortic coarctation. Partial anomalous pulmonary venous return is not commonly associated with bicuspid aortic valves.
4. **B**. The description of the imaging findings is consistent with annuloaortic ectasia, which is most often associated with Marfan syndrome or Ehlers-Danlos syndrome.

Comment

An aneurysm is defined as an abnormal dilation of a vessel. Regarding the ascending aorta, there is some variability in diameter with increasing age, but a diameter of greater than 4 cm is generally considered abnormal. Axial image from contrast enhanced chest computed tomography (CT) shows a very large ascending aortic aneurysm measuring 5.7 cm. A small right pleural effusion is noted.

Aneurysms may be classified based on the integrity of aorta wall (true vs. false), location, and shape. Regarding shape, fusiform aneurysms are characterized by cylindrical dilation of the entire circumference of the aorta, and saccular aneurysms are characterized by a focal outpouching of the aorta. Fusiform aneurysms are most associated with atherosclerosis, whereas saccular aneurysms are most often traumatic or infectious in etiology.

Thoracic aortic aneurysms are less common than abdominal aortic aneurysms. Up to one fourth of thoracic aortic aneurysms coexist with an abdominal aortic aneurysm Although aneurysmal dilation of the ascending aorta is frequently caused by atherosclerosis, this process usually involves other portions of the aorta as well. Annuloaortic ectasia refers to the presence of dilated sinuses of Valsalva with effacement of the sinotubular junction, resulting in a pear-shaped ascending aorta that tapers to a normal- caliber aortic arch. This disorder may be idiopathic or associated with connective tissue disorders such as Ehlers-Danlos and Marfan's syndromes. Syphilis, once a relatively common cause of ascending aortic aneurysms, is now rare. Ascending aortic aneurysms may also occur in the setting of bicuspid aortic valves, irrespective of any functional valvular flow abnormality (stenosis or regurgitation) suggesting an inherent weakness of the aortic wall in these patients.

The major complication of aneurysms is rupture. The risk for rupture is related to the size of the aneurysm. For this reason, elective surgical repair is generally recommended when aneurysms exceed 5 to 6 cm in diameter.

REFERENCES

Agarwal PP, Chughtal A, Matzinger F, Karerooni EA. Multidetector CT of thoracic aortic aneurysms. *Radiographics.* 2009;29:537–552.

Thoracic Radiology: The Requisites, 3rd ed, 97–136.

CASE 76

Carcinoid Tumor

1. **D**. Computed tomography (CT) images demonstrate a focal endobronchial tumor in the proximal right lower lobe bronchus with a focus of coarse peripheral calcification. In a young patient, carcinoid tumor is the most likely diagnosis.
2. **B**. The most common benign pulmonary tumor is a hamartoma. The other choices are less common benign tumors of the lung.
3. **C**. Approximately 30% of carcinoid tumors demonstrate calcification.
4. **D**. DIPNECH occurs almost exclusively in middle-aged or elderly women. On CT, the combination of small, well-defined pulmonary nodules (representing carcinoid tumors and tumorlets) in the mid and lower lung zones and substantial air trapping is suggestive of the diagnosis, especially in a patient with refractory asthma-like symptoms.

Comment

Bronchial carcinoid tumors are uncommon neuroendocrine neoplasms that occur centrally (80%) more commonly than peripherally (20%). Affected patients are usually in the third to seventh decade of life and typically present with cough, hemoptysis, and postobstructive pneumonia.

On chest radiographs, carcinoids typically appear as a central, hilar, or perihilar mass that may be associated with postobstructive atelectasis, pneumonia, mucoid impaction, or bronchiectasis. On CT, carcinoids typically demonstrate well-defined margins and slightly lobulated borders. Carcinoids are usually located close to the central bronchi, usually near airway bifurcations. Calcification is observed in approximately 30% of cases on CT but is not usually evident on conventional radiographs. Most lesions demonstrate intense contrast enhancement.

A minority of carcinoids present as a solitary pulmonary nodule (SPN) in the periphery of the lung. Typical carcinoid tumors in the periphery of the lungs usually grow at a slow rate. Atypical carcinoids, which account for 10% of all carcinoids, occur most often in the lung periphery. These lesions are usually large at the time of presentation and grow at a faster rate than typical carcinoids. Although typical carcinoids rarely metastasize, atypical carcinoids exhibit metastases in up to half of patients.

Therapy of carcinoid tumors consists of surgical resection, with a more aggressive surgical approach for atypical lesions. Adjuvant chemotherapy has also been employed with some success in patients with advanced atypical carcinoid tumors. Typical carcinoids have an excellent prognosis, with a 5-year survival of approximately 90%. In contrast, atypical carcinoids are associated with a 5-year survival of approximately 70%.

Because carcinoid tumors have a high number of somatostatin receptors, scintigraphic imaging with the radiolabeled somatostatin analogue octreotide may be helpful for detecting occult tumors. Conversely, fluorodeoxyglucose–positron emission tomography (FDG-PET) imaging is less useful in this setting because of a high rate of false-negative results for typical carcinoid tumors.

REFERENCES

Benson RE, Rosado-de-Christenson ML, Martínez-Jiménez S, Kunin JR, Pettavel PP. Spectrum of pulmonary neuroendocrine proliferations and neoplasms. *Radiographics.* 2013 Oct;33(6):1631–1649.

Little BP, Junn JC, Zheng KS, Sanchez FW, Henry TS, Veeraraghavan S, Berkowitz EA. Diffuse idiopathic pulmonary neuroendocrine cell hyperplasia: imaging and clinical features of a frequently delayed diagnosis. *AJR Am J Roentgenol.* 2020 Dec;215(6):1312–1320.

Thoracic Radiology: The Requisites, 3rd ed, 391–404

CASE 77

Boerhaave Syndrome

1. A, B, and C. The chest radiograph (Fig. 77.1) demonstrates a large amount of ectopic gas centered within the inferior aspect of the mediastinum. Small pleural effusions with bibasilar atelectasis are also present. Axial contrast enhanced chest computed tomography (CT) image (Fig. 77.2) demonstrates a large amount of pneumomediastinum around the distal esophagus and aorta as well as small pleural effusions in this patient with Boerhaave syndrome. The differential diagnosis for pneumomediastinum includes forceful exhalation against a closed glottis, asthma, esophageal or large airway injury, and extension of retroperitoneal or retropharyngeal gas. Extension of air from a pneumothorax into the mediastinum is not common. The most likely diagnosis given the concentration of gas around the dilated esophagus is esophageal rupture in this patient with history of vomiting, the Boerhaave syndrome.

2. B. Pneumomediastinum in the setting of asthma is thought to be due to the Macklin effect. In the setting of small airway obstruction, alveolar rupture allows gas to track along the pulmonary interstitium centrally into the hila and eventually the mediastinum.

3. D. Esophageal rupture in the setting of Boerhaave syndrome typically occurs in the left lower aspect of the esophagus.

4. C. Mediastinitis is the most serious complication of esophageal rupture with high mortality reported. Treatment ranges from medical management to endoscopic therapy and/or surgery depending on the severity of the rupture and whether it is contained. However, in all cases, nothing should be allowed by mouth and the patient should be placed on broad-spectrum intravenous antibiotics, proton pump inhibitor, and any localized fluid collections drained. Empyema particularly in the left pleural space is not uncommon.

Comment

Esophageal perforation is a common cause of acute mediastinitis and may occur secondary to a variety of mechanisms. Boerhaave syndrome refers to transmural perforation of the distal esophagus that results from repeated episodes of vomiting. Rupture typically occurs posteriorly, near the left diaphragmatic crus. Patients with esophageal perforation typically present with symptoms of fever, leukocytosis, dysphagia, and retrosternal chest pain, which often radiates into the neck. Pneumomediastinum is a frequent chest radiographic finding as in this case. It can be subtle, and air may be difficult to appreciate on the standard chest radiograph. Air or gas in the soft tissues of the neck can be a helpful sign. Additional chest radiographic findings may include diffuse mediastinal widening, pneumothorax, pleural effusion, and empyema. When the diagnosis of esophageal perforation is delayed, additional complications may include mediastinal abscess, esophagopleural fistula, and esophagobronchial fistula.

A diagnosis of suspected esophageal perforation can be made following the administration of water-soluble contrast medium. Such a study demonstrates extravasation of contrast at the site of perforation, but false negatives occur in up to 10% of cases. CT may be helpful in cases for which fluoroscopy is nondiagnostic. It may also be helpful to delineate the location and extent of fluid collections in cases that have progressed to mediastinal abscess formation and empyema. It is important to be aware A delay of greater than 24 hours in the diagnosis of this complication is associated with high morbidity and mortality rates. Thus, prompt diagnosis and treatment are critical.

REFERENCES

Young CA, Menias CO, Bhalla S, Prasad SR. CT features of esophageal emergencies. *Radiographics*. 2008 Oct;28(6):1541–1553.

Katabathina VS, Restrepo CS, Martinez-Jimenez S, Riascos RF. Nonvascular, nontraumatic mediastinal emergencies in adults: a comprehensive review of imaging findings. *Radiographics*. 2011 Jul–Aug;31(4):1141–1160.

Norton-Gregory AA, Kulkarni NM, O'Connor SD, Budovec JJ, Zorn AP, Desouches SL. CT esophagography for evaluation of esophageal perforation. *Radiographics*. 2021 Mar–Apr;41(2):447–461.

Thoracic Radiology: The Requisites, 3rd ed, 97–136, 226–237.

CASE 78

Bronchiectasis

1. A, B, and C. The axial CT image demonstrates findings consistent with bronchiectasis. The differential diagnosis would include nontuberculous mycobacterial pneumonia, allergic bronchopulmonary aspergillosis, and cystic fibrosis. There is no evidence of pulmonary fibrosis to suggest usual interstitial pneumonitis. Traction bronchiectasis is a feature of pulmonary fibrosis but other findings of fibrosis such as reticulation, architectural distortion, and/or honeycombing are absent.

2. D. In the setting of severe bronchiectasis, differentiation of bronchiectasis from cystic lung disease may be difficult. A helpful CT postprocessing technique is minimum intensity projection. With the use of thick minimum intensity projection slices, the continuity of cystic air spaces with more normal appearing central bronchi is readily apparent in cases of bronchiectasis.

3. A. Cylindrical, varicoid, and cystic (saccular) bronchiectasis are all subtypes of bronchiectasis Spherical bronchiectasis is not a subtype.

4. B. Up to 5% of adults with cystic fibrosis will develop hepatic cirrhosis. With the increase in life span of patients with cystic fibrosis, morbidity and mortality from chronic liver disease is likely to increase.

Comment

The term *bronchiectasis* refers to abnormal, irreversible dilation of the bronchi. The definitive pathologic description of bronchiectasis was reported by Reid and is based on the morphology of the bronchi and the number of bronchial subdivisions that are present. In cylindrical bronchiectasis, the bronchi are minimally dilated and have a straight, regular contour (Fig. 78.2). The average number of bronchial subdivisions from the hilum to the lung periphery is 16 (17 to 20 is normal). In varicoid bronchiectasis, the bronchi demonstrate a beaded appearance with sequential dilatation and constriction (Fig. 78.3). The average number of bronchial divisions is 8. In cystic bronchiectasis, the bronchi have a ballooned appearance (Fig. 78.4). The average number of bronchial divisions is only 4.

Bronchiectasis can be distinguished from cystic lung disease by applying the following imaging criteria:

1. When dilated bronchi course perpendicular to the scanning plane, a pulmonary artery or arteriole will always course adjacent to it (signet ring sign). In contrast, true lung cysts, such as those associated with LAM, are located randomly in the lung parenchyma.

2. Dilated bronchi course parallel to the scanning plane, you will observe that the cystic spaces connect with one another.

3. Cystic bronchiectasis is often associated with air-fluid levels, a finding that is not generally observed in cystic lung disease.

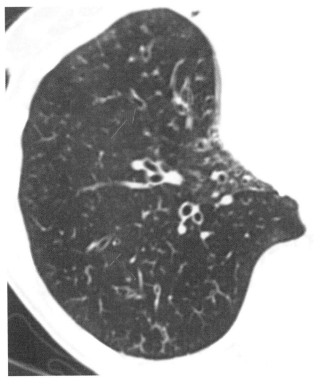

Fig. 78.2

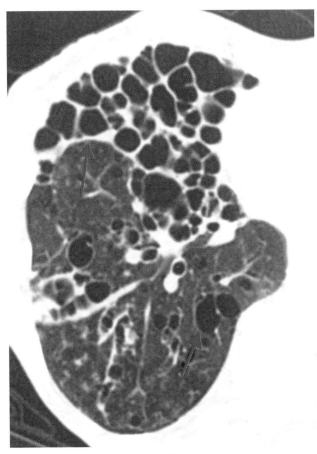

Fig. 78.4

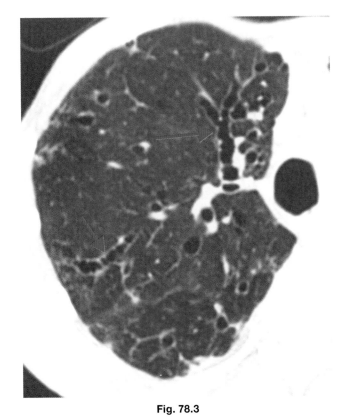

Fig. 78.3

REFERENCES

Milliron B, Henry TS, Veeraraghavan S, Little BP. Bronchiectasis: Mechanisms and imaging clues of associated common and uncommon diseases. *Radiographics.* 2015 Jul–Aug;35(4):1011–1030.

Thoracic Radiology: The Requisites, 3rd ed, 137–158.

CASE 79

Giant Bulla

1. A and B. The imaging findings are highly suggestive of very large bulla. Although, a right-sided pneumothorax could mimic this appearance. However, the absence of a distinct visceral pleural line as well as gradual attenuation of lung vessels at the junction of the superior aspect of the right lung and mid aspect of the right lung are much more suggestive of a bulla rather than a pneumothorax. A portion of the inferior wall of the bulla can be identified inferiorly and medially.

2. B. A bulla is defined as a gas containing space in the lung ≥ 1 cm with a thin well-defined wall. Both bullae and blebs represent subpleural cystic air spaces, which are usually well-defined.

3. D. Of the listed modalities, chest CT is the most sensitive tool to detect early emphysema.

4. D. Although basilar predominant panlobular emphysema is almost always associated with alpha-1 antitrypsin deficiency, in a minority of patients, previous IV Ritalin use is the underlying cause of this pattern.

Comment

The chest radiograph in this case demonstrates a large area of absent pulmonary vessels in the right lung with sparing of the right base It displaces the remainder of the lung inferiorly and appears to have a well-defined wall inferiorly and medially. A large pneumothorax is a consideration. However, the absence of a visceral pleural line and gradual transition from the normal lung parenchyma to an area of absent pulmonary vessels demarcated by a wall indicates the presence of a large bulla rather than a pneumothorax.

Bullae may develop in association with any type of emphysema, but they are most commonly associated with paraseptal and centrilobular emphysema. However, they are not always associated with diffuse emphysema. Bullae usually enlarge over months to years, but the growth rate is quite variable. Occasionally, bullae can become quite large and may be focal in distribution. Large bullae may compromise respiratory function. The resulting syndrome has been referred to by various terms, including bullous emphysema, vanishing lung syndrome, and primary bullous disease of the lung. This entity occurs most often in young men and is characterized by large, progressive upper lobe bullous disease. Although it may occur in nonsmokers, most affected patients are smokers.

Computed tomography (CT) is the preferred modality for the assessment of patients with suspected bullous emphysema. CT is helpful for delineating the number, size, and location of bullae. It can also assess the degree of compression of underlying normal lung and determine the presence and severity of emphysema in the remaining portion of the lung parenchyma.

In symptomatic patients, surgical resection of bullae can result in marked improvement in pulmonary function. The greatest benefit from surgery is observed in patients with a large bulla (occupying 50% or more of a hemithorax) and a moderate reduction in forced expiratory volume in 1 second (FEV1). In contrast, patients with severe generalized emphysema tend to do poorly and are thus not ideal candidates for bullectomy.

REFERENCES
Lynch DA, Austin JH, Hogg JC, Grenier PA, Kauczor HU, Bankier AA, Barr RG, Colby TV, Galvin JR, Gevenois PA, Coxson HO, Hoffman EA, Newell Jr JD, Pistolesi M, Silverman EK, Crapo JD. CT-definable subtypes of chronic obstructive pulmonary disease: a statement of the Fleischner Society. *Radiology*. 2015 Oct;277(1):192–205.
Thoracic Radiology: The Requisites, 3rd ed, 19–60, 391–404.

CASE 80

RML and RLL atelectasis

1. **D.** The posteroanterior (PA) radiograph demonstrates a focal opacity in the central and inferior aspect of the right lung with obscuration of the right hemidiaphragm and right heart border. The upper border is sharply defined, and that border extends medial to the interlobar artery in the right hilum. The upper border is produced by the depressed minor fissure laterally and the major fissure medially (arrow) (the minor fissure can never extend medial to the lateral border of the interlobar artery so the lower lobe must be collapsed.) There is mild right lung volume loss suggested by rightward shift in the mediastinum and trachea. These findings are typical of combined right middle and right lower lobe collapse.
2. **C.** Obstruction of the bronchus intermedius would cause combined right middle and right lower lobe atelectasis. The bronchus intermedius arises from the right mainstem bronchus distal to the takeoff of the right upper lobe bronchus.
3. **D.** Although all listed answer choices could cause complete right lung atelectasis, in a recently intubated patient, mucous plugging is most likely. If the endotracheal tube is advanced too far, it most often extends into the right mainstem bronchus rather than the left mainstem bronchus due to the right mainstem bronchus's more obtuse angulation

relative to the trachea; this would result in left lung atelectasis rather than right lung atelectasis. In the outpatient setting, complete left lung atelectasis is very secondary to a central lung carcinoma.
4. **D.** Hepatocellular carcinoma does not commonly metastasize to the central airways. Common distant primary malignancies which metastasize to the trachea and central bronchi include melanoma, renal cell carcinoma, breast cancer, and colon cancer.

Comment

The radiographic appearance is typical of combined right middle and lower lobe collapse (Fig. 80.1). There is a well-defined opacity in the central aspect of the right lung with associated silhouetting of the right hemidiaphragm and right heart border with right lung volume loss. The sharp upper border is produced by the minor and major fissures which are both depressed.

Combined right middle and lower lobe collapse can occur when a tumor obstructs the bronchus intermedius. This combination occurs more frequently than combined right upper and right middle lobe collapse because the bronchi to these lobes are remote from one another. When the latter combination occurs, the appearance is identical to left upper lobe collapse.

In this patient, the combined lobar collapse occurred secondary to endobronchial metastatic disease. Also note the presence of pulmonary metastases, best visualized in the left lung. Endobronchial metastases are uncommon and are found in less than 5% of patients at autopsy. Presenting symptoms may include cough, wheeze, and hemoptysis. Coughing may infrequently result in expectoration of tumor fragments; rarely, this is the first indication of metastatic disease.

Radiographic findings in the setting of partial airway obstruction include oligemia and air trapping. In the setting of complete bronchial obstruction, findings include lobar, segmental, or subsegmental atelectasis and postobstructive pneumonitis. A hilar or central mass may also be evident.

REFERENCES
Seo JB, Im JG, Goo JM, et al. Atypical pulmonary metastases: spectrum of radiologic findings. *Radiographics*. 2001;21:403–417.
Thoracic Radiology: The Requisites, 3rd ed, 19–60.

CASE 81

Lipoma

1. **A and C.** Axial image from a non-contrast chest CT demonstrates a large fatty mass in the left axilla. Coronal noncontrast T1-weighted MRI demonstrates diffuse hyperintense signal throughout the mass which extends superiorly into the neck characteristic of a lipoma. The imaging findings are essentially diagnostic of a lipoma. There is a small amount of wispy soft tissue within this lesion; therefore, liposarcoma could be considered in the differential diagnosis but is much less likely.
2. **D.** On T1 weighted MRI, non-proteinaceous or hemorrhagic fluid is usually T1 hypointense. The other listed materials (fat, melanin, methemoglobin) are all T1 hyperintense.
3. **C.** The greater degree of soft tissue within a fatty mass, the greater the likelihood of liposarcoma.
4. **C.** Lipomatous hypertrophy of the interatrial septum represents a benign fatty infiltration of the atrial septum. This lesion is typically dumbbell shaped that classically spares the fossa ovalis. Though this lesion is usually asymptomatic, it may be a cause of symptomatic arrhythmias and vascular obstruction. In 80% of patients, there is increased FDG uptake on PET-CT, likely because of metabolically active brown fat.

Comment

The CT and MRI images demonstrates a fatty mass in the left axilla that contains a minimal amount of soft tissue attenuation material. T1 hyperintensity is typical of fatty lesions. The mass extends into the lower aspect of the left neck.

Lipomas may occur in a variety of locations in the thorax, including the mediastinum, chest wall, extrapleural space, esophagus, heart, airway, and rarely, the lung parenchyma. Although lipomas typically appear as well-marginated lesions characterized by homogeneous fat attenuation, soft tissue elements may be observed. In such cases, it may not be possible to distinguish lipoma from thymolipoma or low-grade liposarcoma. The pliability and lack of invasiveness of lipomas may aid in their differentiation from liposarcomas; for example, lipomas typically drape around adjacent vessels, ribs, and mediastinal structures without invading them. Liposarcomas typically contain a larger soft tissue component, have irregular margins, and frequently invade adjacent mediastinal and chest wall structures. Thus, the presence of well-defined margins and lack of invasiveness favor a diagnosis of lipoma over liposarcoma.

REFERENCES

Gaerte SC, Meyer CA, Winer-Muram HT, et al. Fat-containing lesions of the chest. *Radiographics*. 2002;22:S61–S78.

Thoracic Radiology: The Requisites, 3rd ed, 159–192.

CASE 82

Apical Cap Secondary to Extrapleural Hematoma

1. **A and D**. Blood from intercostal vessel injury, rib fracture, or dissecting mediastinal hematoma (ruptured aorta) can accumulate between the parietal pleura and ribs, forming an apical cap. Most acute hemothoraces accumulate dependently. However, pleural blood could cause an apical cap if the patient had pre-existing pleural adhesions. Pulmonary contusion manifests as lung consolidation or ground-glass opacity in a nonanatomic distribution. Asbestos-related pleural thickening usually extends to the costophrenic angle. The apical pleura is typically spared. The cap in this case is longer in dimension than a classic pleural plaque.
2. **C**. Bone destruction adjacent to a pleural cap is most suggestive of a primary lung carcinoma (superior sulcus tumor). Hilar lymphadenopathy and pleural effusion can be caused by extrathoracic tumor metastases or inflammation. Mediastinal widening may be produced by infection (mediastinitis) or hematoma both of which can track into the apical extrapleural space.
3. **C**. Many patients develop apical fibrosis and pleural scarring with age. Most of these patients are asymptomatic. The apical caps usually have irregular margins, are less than 5 mm thick, and are typically symmetric. The prevalence increases with age. Apical caps from extension of mediastinal hematoma are typically unilateral and more commonly occur on the left. These may be the result of a traumatic aortic injury. Radiation for breast carcinoma typically is limited to the anterior chest wall. Radiation to these areas can causes fibrosis in the adjacent ipsilateral lung apex and result in a unilateral apical cap. Head and neck carcinomas often metastasize to cervical and supraclavicular lymph nodes and can produce an apical cap when the lymph node metastases are large. These metastases are more likely to be unilateral than bilateral. Also, radiation to the ipsilateral neck in such cases may also produce an apical cap.

4. **A**. CT of the chest can best characterize the abnormality and delineate its full extent. Although MRI can provide a lot of information, a CT scan is a better first-line test to further characterize the abnormality because of its superior spatial resolution and ability to rapidly image the entirety of the chest and neck. Ultrasound may be useful to assess pleural and extrapleural abnormalities, but it is limited in its ability to fully delineate the extent of disease. Furthermore, deep tissues may not be visible. FDG-PET does not have a role in evaluating the acutely ill patient.

Comment

Differential Diagnosis

AP radiograph (Fig. 82.1) shows a left apical cap. There is a subtle displaced fracture of the left first rib, indicating that extrapleural hematoma or loculated hemothorax is the most likely cause. Coronal reformatted contrast-enhanced CT image (Fig. 82.2) confirms the presence of blood in the upper left hemithorax. The blood abuts the inner margin of the adjacent ribs, indicating an extrapleural location. The relatively smooth margins and the presence of an acute rib fracture argue against neoplasm.

Discussion

The term *apical cap* has been used to describe the presence of opacity located in or adjacent to the extreme apex of the lung on chest radiographs (see Fig. 82.1). On chest radiographs of normal, asymptomatic patients, biapical smooth or irregular opacities located at the apices of the lungs, usually measuring less than 5 mm in diameter, are often present. The lower margin is usually sharply delineated but often has an undulating border. Apical caps are thought to represent the result of nonspecific subpleural scarring and apical pleural thickening, and they are usually of no clinical significance. The prevalence of apical caps increases with age. This finding when isolated does not represent old healed granulomatous disease (i.e., tuberculosis).

A variety of entities can result in an enlarged apical cap. The various causes of a unilateral enlarged cap include lymphoma or abscess extending down from the neck, primary lung carcinoma (superior sulcus or Pancoast tumor), and mediastinitis or hematoma tracking into the apical extrapleural space. Regarding bilaterally enlarged apical caps, they may be associated with radiation fibrosis (e.g., for Hodgkin lymphoma), mediastinal lipomatosis, and vascular abnormalities such as coarctation of the aorta with enlarged collateral vessels.

In this case, the presence of a smoothly marginated enlarged left apical cap is the result of an extrapleural hematoma. The apical cap is smoothly marginated, reflecting the extrapleural location. Extrapleural hematomas typically do not require treatment. Active intercostal arterial bleeding may be treated with embolization. It is important to distinguish hemothorax from extrapleural hematoma, as the former usually requires percutaneous drainage to avoid the subsequent development of a fibrothorax.

REFERENCES

McLoud TC, Isler RJ, Novelline RA, et al. The apical cap. *AJR Am J Roentgenol*. 1981;137:299–306.

Thoracic Radiology: The Requisites, 3rd ed, 159–192.

CASE 83

Bleomycin Lung Toxicity

1. **A and D**. Bleomycin lung toxicity, and fungal infection can present as patchy consolidation in a patient on chemotherapy. Congestive heart failure typically presents with diffuse lung edema and pleural effusions. Collagen vascular disease is usually not associated with peripheral consolidation.
2. **A**. Approximately 4% of patients receiving bleomycin develop lung toxicity.
3. **A**. Although bleomycin is used to treat some patients with lymphoma, lymphoma itself does not increase a patient's risk of bleomycin induced lung toxicity. Concurrent radiotherapy, renal insufficiency, and advanced age all raise a patient's risk for developing bleomycin induced lung toxicity.
4. **C**. Most patients improve within a few weeks, not a few days, although a small number of patients may take much longer to recover, including up to two years. Bleomycin must be discontinued to prevent worsening lung injury, and most patients are treated with corticosteroids, which are slowly tapered as the patient's clinical condition improves.

Comment

Differential Diagnosis

Axial and coronal computed tomography (CT) images show patchy peripheral consolidation in the right lung. Consolidation in a patient treated with chemotherapy can result from infection or drug reaction.

Discussion

Bleomycin is an antitumor agent that is used to treat lymphomas, testicular carcinomas, and certain squamous cell carcinomas. Lung toxicity occurs in approximately 4% of patients and is the principal dose-limiting factor for this agent. Fibrosis is the most serious pulmonary complication but organizing pneumonia reaction and acute hypersensitivity reaction can occur.

Affected patients typically present with an insidious onset of dyspnea, nonproductive cough, and occasional fever. Pulmonary function tests reveal a decreased DLco, a sensitive measure for early bleomycin lung injury.

Chest radiographs may be normal or might show reticular opacities in a basilar and subpleural distribution. Peripheral and peribronchial consolidation can also develop. Thin section CT is more sensitive than radiographs for detecting lung abnormalities and can show characteristic findings even when the chest radiograph is normal. Consolidation (Figs. 83.1 and Fig. 83.2) can represent drug-induced organizing pneumonia, which can also be mass like or nodular in appearance. Nodules can vary in size from 5 mm to 3 cm. Infection, particularly fungal infection is the other major diagnosis to consider. Organizing pneumonia is usually subpleural in a peripheral distribution and/or in a peribronchial distribution. In contrast to metastases, air bronchograms are often present within the nodules.

Early detection of bleomycin-induced lung injury is important because prompt discontinuation of bleomycin can result in improved lung function and healing in patients with early stages of disease. In patients with more-advanced disease, the prognosis is variable. Although some patients respond to steroids, others develop progressive fibrosis, which can lead to respiratory failure and death.

REFERENCES
Rossi SE, Erasmus JJ, McAdams HP, et al. Pulmonary drug toxicity: radiologic and pathologic manifestations. *Radiographics*. 2000;20:1245–1259.
Thoracic Radiology: The Requisites, 3rd ed, 355–376.

CASE 84

Primary Lung Adenocarcinoma With N2 Nodal Disease

1. **A, B, and D**. The radiograph shows right hilar and right paratracheal lymphadenopathy, which can result from primary lung carcinoma or metastases, including renal cell carcinoma and testicular carcinoma among others. Primary tuberculosis can also present with hilar and mediastinal lymphadenopathy, although this appearance is more common in children than adults. Silicosis can lead to hilar and mediastinal lymphadenopathy. However, no underlying pneumoconiotic nodules are present on the standard radiograph. Also, lymphadenopathy in silicosis is usually bilateral in distribution.
2. **C**. N2 denotes metastasis to ipsilateral mediastinal or subcarinal lymph nodes. N0 denotes no lymph node metastasis, N1 denotes ipsilateral intrapulmonary, bronchial, or hilar lymph node metastasis, and N3 denotes any supraclavicular, scalene, or contralateral mediastinal or hilar lymph node metastasis.
3. **D**. Combined with T1-3, N1 disease determines the designation of stage IIIA. The patient is staged as IIIB when N2 disease occurs with a T3 or T4 lesion. Any axillary lymph node metastasis is staged as M1. In the absence of a T3 or T4 lesion and no distant metastases, some patients with N2 lymph node metastases may be candidates for surgical resection typically after neoadjuvant chemotherapy. FDG-PET is sensitive for lymph node metastases and is superior to computed tomography (CT), but the false positive rate is high. Surgical or bronchoscopic (EBUS) nodal biopsy is usually required for adequate nodal staging.
4. **C**. Ipsilateral pleural metastasis is staged as M1a and is therefore a contraindication for resection. Chest wall invasion is staged as T3 and is potentially resectable. A tumor metastasis to the same lobe is staged as T3 and potentially resectable. A central lesion resulting in obstructive pneumonia of the entire lung is staged as T2 and may be resectable.

Comment

Differential Diagnosis

The PA chest radiograph (Fig. 84.1) shows right hilar enlargement and a right lower paratracheal mass, consistent with lymphadenopathy. Contrast-enhanced CT image shows right hilar (Fig. 84.2) and right lower paratracheal (Fig. 84.3) lymphadenopathy. The differential diagnosis is broad but most commonly would include primary lung carcinoma, metastases (testicular and renal, especially), lymphoma, and granulomatous infections such as tuberculosis and histoplasmosis.

Discussion

In patients with non–small cell lung cancer, the nodal status provides important information for determining prognosis and planning appropriate therapy. Lymph nodes are categorized into seven specific zones: supraclavicular, upper, aorticopulmonary, subcarinal, lower, hilar-interlobar, and peripheral. No changes were made for the N designation in the 8th edition of the TNM classification system. According to the TNM classification system, nodal involvement is graded from N0 to N3 as follows:

- N0 = no demonstrable metastases to regional lymph nodes
- N1 = metastasis to lymph nodes in the ipsilateral peripheral or hilar-interlobar regions
- N2 = metastasis to ipsilateral mediastinal nodes (upper, aorticopulmonary, lower or subcarinal)

- N3 = metastasis to any supraclavicular nodes, or to contralateral mediastinal (upper, aorticopulmonary, lower), hilar-interlobar, or peripheral regions.

CT and magnetic resonance imaging (MRI) play an important but limited role in the assessment of the nodal status in patients with lung carcinoma. These imaging studies rely primarily on anatomic features of lymph nodes, most notably lymph node size. Short axis diameter >1 cm is generally considered abnormal. This strategy is associated with sensitivities in the range of 60% to 79% and specificities in the range of 60% to 80%. Thus, for staging purposes, enlarged nodes must be evaluated by biopsy. The primary role of these imaging examinations is to identify the location of enlarged nodes. This information allows appropriate biopsy procedures to be planned.

In recent years, FDG-PET imaging has been shown to be superior to CT and MRI in the assessment of mediastinal lymph node metastases. This technique relies on physiologic (glucose metabolism) rather than anatomic features to identify abnormal lymph nodes. Thus, it has the potential to identify neoplastic involvement within small nodes and to distinguish enlarged, hyperplastic nodes from neoplastic ones. However, the number of false-positive and false-negative studies (particularly in small nodes with microscopic metastases) requires that lymph node sampling still be performed in most cases.

REFERENCES

Sharma A, Fidias P, Hayman LA, et al. Patterns of lymphadenopathy in thoracic malignancies. *Radiographics*. 2004;24:419–434.

Carter BW, Lichtenberger 3rd JP, Benveniste MK, de Groot PM, Wu CC, Erasmus JJ, Truong MT. Revisions to the TNM staging of lung cancer: rationale, significance, and clinical application. *Radiographics*. 2018 Mar–Apr;38(2):374–391.

Thoracic Radiology: The Requisites, 3rd ed, 19–60, 450–459.

CASE 85
Superior Vena Cava Syndrome from Lung Cancer

1. A. Lung cancer can invade or metastasize to the mediastinum and compress or occlude the superior vena cava. Although there are numerous dilated vessels in the right hemithorax, they contain undiluted contrast, which indicates that they are in continuity with the vein into which the contrast was administered and not deriving flow from an arteriovenous malformation, which should have blood mixed with contrast. Extravasated contrast collects in the soft tissues and does not fill multiple vessels.
2. C. Lung cancer is a common disease and often results in direct mediastinal invasion or mediastinal adenopathy both of which can cause SVC obstruction. Long-term intravenous devices such as pacemaker leads can cause SVC stenosis or thrombosis. However, these devices are not the most common causes of SVC syndrome. Fibrosing mediastinitis is associated with SVC syndrome but is a relatively rare disease. Radiation therapy can cause fibrosis in the mediastinum and result in SVC stenosis, but its occurrence is unusual.
3. D. Dural venous sinus thrombosis is not a typical manifestation of SVC syndrome. Impaired venous return from the head and neck can result in head and face edema, extremity edema, and visual disturbances.
4. D. Targeted radiation therapy to the mediastinum can lead to rapid improvement of the symptoms of SVC syndrome. Chemotherapy may be useful in chemosensitive tumors; however, it is not the preferred first-line treatment for SVC syndrome related to non–small cell lung carcinoma. Surgical resection is generally not indicated because patients with

SVC syndrome related to non–small cell lung carcinoma generally have unresectable disease. Surgical bypass may be used in some cases for palliation where other therapies have failed. SVC stenting may be useful in some patients who fail initial therapy. However, data are somewhat limited.

Comment
Differential Diagnosis

Contrast-enhanced CT image (Fig. 85.1) shows a soft tissue mass infiltrating the mediastinum with obliteration of the superior vena cava. Numerous chest wall and mediastinal collateral vessels are present filled with undiluted contrast. The infiltrating soft tissue mass is most consistent with lung carcinoma. Other neoplastic causes would include lymphoma and thymic carcinoma. Fibrosing mediastinitis can also cause SVC syndrome. This most commonly presents with a large, partially calcified nodal mass in the mediastinum.

Discussion

Superior vena cava (SVC) syndrome is caused by obstruction of the SVC by external compression, intraluminal thrombosis, neoplastic infiltration, or a combination of these processes. Most cases result from neoplasm, most commonly lung carcinoma (especially small cell carcinoma). Lymphoma, thymic carcinoma, and metastatic carcinoma are additional malignant causes. There are a variety of benign causes, including long-term intravenous devices (e.g., Hickman catheters and permanent pacemakers) and fibrosing mediastinitis.

Chest radiographs often show a mass in the right paratracheal region that may be accompanied by distention of the azygos vein. In the setting of fibrosing mediastinitis, the right paratracheal mass is often an enlarged calcified node. In patients who develop thrombosis of the SVC because of an indwelling catheter, lateral displacement of the catheter may be apparent.

Computed tomography (CT) or magnetic resonance imaging (MRI) can confirm the diagnosis of SVC obstruction. On CT, the diagnosis is based on decreased or absent contrast opacification of the SVC in conjunction with opacification of collateral vessels. Both findings are necessary to make a reliable diagnosis. Contrast-enhanced CT with multiplanar reformation and 3D reconstructions is highly accurate at detecting the presence and level of SVC obstruction. It is also valuable in determining the cause of obstruction and for delineating the collateral venous circulation. The presence of collateral venous vessels should prompt a search for a central venous obstruction.

Treatment for SVC syndrome related to lung cancer is primarily with radiation therapy. Chemotherapy may be used in some patients especially those with small cell carcinoma. Surgical bypass is generally reserved for patients with benign causes of SVC obstruction or for palliation in those who fail radiation and chemotherapy for malignancy.

REFERENCES

Eran S, Karaman A, Okur A. The superior vena cava syndrome caused by malignant disease: imaging with multidetector row CT. *Eur J Radiol*. 2006;59:93–103.

Carter BW, Lichtenberger 3rd JP, Benveniste MK, de Groot PM, Wu CC, Erasmus JJ, Truong MT. Revisions to the TNM staging of lung cancer: rationale, significance, and clinical application. *Radiographics*. 2018 Mar–Apr;38(2):374–391.

Thoracic Radiology: The Requisites, 3rd ed, 450–459.

CASE 86

Diffuse Alveolar Hemorrhage From Vasculitis

1. **A and C.** The differential diagnosis for widespread consolidation in the acutely ill patient includes pulmonary hemorrhage, pulmonary edema, diffuse infectious pneumonia, massive aspiration, and acute lung injury. Langerhans cell histiocytosis is a smoking related disease characterized by upper lung predominant nodules and cysts. Silicosis is characterized by well-defined nodules with an upper lobe predominance with or without progressive massive fibrosis. Acute silicosis however can produce diffuse lung disease which is mostly ground glass in appearance. The pathology is that of alveolar proteinosis.
2. **C.** Pulmonary vasculitis is the most common cause of diffuse alveolar hemorrhage. Hemophilia is rare. Drug induced pulmonary hemorrhage is rare and can occur with therapeutic drugs such as erlotinib or illicit drugs such as crack cocaine. Infection rarely causes diffuse alveolar hemorrhage.
3. **B.** The most common lung manifestation of microscopic polyangiitis is diffuse alveolar hemorrhage. Diffuse alveolar hemorrhage related to granulomatosis with polyangiitis (Wegener's granulomatosis) only occurs in 10% to 15% of patients. Diffuse alveolar hemorrhage from eosinophilic granulomatosis with polyangiitis (formerly Churg-Strauss syndrome) is rare. Takayasu arteritis primarily affects the aorta and its branches. Large pulmonary artery involvement does occur, but diffuse alveolar hemorrhage is not a feature.
4. **A.** The diagnosis of diffuse alveolar hemorrhage is confirmed by bronchoalveolar lavage, which shows progressive increase in return of blood in lavage fluid. Transbronchial and surgical biopsy can show hemosiderin-laden macrophages or areas of hemorrhage but are not the best choices for diagnosis. Sputum analysis has low yield and may show red blood cells but does not confirm diffuse alveolar hemorrhage.

Comment

Differential Diagnosis

The portable anteroposterior (AP) radiograph (Fig. 86.1) shows diffuse lung consolidation. Computed tomography (CT) shows dense bilateral consolidation posteriorly and patchier ground-glass opacity anteriorly (Fig. 86.2). The differential diagnosis for diffuse lung opacity in the acutely ill patient is broad and includes diffuse pneumonia from infection, cardiogenic and non-cardiogenic edema, hemorrhage, massive aspiration, or acute lung injury. Hemoptysis, when present, and decreased hematocrit favor diffuse alveolar hemorrhage.

Discussion

Diffuse alveolar hemorrhage (DAH) is characterized by bleeding into the alveolar spaces and results from disruption of the alveolar-capillary basement membrane. The clinical presentation is acute, and patients usually present with cough, fever, dyspnea, and hemoptysis. However, approximately one-third of patients with DAH do not have hemoptysis. Although a wide variety of insults can lead to DAH, the histopathologic injury can be grouped into capillaritis, bland hemorrhage, and diffuse alveolar damage (DAD).

Capillaritis can result from systemic vasculitis (especially anti-neutrophil cytoplasmic antibody associated), anti-glomerular basement membrane antibodies, collagen vascular disease, or be idiopathic. Causes of DAD are numerous and include infection, systemic sepsis, reaction to drugs, trauma, and collagen vascular disease. Bland DAH may develop secondary to left heart failure, anticoagulation, and hemorrhagic disorders.

Radiographic findings of DAH vary by the extent and severity of DAH. Radiographs of patients with mild DAH may be normal or near normal, while those of patients with severe disease may show extensive consolidation. CT findings are similar, ranging from mild ground-glass opacity to extensive multilobar consolidation. The distribution of opacities tends to be more central and perihilar, but the findings are often indistinguishable from other causes of diffuse lung opacity such as edema, infection, and alveolar damage.

Bronchoalveolar lavage is the reference standard for establishing a diagnosis of DAH. Increased blood products in returned lavage fluid is diagnostic of DAH. Hemosiderin-laden macrophages can also be identified in lavage fluid. Treatment includes management of underlying causes (when known) and supportive therapy as needed.

REFERENCES
Krause ML, et al. Update on diffuse alveolar hemorrhage and pulmonary vasculitis. *Immunol Allergy Clini North Am.* 2012 Nov;32(4):587–600.
Thoracic Radiology: The Requisites, 3rd ed, 238–258, 335–354.

CASE 87

Usual Interstitial Pneumonia (UIP) Caused by Idiopathic Pulmonary Fibrosis (IPF)

1. **B.** Subpleural and basal predominant reticulation with honeycombing is highly diagnostic of usual interstitial pneumonia. Desquamative interstitial pneumonia is characterized by extensive ground-glass opacity, sometimes with accompanying mild fine reticulation and occasional small cysts. Nonspecific interstitial pneumonia is usually characterized by ground-glass opacity with or without reticulation in basal and peribronchial distribution. Lymphoid interstitial pneumonia can be quite variable but is usually characterized by ground-glass opacity, nodules, and cysts.
2. **D.** For patients with a definite UIP pattern of fibrosis on CT, biopsy is rarely warranted. Surgical biopsy is not without risk and rarely will change the diagnosis with this pattern. Transbronchial and CT-guided needle biopsy are not sufficient to make a pathologic diagnosis of UIP, primarily because of the small sample size and relative peripheral location of fibrosis. A multidisciplinary approach to diagnosis is important with involvement of the radiologist, pulmonologist, and pathologist.
3. **A.** A usual interstitial pneumonia (UIP) pattern of fibrosis is most strongly associated with rheumatoid arthritis. Nonspecific interstitial pneumonia (NSIP) is the most common pattern of diffuse lung disease in patients with progressive systemic sclerosis. NSIP and organizing pneumonia are the most common patterns of diffuse lung disease in patients with polymyositis. Lymphoid interstitial pneumonia (LIP) is associated with Sjögren syndrome.
4. **D.** Asbestos can result in pulmonary fibrosis (asbestosis), typically with a usual interstitial pneumonia (UIP) pattern of fibrosis. Coal and silica cause pneumoconiosis characterized by small perilymphatic nodules predominantly in the upper lungs. Nodules can coalesce to form large opacities, termed progressive massive fibrosis. Beryllium causes a granulomatous response in the lungs indistinguishable from sarcoidosis.

Comment

Differential Diagnosis

Axial (Figs. 87.1 and 87.2) and coronal reformatted (Fig. 87.3) CT images show subpleural and basal predominant reticulation with honeycombing and traction bronchiectasis, consistent with UIP pattern of pulmonary fibrosis. This pattern on CT is highly specific for UIP and most commonly represents IPF.

Discussion

UIP is a pattern of chronic diffuse lung injury characterized by restrictive physiology and reduced diffusing capacity. Most patients with UIP have no identifiable cause, termed IPF. Other causes of UIP histology and CT pattern include collagen vascular disease (particularly rheumatoid arthritis), familial fibrosis, drug toxicity, and asbestos exposure (asbestosis). Older age and male sex are risk factors for IPF. Patients present with progressive dyspnea, dry cough, restrictive pulmonary physiology, and reduced diffusion capacity. Digital clubbing may be present, and coarse end expiratory crackles are heard on expiration, particularly in the lower lung zones.

The diagnosis of UIP is usually made by chest CT when the characteristic pattern of subpleural and basal predominant reticulation with honeycombing is present. In most cases, this CT pattern and clinical evaluation alone are enough to establish a diagnosis of IPF. Occasionally, a surgical lung biopsy may be required either because of confounding findings on chest CT or clinical evaluation. Histopathologically, UIP is characterized by spatially and temporally heterogeneous areas of fibrosis and lobular collapse with characteristic fibroblastic foci at the leading edge of fibrosis. Microscopic honeycombing may be present, and inflammation is minimal or absent.

UIP, regardless of cause, is associated with a poor prognosis. Many patients with IPF die of their disease within 3 to 4 years of diagnosis. Complications include progressive respiratory decline, acute exacerbations, and lung cancer. Treatment options for IPF are limited to two novel drugs, which have been shown to improve progression free survival but not overall survival

REFERENCES
Ryu JH, Moua T, Daniels CE, et al. Idiopathic pulmonary fibrosis: evolving concepts. *Mayo Clin Proc.* 2014 Aug;89(8):1130–1142.
Raghu G, Remy-Jardin M, Myers JL, et al. American Thoracic Society, European Respiratory Society, Japanese Respiratory Society, and Latin American Thoracic Society. Diagnosis of idiopathic pulmonary fibrosis: an official ATS/ERS/JRS/ALAT clinical practice guideline. *Am J Respir Crit Care Med.* 2018 Sep 1;198(5):e44–e68.
Thoracic Radiology: The Requisites, 3rd ed, 355–376.

CASE 88

Intramuscular Hematoma From Supratherapeutic Warfarin Therapy

1. **A and C.** Foci of high attenuation in an intramuscular mass are typical in acute hematomas. An intramuscular metastasis such as renal cell carcinoma can spontaneously hemorrhage, as well. Soft tissue abscesses will have a low attenuation central portion. High attenuation foci are not typical. Elastofibromas occur inferior to the scapular tip and usually feature soft tissue and fat attenuation.
2. **B.** High attenuation, noncalcified foci within a heterogeneous collection are typical of blood products. Some tumors contain high attenuation foci, but most are equal or slightly lower attenuation than skeletal muscle. The foci of high attenuation

are only moderately greater than those of skeletal muscle, making calcium very unlikely. Fat is of low attenuation.
3. **A.** Intramuscular hematoma is not a risk factor for malignant degeneration. Intramuscular hematoma can impede blood flow to the affected muscle and result in ischemic myopathy. Neuropathy can result from an intramuscular hematoma chronically compressing peripheral nerves. Intramuscular hematoma can cause pressure necrosis of adjacent bone, especially when the hematoma is quite large.
4. **D.** Spontaneous intramuscular hematoma can be a complication of hemophilia. Aspirin prolongs bleeding time but does not predispose to spontaneous intramuscular hematoma. Extravasation of IV contrast medium can occur during power injection but does not cause spontaneous intramuscular hematoma. Vitamin K supplementation would interfere with warfarin therapy, reducing its anticoagulation effect.

Comment

Differential Diagnosis

Anteroposterior (AP) chest radiograph demonstrates hazy opacification of the left hemithorax with enlargement of the soft tissues in the left lateral chest wall (Fig. 88.1). The CT image shows a large, well-marginated, heterogeneous left posterolateral chest wall mass centered within the musculature (Fig. 88.2). The high-attenuation foci in this mass on unenhanced CT represent blood products and are consistent with acute intramuscular hematoma, a complication of supratherapeutic warfarin therapy. One could consider a hemorrhagic metastasis, such as renal cell carcinoma.

Discussion

Cross-sectional imaging studies can be helpful in the identification of the site and extent of intramuscular hematomas in patients with either traumatic injury or spontaneous hemorrhage. Because of its relative low cost and lack of ionizing radiation, ultrasonography is usually the preferred test for this purpose. In patients with large hematomas, CT and magnetic resonance imaging (MRI) are occasionally helpful in determining the extent and the age of hemorrhage and identifying the effect of the hemorrhage on adjacent organs.

Therapy is usually supportive. However, large hematomas may require surgical intervention if ischemic injury or neuropathy is suspected. Myositis ossificans can occur in up to 10% of patients with intramuscular hematoma and can cause pain and decreased function.

REFERENCES
McKenzie G, Raby N, Ritchie D. Pictorial review: Non-neoplastic soft tissue masses. *Br J Radiol.* 2009 Aug;82(981):775–785.
Thoracic Radiology: The Requisites, 3rd ed, 159–192.

CASE 89

Scimitar Syndrome

1. **A and C.** The large curvilinear opacity in the right lower lung is most likely a vascular structure, likely an anomalous pulmonary vein. A vein draining a pulmonary arteriovenous malformation is likely without identification of a similar size artery feeding the malformation. Congenital pulmonary airway malformation is typically not associated with a large vascular anomaly, and the mucocele of bronchial atresia usually has a smaller diameter.
2. **B.** Because the pulmonary vein drains into the right atrium, a left-to-right shunt is most likely present. A left-to-left shunt

occurs when an anomalous pulmonary vein drains to the left atrium. A right-to-right shunt would occur when a pulmonary artery drained into another artery or the right atrium. A right-to-left shunt occurs with a pulmonary arteriovenous malformation, where blood bypasses the normal pulmonary capillary bed.

3. **B**. Scimitar syndrome is associated with a host of congenital abnormalities, and hypoplastic lung with abnormal airway branching is the most common. There is no apparent increased incidence of lung cancer, kidney abnormalities, or muscular dystrophy.

4. **D**. Scimitar syndrome in an *asymptomatic* adult is generally an incidental finding that requires no management. Resection, endovascular coiling, or bronchoscopy are not indicated for this patient.

Comment

Differential Diagnosis

Posteroanterior (PA) chest radiograph (Fig. 89.1) shows a large, curvilinear structure coursing from the right infrahilar region to the medial right lung base, reflecting the scimitar vein, named because of its likeness to a Turkish sword. The right lung is slightly hypoplastic, and the right main bronchus is smaller than usual. Coronal maximum intensity projection (MIP) from magnetic resonance (MR) angiogram of the chest (Fig. 89.2) shows the curvilinear structure draining into the suprahepatic inferior vena cava. Differential considerations would include pulmonary vein varix or meandering pulmonary vein. Differential causes for the slightly hypoplastic right hemithorax could include pulmonary underdevelopment, interruption of the right pulmonary artery, pulmonary vein stenosis, and Swyer-James-MacLeod syndrome.

Discussion

Scimitar syndrome (venolobar syndrome) is a form of partial anomalous pulmonary venous drainage, where the scimitar vein drains all or part of the ipsilateral lung into the systemic venous circulation, typically the inferior vena cava. In two-thirds of cases, the scimitar vein drains the entire lung and in one-third of cases, only the inferior half of the lung drains through the scimitar vein. In addition to anomalous venous drainage, other anomalies are present to varying extents. Hypoplasia of the ipsilateral lung occurs in nearly all cases with varying degrees of abnormal lobation, airway branching, and dextroposition of the heart. The ipsilateral pulmonary artery is usually smaller than normal, and systemic arterial supply to a portion of the affected lung occurs in up to two-thirds of patients. Other defects include secundum type atrial septal defect, diaphragmatic hernia, and horseshoe lung. The pathogenesis of scimitar syndrome is unclear, and the developmental abnormalities that lead to the anomalous anatomy are not well described.

Scimitar syndrome has two distinct clinical manifestations. The infantile form has a high association with significant congenital cardiovascular anomalies including ventricular septal defect, aortic coarctation and hypoplasia, tetralogy of Fallot, truncus arteriosus, and abnormal origin of the left coronary artery. Because of the associated malformations, mortality and morbidity rates are high.

In contrast to the infantile form, the adult form of scimitar syndrome is often asymptomatic or presents only with milder symptoms from shunting or other anomalies. Asymptomatic patients typically do not require treatment.

Computed tomography (CT) or MR angiography can better delineate the anatomy of scimitar syndrome. MR has the advantage of being able to quantify shunts whereas CT can better delineate lung abnormalities.

REFERENCES
Gudjonsson U, Brown JW. Scimitar syndrome. *Semin Thorac Cardiovasc Surg Pediatr Card Surg Annu.* 2006:56–62.
Thoracic Radiology: The Requisites, 3rd ed, 193–209.

CASE 90

Pericardial Effusion

1. **A and B**. Myocardial infarction with left ventricular failure is the most common cause of pericardial effusion. Serositis related to systemic lupus erythematosus and other collagen vascular diseases can cause pleural and pericardial effusion. Pericardial effusion is not a typical finding of relapsing polychondritis, which primarily affects the trachea and bronchi. Acute pulmonary embolism can cause pleural effusion, but pericardial effusion does not occur.

2. **D**. The lateral view shows a low-density vertical line behind the sternum (mediastinal fat) and another low-density vertical line posterior to it (epicardial fat). These two lines are separated by fluid density which represents the pericardial effusion. The appearance resembles an Oreo cookie.

3. **C**. Cardiac MRI is extremely sensitive for detecting pericardial effusions. The entire pericardium can be imaged in multiple planes. Chest radiographs have very low sensitivity for pericardial effusion, especially with volumes less than 200 mL. Transthoracic and transesophageal echocardiography are highly sensitive for pericardial effusion but can miss effusions loculated posteriorly because of limited acoustic windows.

4. **D**. Dressler syndrome refers to pleural and pericardial effusions, which develop 2 to 10 weeks after acute myocardial infarction. Dressler syndrome is not related to rheumatoid arthritis, viral myocarditis, and radiation induced injury.

Comment

Differential Diagnosis

The posteroanterior (PA) radiograph shows and enlarged cardiac silhouette (Fig. 90.1). The lateral radiograph shows a vertically oriented soft tissue stripe anterior to the heart bordered by two stripes of fat attenuation (Fig. 90.2), representing a pericardial effusion. Unenhanced computed tomography (CT) image (Fig. 90.3) shows the full extent of the pericardial effusion and illustrates the anterior mediastinal and epicardial fat, which enable the effusion to be visible on the lateral radiograph. Pleural effusions are also present. The differential diagnosis for pericardial effusion is broad and includes infection, trauma, radiation therapy, drug toxicity, collagen vascular diseases, metabolic disorders, and neoplasms.

Discussion

The lateral radiograph shows a curvilinear retrosternal stripe bracketed by fat attenuation, also referred to as the double-lucency, sandwich or Oreo cookie sign. This sign refers to widening (>4 mm) of the soft tissue opacity of the pericardium between the lucent stripes that represent fat located anterior (mediastinal) and posterior (epicardial) to the pericardium. This sign has a relatively low sensitivity but a high specificity for detecting pericardial effusion.

Chest radiography is associated with a relatively poor sensitivity for detecting pericardial effusions. It has been estimated that 200 mL of pericardial fluid must be present to reliably make the diagnosis radiographically. In contrast, CT and echocardiography are highly sensitive for detecting pericardial effusion and is the studies of choice for screening patients with suspected pericardial effusion. MRI may be helpful for characterizing complex pericardial fluid collections. Furthermore, MRI provides detailed imaging of the entire pericardium in contrast to echocardiography, which can be limited by acoustic windows.

The most common cause of pericardial effusion is myocardial infarction with left ventricular failure. Dressler syndrome refers to the development of pericardial and pleural effusions 2 to 10 weeks following acute myocardial infarction. Such effusions can be hemorrhagic, particularly in patients who have received anticoagulation therapy.

Large pericardial effusions can require drainage to prevent or relieve cardiac tamponade. Some effusions will resolve without treatment. Pericardial thickening can result in constrictive pericarditis.

REFERENCES

Kligerman S. Imaging of Pericardial Disease. *Radiol Clin North Am.* 2019 Jan;57(1):179–199.

Thoracic Radiology: The Requisites, 3rd ed, 226–237.

CASE 91

Idiopathic Bronchiectasis

1. **A and B**. Ciliary dyskinesia predisposes patients to recurrent sinopulmonary infections, and bronchiectasis can result from recurrent airway inflammation. Allergic bronchopulmonary aspergillosis occurs primarily in patients with asthma and cystic fibrosis and leads to bronchiectasis because of chronic bronchial inflammation. Traction bronchiectasis and bronchiolectasis can develop in the setting of interstitial fibrosis. However, this is a secondary phenomenon and not related to an intrinsic bronchial abnormality. In addition, the dilated peripheral airways will be within areas of fibrosis. These ectatic airways may appear varicose in morphology. Lymphangioleiomyomatosis is characterized by the development of lung cysts with smooth, thin walls. Bronchiectasis is not a component of the disease. Cigarette smoking leads to chronic airway inflammation and bronchial wall thickening but generally does not result in bronchiectasis.

2. **D**. Infection is the most common cause of bronchiectasis, especially infections during childhood. Congenital bronchiectasis is uncommon and is often the result of deficiency in bronchial cartilage (e.g., Williams-Campbell syndrome). Interstitial pneumonia is uncommon and can be associated with traction bronchiectasis in areas of fibrosis. Lymphangioleiomyomatosis is characterized by the development of lung cysts with smooth, thin walls. Bronchiectasis is not a component of the disease.

3. **C**. Bronchial wall thickening is a nonspecific finding on computed tomography (CT) and can be encountered in processes such as bronchitis, lymphangitic carcinomatosis, and lung edema. Bronchial diameter greater than that of the adjacent artery, lack of normal bronchial tapering, and bronchi visible in peripheral 1 cm of lung are considered direct signs of bronchiectasis.

4. **D**. Pleural effusion is not a direct consequence of bronchiectasis. However, a parapneumonic effusion can develop from bronchiectasis-related pneumonia. Bronchiectasis is one of the most common causes of hemoptysis. The chronically inflamed bronchi are often friable and prone to hemorrhage. Atelectasis from bronchiectasis can result from mucoid impaction, poor clearance of secretions, and bronchomalacia. Chronic bronchiectasis limited to a lobe may result in complete atelectasis of that lobe without bronchial obstruction. Dilated air bronchograms are a prominent feature. Poor mucociliary clearance in dilated and inflamed bronchi predisposes affected patients to recurrent pneumonia.

Comment

Differential Diagnosis

Axial (Fig. 91.1) and coronal (Fig. 91.2) CT images show mild bronchiectasis characterized by cylindrical dilation of peripheral airways, bronchial wall thickening, and mucus plugging. Also note the presence of tree-in-bud opacities and mosaic attenuation, reflecting associated small airways disease. The causes of bronchiectasis are myriad and include infection (including atypical mycobacterial), immune deficiency, ciliary dyskinesia, congenital cartilage deficiency in the airways, chronic aspiration, allergic bronchopulmonary aspergillosis, cystic fibrosis, small airways disease, and others.

Discussion

Bronchiectasis is defined as abnormal, irreversible dilation of the bronchi. Bronchiectasis can arise secondary to a wide variety of congenital and acquired abnormalities. Cystic fibrosis is the most common associated congenital abnormality, and prior infection, especially childhood infections, is the most common acquired abnormality.

Chest radiographs are often normal in patients with mild degrees of bronchiectasis but occasionally reveal parallel, thickened bronchial walls, also referred to as a tram-track appearance. With cystic bronchiectasis, radiographs can reveal clusters of air-filled cysts, often with fluid levels. CT is highly sensitive and specific for diagnosing bronchiectasis. Findings include a bronchial wall diameter greater than its adjacent artery (resulting in a signet-ring sign when the dilated bronchus and accompanying artery are viewed in cross section), identification of bronchi within the peripheral centimeter of the lung, lack of normal bronchial tapering, bronchial wall thickening, and strings or clusters of cysts. Because bronchial wall thickening may also be seen in other forms of airway disease, it should not be used as a sole criterion for diagnosing bronchiectasis.

Complications of bronchiectasis include recurrent infections, hemoptysis, mucus impaction, and atelectasis. Patients are usually treated conservatively with antibiotics as needed. Severe hemoptysis can require bronchial artery embolization or resection of affected lung.

REFERENCES

Bonavita J, Naidich DP. Imaging of bronchiectasis. *Clin Chest Med.* 2012;Jun;33(2):233–248.

Milliron B, Henry TS, Veeraraghavan S, Little BP. Bronchiectasis: mechanisms and imaging clues of associated common and uncommon diseases. *Radiographics.* 2015 Jul–Aug;35(4):1011–1030.

Thoracic Radiology: The Requisites, 3rd ed., pp. 137–158.

CASE 92

Achalasia

1. **B and D**. Achalasia results in esophageal obstruction and dysmotility. The esophagus proximal to the hypertonic segment can be filled with air, liquid, or food debris. Esophageal carcinoma can cause esophageal obstruction, leading to proximal distension and retained food, liquid, and gas. However, the degree of esophageal dilation illustrated in this case is rare in esophageal carcinoma and usually indicates a more chronic condition.

Tumor cells can also invade the nerves of the lower esophageal sphincter, preventing normal relaxation during swallowing (pseudoachalasia). Most esophageal duplication cysts are fluid filled and typically are round, masslike structures. Resultant high-grade obstruction would be highly unusual. An esophageal diverticulum is a focal outpouching or round paraesophageal mass and does not cause diffuse dilation of the esophagus.

2. **A.** The tubular nature of the gas-filled structure is typical of the esophagus. Although an enlarged azygos vein displaces the azygoesophageal contour, it does not contain gas. The gas-filled structure extends above the expected location of the azygos arch is at the level of the tracheobronchial angle. The right atrium is not enlarged. Its contours are anterior to the azygoesophageal recess. The left atrium is normal in this patient.

3. **C.** An esophagram can provide information regarding esophageal motility, unlike the other tests which are listed. A CT can show esophageal dilation, thickening, and narrowing, but it cannot evaluate esophageal motility. MRI has a very limited role in the evaluation of esophageal disorders. The lateral radiograph can provide further support that the abnormal structure is the esophagus, but it will not provide any functional information.

4. **A.** Progressive systemic sclerosis (scleroderma) typically results in dilation of the esophagus and dysmotility with a patulous lower esophageal sphincter. Achalasia results from failure of the lower esophageal sphincter to relax. Chagas disease is caused by *Trypanosoma cruzi*, which can invade and destroy the nerve plexus responsible for relaxation of the lower esophageal sphincter. It occurs primarily in South America. Tumor invasion of the nerve plexus responsible for relaxation of the lower esophageal sphincter (pseudoachalasia) can mimic achalasia.

Differential Diagnosis

The posteroanterior (PA) chest radiograph (Fig. 92.1) shows a dilated, tubular structure containing a fluid level coursing through the mediastinum and displacing the normal azygoesophageal contour, representing the esophagus. Achalasia is the most likely cause of severe esophageal dysmotility and dilation. Other causes include Chagas disease, pseudoachalasia (neoplastic invasion of the nerves of the lower esophageal sphincter), and progressive systemic sclerosis (scleroderma).

Discussion

The azygoesophageal interface is produced by the juxtaposition of aerated lung in the right lower lobe and the soft tissue opacity of the right lateral margin of the azygos vein, esophagus, or both. On normal chest radiographs, the azygoesophageal interface begins at the level of the azygos arch and extends inferiorly to the level of the diaphragm. It normally produces a concave slope as it curves slightly toward the left. Abnormalities of either the azygos vein (e.g., azygos continuation of the inferior vena cava) or esophagus (e.g., achalasia) can result in rightward displacement of this interface. Subcarinal masses such as bronchogenic cysts and lymph node enlargement can also result in focal rightward displacement of the azygoesophageal interface, usually producing a rightward convexity in the subcarinal region.

The chest radiograph (Fig. 92.1) shows diffuse, marked rightward displacement of the azygoesophageal contour. When an air-filled, distended esophagus displaces the azygoesophageal contour, a stripe is formed rather than an interface. This patient has a history of achalasia. In most patients with this disorder, the esophagus contains a large amount of retained secretions. Therefore, the radiograph typically shows a displaced azygoesophageal interface rather than a stripe. Retained secretions

and food can also result in a discrete fluid level within the distended esophagus.

Treatment for achalasia includes a Heller myotomy to release the lower esophageal sphincter. Some patients require balloon dilation. Secondary gastroesophageal reflux can develop after myotomy.

REFERENCES
Whitten CR, Khan S, Munneke GJ, Grubnic S. A diagnostic approach to mediastinal abnormalities. *Radiographics*. 2007;27:657–671.
Thoracic Radiology: The Requisites, 3rd ed., pp. 19–60, 97–136.

CASE 93
Cavity Caused by Coccidioidomycosis

1. **A and C.** Granulomatosis with polyangiitis (Wegener's) can cause lung nodules and cavities. Cavities often have thick irregular walls; however, with clearing, the walls can become thin. A solitary cavitary lesion is a common manifestation of chronic coccidioidomycosis. Cavities can form in advanced sarcoidosis but usually do so in the setting of traction bronchiectasis and fibrosis. There are no findings on the images to suggest sarcoidosis. Septic infarcts are usually multiple, peripheral and predominate in the lower lobes. They can cavitate and usually have thick walls and the broad surface usually abuts the pleura. Most are smaller than the cavity in this patient.

2. **D.** *Coccidioides* is endemic to the American Southwest in addition to Mexico, Central America, and South America.

3. **B.** Lung cavities are typical of the chronic form of coccidioidomycosis and not the acute pneumonic form. Most infected patients are asymptomatic, and disseminated disease is rare. Most patients with the pneumonic form have spontaneous resolution of their infection.

4. **B.** Most patients with disseminated coccidioidomycosis have multiple tiny nodules, typically 5 to 10 mm in diameter. Multifocal lung consolidation, diffuse ground-glass opacity, and septic pulmonary infarcts are not typical features of disseminated coccidioidomycosis.

Comment
Differential Diagnosis

The posteroanterior (PA) radiograph (Fig. 93.1) shows an ovoid mass just lateral to the left hilum. Cavitation is more conspicuous on computed tomography (CT) (Fig. 93.2). Note the thick wall of the cavity but the rather smooth interior. Some satellite nodules are also present. Malignant neoplasm and infection should be strongly considered. Granulomatosis with polyangiitis can also present as a cavitary lesion but more often lesions are multiple.

Discussion

Coccidioidomycosis infection is caused by inhalation of spores of *Coccidioides immitis* or *Coccidioides posadasii*, soil inhabitants endemic to desert areas. Although most patients are asymptomatic following exposure, some experience a mild, flulike illness.

Radiographic findings vary depending on the stage of infection. Following initial inhalation of the spores, there is a local pneumonic response, which is characterized radiographically as an area of consolidation. Such consolidation usually involves less than an entire lobe, is often located in the lower lobes, and usually resolves spontaneously without therapy.

Chronic pulmonary coccidioidomycosis is characterized radiographically by solitary or multiple pulmonary nodules and cavities.

Such cavities, as shown in this case, can have variable wall thickness and are usually radiologically indistinguishable from other causes of cavitary lesions. In a minority (10% to 15%) of patients, coccidioidomycosis is associated with characteristic thin walled (grape skin) cavities. Such cavities can rapidly change in size, presumably due to a check-valve communication with the bronchial tree.

Disseminated coccidioidomycosis is rare; it appears radiographically as multiple nodules. The nodules usually range in size from 5 mm to 1 cm in diameter, but smaller miliary nodules are observed in some cases. The course of disseminated coccidioidomycosis is variable: it may be chronic and insidious or rapidly fatal. The infection is usually fatal in patients who are immunocompromised.

Like other infections, coccidioidomycosis can cause a false-positive result on fluorodeoxyglucose–positron emission tomography (FDG-PET) studies. This can occur in the acute or chronic phase of infection. Most patients require no treatment. Antifungal therapy may be used in patients whose disease fails to clear spontaneously.

REFERENCES
Lindell RM, Hartman TE:. Fungal infections. In: Müller NL, Silva CI, eds. *Imaging of the Chest*. Philadelphia: Saunders; 2008:362–365.
Kunin JR, Flors L, Hamid A, Fuss C, Sauer D, Walker CM. Thoracic endemic fungi in the United States: importance of patient location. *Radiographics*. 2021 Mar–Apr;41(2):380–398.
Thoracic Radiology: The Requisites, 3rd ed., pp. 289–309.

CASE 94

Hydrostatic Pulmonary Edema

1. **A and C**. Hydrostatic pulmonary edema (edema secondary to congestive heart failure or volume overload) is the most common cause of interlobular septal thickening. Smooth interlobular septal thickening is not a typical feature of usual interstitial pneumonia, which is characterized by irregular lines (reticulation), reflecting interstitial fibrosis. Smooth interlobular septal thickening is not a typical finding of sarcoidosis. However, small nodules may be present along the interlobular septa in patients with sarcoidosis.

2. **A**. Kerley B lines on the chest radiograph correspond to thickened interlobular septa on CT. Other chest radiographic findings include thickening of the interlobar fissures that is due to edema in or thickening of the subpleural interstitium on both sides of the fissure. Bronchovascular bundle thickening on the chest radiograph corresponds to edema in or thickening of the peribronchovascular interstitium. Fluffy lung consolidation does not correspond to interlobular septal thickening on CT.

3. **A**. HRCT requires the use of thin collimation (≤1.5 mm). Prone imaging may be used in some patients as part of an interstitial lung disease protocol. Multiplanar reformations can be generated from volumetric CT imaging. However, they are not a required component of HRCT. A high spatial frequency reconstruction kernel provides edge sharpening, better delineating the small bronchopulmonary structures on HRCT.

4. **B**. Repeat chest imaging, either with a radiograph or CT, following diuresis can easily confirm whether septal thickening is the result of hydrostatic edema. FDG-PET might show uptake throughout the lung if the septal thickening reflects diffuse lymphangitic carcinomatosis. However, the results are nonspecific. Transbronchial biopsy and surgical biopsies are of course invasive. They may be a good option if septal thickening persists despite diuresis, and the clinical presentation suggests chronic interstitial lung disease.

Comment

Differential Diagnosis

The primary differential diagnosis for smooth interlobular septal thickening is pulmonary edema and lymphangitic carcinomatosis. Edema tends to be symmetric and gravitationally dependent, whereas lymphangitic carcinomatosis more often is randomly distributed. Pleural effusions can be present with either condition. Other causes of septal thickening include pulmonary venous obstruction, storage diseases and amyloidosis, as well as lymphatic and lymphoproliferative disorders. Septal thickening can also be a secondary finding in patients with infection and pulmonary hemorrhage.

Discussion

Although the diagnosis of congestive heart failure is usually made on the basis of typical clinical and radiographic findings, occasionally patients with unsuspected congestive heart failure are imaged with HRCT of the chest in search of a cause of dyspnea. Hydrostatic edema is also an occasional incidental finding in patients who are being scanned for other purposes. Thus, it is important to be aware of the typical HRCT features of hydrostatic edema.

On CT of patients with hydrostatic edema (Fig. 94.1), a combination of ground-glass opacity, smoothly thickened septal lines, peribronchovascular interstitial thickening, increased vascular caliber, and thickened fissures may be present. Small pleural effusions, often on the right, are also often present. Signs of fibrosis such as honeycombing, traction bronchiectasis, and architectural distortion are absent. Interestingly, patients with acute congestive heart failure have also been reported to have occasionally enlarged mediastinal lymph nodes which are edematous and haziness of the mediastinal fat also caused by edema.

Correlation between imaging findings and clinical data is usually sufficient to confirm the diagnosis. When the diagnosis is in doubt clinically, a follow-up study after diuresis is occasionally helpful to confirm resolution of abnormalities and to exclude chronic interstitial lung disease.

REFERENCES
Storto ML, Kee ST, Golden JA, Webb WR. Hydrostatic pulmonary edema: high-resolution CT findings. *AJR Am J Roentgenol*. 1995;165:817–820.
Thoracic Radiology: The Requisites, 3rd ed., pp. 226–237.

CASE 95

Internal Mammary Lymph Node Enlargement

1. **B and C**. Lymphoma and breast carcinoma are common causes of internal mammary lymphadenopathy. Aortic coarctation can cause enlargement of the internal mammary (thoracic) vessels, resulting in a lobulated retrosternal opacity. However, the aorta is normal in this patient, and aortic coarctation would not account for anterior mediastinal abnormality. Although lymphadenopathy is a common manifestation of tuberculosis, involvement of the internal mammary lymph nodes is uncommon in the absence of disseminated disease.

2. **B**. Ipsilateral axillary lymph nodes are the most common site of lymph node metastases in patients with breast carcinoma. Internal mammary lymph nodes are a common site of lymph node metastases in breast cancer, but they are not the most common. Hilar and mediastinal lymph nodes are less-common sites of lymph node metastases from breast carcinoma.

3. **B**. Internal mammary lymph nodes are apparent on the lateral chest radiograph only when they are quite large.

4. **C.** Primary mediastinal lymphoma, which is confined to the anterior mediastinum, is most commonly diffuse large B cell lymphoma (also referred to as *Primary mediastinal B cell lymphoma*). This is a relatively recently described tumor which can closely resemble Hodgkin disease. Classical Hodgkin lymphoma can occur in the anterior mediastinum but is less common. Follicular lymphoma less commonly is isolated to the anterior mediastinum. Small lymphocytic lymphoma is usually systemic affecting the spleen and multiple lymph node stations throughout the body.

Comment

Differential Diagnosis

The lateral radiograph (Fig. 95.1) shows a lobulated opacity filling the retrosternal clear space. Contrast-enhanced computed tomography (CT) image (Fig. 95.2) shows bilateral internal mammary lymphadenopathy and a soft tissue mass in the anterior mediastinum. Although breast carcinoma metastases are the most common cause of internal mammary lymphadenopathy, lymphoma would be more common in this male patient.

Discussion

Enlarged internal mammary lymph nodes are generally not visible on chest radiographs until they are considerably enlarged. On a posteroanterior (PA) chest radiograph of a patient with enlarged internal mammary nodes, a focal parasternal opacity, which is usually seen at the level of the first three intercostal spaces and less commonly at the fourth or fifth level, may be present. On a lateral radiograph, a lobulated retrosternal opacity may be present, as in this case. A lobulated retrosternal opacity may also be present in patients with dilated internal mammary vessels. For example, coarctation of the aorta is associated with collateral internal mammary arteries, and superior vena cava obstruction is associated with collateral internal mammary veins. The former is associated with a characteristic appearance of the aorta and occasional rib notching, and the latter is usually associated with a large mass in the right paratracheal region.

REFERENCES

Sharma A, Fidias P, Hayman LA, et al. Patterns of lymphadenopathy in thoracic malignancies. *Radiographics*. 2004;24:419–434.

Thoracic Radiology: The Requisites, 3rd ed., pp. 97–136.

CASE 96

CT-Guided Transthoracic Needle Biopsy Procedure

1. **B.** Emphysema is the greatest risk factor for developing pneumothorax following transthoracic needle biopsy of the lung. Approximately 50% of patients with emphysema will develop pneumothorax following biopsy in contrast to approximately 20% to 30% of patients without emphysema. Older age and lower lobe location do not significantly affect pneumothorax rate. Biopsy of subpleural lesions is less likely to result in pneumothorax because the needle may not pass through aerated lung.

2. **D.** The sensitivity of transthoracic needle biopsy for malignant lesions is greater than 90%. There is no significant difference between core needle biopsy and fine needle aspiration in most cancers. However non-solid nodules have a higher yield with core needle biopsies.

3. **B.** Up to 30% of patients undergoing transthoracic needle biopsy will develop a pneumothorax. Most pneumothoraces resolve without treatment. Mild perilesional hemorrhage

is common, but hemoptysis only occurs in up to 10% of patients. Air embolism and biopsy track seeding with tumor cells are extremely rare complications.

4. **C.** Use of a cutting needle for core needle biopsy improves the diagnostic yield of transthoracic needle biopsy (TTNB) for a specific benign diagnosis. Increasing volume of aspirate will not likely improve the diagnostic yield of TTNB for a benign lesion. On-site cytopathology can be useful for improving the diagnostic yield of fine needle aspiration for malignant lesions. However, establishing a benign diagnosis based on fine-needle aspiration alone can be very difficult. Use of CT fluoroscopy does not improve the diagnostic yield of TTNB for benign lesions.

Comment

The CT image (Fig. 96.1) shows a TTNB procedure. The CT image confirms the intralesional location of the biopsy needle.

Regarding planning a TTNB procedure, a prebiopsy CT scan should be obtained. The shortest, most vertical route should be chosen, and the path of the needle should avoid interlobar fissures, pulmonary vessels, bullae, and areas of severe emphysema.

TTNB is a relatively safe and accurate procedure for obtaining biopsy specimens of lung nodules and masses. The sensitivity for malignant nodules is greater than 90%, and the accuracy for differentiating among various cell types of lung cancer is roughly 80%. A major limitation of TTNB using fine-needle aspiration is a relatively low sensitivity (10%–40%) for making a specific benign diagnosis. However, this can be significantly improved by using core needle biopsy devices. Such devices provide histologic specimens, which improve the accuracy of diagnosing benign entities such as granulomas, hamartomas, and organizing pneumonia.

It is important to remember that a biopsy for negative malignancy is not diagnostic unless a specific benign diagnosis has been established. Indeed, about 30% of lesions with nonspecific negative biopsy results ultimately prove to be malignant. Thus, when faced with nonspecific negative biopsy result, one should consider repeating the biopsy with a core needle biopsy. Alternatively, with on-site cytopathology, FNA can be performed through a guide needle, and if the FNA specimen is insufficient, core needle biopsy can be formed at the same time. With the increasing importance of molecular markers for cancer diagnosis and treatment, core needle biopsy becomes more important for tissue sampling. Core needle biopsy is also recommended for biopsy of lesions with a suspected diagnosis of lymphoma to provide sufficient tissue for classification of lymphoma.

REFERENCES

Cham MD, Lane ME, Henschke CI, Yankelevitz DF. Lung biopsy: special techniques. *Semin Respir Crit Care Med*. 2008;Aug;29(4):335–349.

Thoracic Radiology: The Requisites, 3rd ed., pp. 460–472.

CASE 97

Bronchial Atresia

1. **A and C.** Pulmonary carcinoids can grow in a bronchial lumen and result in mucoid impaction and a bronchocele (a circumscribed dilation of a bronchus). Typically, an endobronchial mass expanding the airway is visible. Bronchial atresia can result in mucoid impaction and bronchocele formation. Constrictive bronchiolitis affects the small airways and results in diffuse or heterogeneous low-attenuation lung from air trapping. This is present in the upper lobe in this case, but constrictive bronchiolitis is not associated with a bronchocele. Lung abscesses are typically round and contain liquid with

or without gas. A lung abscess would not explain the adjacent hyperlucency and the walls of abscesses are usually thick.

2. **D**. Air can enter lung distal to an obstruction through the canals of Lambert and pores of Kohn. Bronchopleural fistula results in air entering the pleural space from adjacent, usually inflamed, or necrotic, lung. An anomalous bronchus usually does not provide aeration to lung distal to a mucocele.

3. **A**. The left upper lobe, especially the apicoposterior segment, is the most common site of bronchial atresia. However, bronchial atresia can affect any lobe and rarely can be multi-segmental or multilobar.

4. **C**. Most patients with bronchial atresia require no treatment. Resection is rarely indicated. There is no role for endobronchial therapy.

Comment

Differential Diagnosis

Axial and coronal (Figs. 97.1 and 97.2) computed tomography (CT) images show a tubular structure in the left upper lobe containing an air-fluid level. The part of the lung supplied by this bronchus is hyperlucent due to air trapping. This appearance is most consistent with bronchial atresia. Endobronchial neoplasms can also cause bronchocele formation. The differential diagnosis of bronchial atresia (BA) includes other causes of mucoid impaction including allergic bronchopulmonary aspergillosis (ABPA), benign and malignant endobronchial tumors (carcinoid, or rarely lung cancer), cystic bronchiectasis related to previous infection, and tuberculous bronchostenosis.

Discussion

BA is a rare and benign condition characterized by focal atresia of a segmental, subsegmental, or lobar bronchus. The left upper lobe, especially the apicoposterior segment, is most commonly involved. The airways distal to the point of atresia are normal but the obstruction to proximal drainage causes accumulation of mucus distal to the point of atresia, with resultant mucoid impaction and formation of a bronchocele. An important associated feature is hyperinflation of the distal lung parenchyma through collateral air drift and air trapping. BA manifests radiologically as a round, ovoid, or branching structure (bronchocele filled with mucus) associated with distal hyperinflation, but it may be overlooked on the chest radiograph. Although its imaging features are characteristic, BA is commonly misdiagnosed, often mistaken for an arteriovenous malformation. Because most cases of BA do not require surgical resection, recognition of its characteristic imaging features is essential for conservative management.

REFERENCES

Kinsella D, Sissons G, Williams MP. The radiological imaging of bronchial atresia. *Br J Radiol*. 1992;65:681–685.

Biyyam D, Chapman T, Ferguson M, et al. Congenital lung abnormalities: embryologic features, prenatal diagnosis, and postnatal radiologic-pathologic correlation. *Radiographics*. 2010;30:1721–1738.

Thoracic Radiology: The Requisites, 3rd ed., pp. 193–209.

CASE 98

Hypersensitivity Pneumonitis

1. **C and D**. The differential diagnosis for ground-glass attenuation centrilobular nodules is primarily hypersensitivity pneumonitis (HP) and respiratory bronchiolitis. HP is much more likely given the extent of nodules and the patient's symptoms. Sarcoidosis and silicosis are characterized by the presence of well-defined nodules in a mid and upper lung predominantly. The nodules are usually solid and located in a perilymphatic distribution.

2. **B**. Both the pulmonary artery and bronchiole are in the central core of the pulmonary lobule. The pulmonary veins are not located in the central core of the pulmonary lobule but in the interlobular septa. Pulmonary lymphatics are located primarily in the interlobular septa as well as in the bronchovascular bundles.

3. **D**. Chronic eosinophilic pneumonia is not associated with cigarette smoking and often occurs in asthmatic patients. Respiratory bronchiolitis, pulmonary Langerhans cell histiocytosis, and desquamative interstitial pneumonia occur primarily in cigarette smokers.

4. **D**. Hypersensitivity pneumonitis results primarily from a cell-mediated delayed-type hypersensitivity reaction (type IV). IgE and cytotoxic antibodies do not play a significant role in the pathogenesis of hypersensitivity pneumonitis. Immune complexes play a smaller role in the pathogenesis of HP.

Comment

Differential Diagnosis

Computed tomography (CT) images (Figs. 98.1 and 98.2) show diffuse centrilobular ground-glass attenuation nodules with some areas of confluent ground-glass opacity. A few low attenuation lobules are present, suggesting a component of air trapping. The leading diagnostic consideration for a CT with this appearance is hypersensitivity pneumonitis. Respiratory bronchiolitis should be considered in a person who smokes, although the extent of ground-glass nodules is typically much less. Occasionally, infection, especially *Pneumocystis jirovecii* can have a similar appearance but confluent ground glass opacities predominate rather than ground glass nodules.

Discussion

The presence of centrilobular ground-glass nodules on computed tomography (CT) should prompt consideration of the diagnosis of nonfibrotic HP. Affected patients typically present with dyspnea and chronic cough, and the clinical picture may be confused with other forms of diffuse lung disease. Often, the radiologist is the first member of the health care team to suggest the possibility of HP, and the clinical team can then investigate the patient's environmental and occupational exposures to seek a causative antigen. Differential diagnostic considerations for centrilobular ground-glass nodules should include respiratory bronchiolitis, a disease that affects cigarette smokers, and, in the proper clinical setting, infection, including *Pneumocystis jirovecii* pneumonia, although this manifestation is less common than others. Centrilobular nodules in hypersensitivity pneumonitis usually are poorly defined and may be associated with patchy areas of ground-glass attenuation. The findings tend to predominate in the upper lung zones, and air trapping may be present on expiratory CT imaging. Treatment of subacute hypersensitivity pneumonitis consists of removing the offending antigen from the patient's environment and often prescribing corticosteroids.

REFERENCES

Hypersensitivity Pneumonitis: A Comprehensive Review. J Investig Allergol Clin Immunol. 2015;25(4):237–250

Thoracic Radiology: The Requisites, 3rd ed., pp. 355–376.

CASE 99

Solitary Pulmonary Nodule: Lung Cancer Screening

1. **A, B, and C**. A small noncalcified lung nodule could represent primary lung carcinoma, a metastasis, or a noncalcified

granuloma. Although infection (typically granulomatous, i.e., tuberculosis [TB] or fungal) can present as multiple or a solitary nodules, primary bacterial infection does not usually present as a well-defined small nodule.

2. **C.** A 7 mm solid nodule on a baseline screening scan would be classified as Lung-RADS 3 (probably benign) category. Lung-RADS 1 includes no nodules or definitely benign nodules. Lung-RADS 2 includes solid nodules at baseline <6 mm. Lung-RADS 3 includes solid nodules ≥6 mm but <8 mm. Lung-RADS 4a includes solid nodules ≥8 to <15 mm at baseline.

3. **A.** The recommended management for a Lung-RADS 3 category is a 6-month follow-up CT. FDG PET/CT is generally reserved for larger lesions, and tissue sampling is only indicated for high-risk lesions.

4. **A.** Nodules that fall in the Lung-RADS 3 category have a 1% to 2% chance of being malignant.

Comment

Differential Diagnosis

Unenhanced CT image (Fig. 99.1) shows a solid, noncalcified 7 mm nodule in the left upper lobe. Most small nodules (less than 8 mm) are benign. However, occasionally a small nodule represents a primary lung carcinoma or small metastasis.

Discussion

Lung CT Screening Reporting and Data System (Lung-RADS) is designed to standardize screening CT reporting and management. The assessment categories include descriptions of nodule morphology, nodule size, and nodule growth as well as the probability of malignancy and estimated prevalence in the screened population. Outside of lung cancer screening, the Fleischner Society recommendations for lung nodule management are most used to manage incidentally detected lung nodules. The Fleischner Society recommendations for solid nodules stratify patients based on risk for lung cancer. In contrast, the Fleischner Society recommendations for subsolid nodules do not stratify patients by risk. Because Lung-RADS was designed specifically for lung cancer screening, all patients are considered at high risk for lung cancer and stratification is based on the size and density of the nodule itself and its behavior.

REFERENCES
Lung CT Screening Reporting and Data System (Lung-RADS™) version 1.1. American College of Radiology. 2019.
MacMahon H, Naidich DP, Goo JM, Lee KS, Leung ANC, Mayo JR, Mehta AC, Ohno Y, Powell CA, Prokop M, Rubin GD, Schaefer-Prokop CM, Travis WD, Van Schil PE, Bankier AA. Guidelines for management of incidental pulmonary nodules detected on CT images: from the Fleischner Society 2017. *Radiology.* 2017;Jul;284(1):228–243.
Thoracic Radiology: The Requisites, 3rd ed., pp. 441–449.

CASE 100

Post-Intubation Tracheal Stenosis

1. **B and C.** Focal narrowing of the subglottic trachea is a complication of endotracheal intubation. Subglottic tracheal narrowing is a common complication of granulomatosis with polyangiitis (Wegener's granulomatosis). Double aortic arch can cause tracheal narrowing, but this typically occurs in a more caudad location. No right aortic arch is identified on the images provided. Mounier-Kuhn

syndrome is associated with tracheobronchomegaly and not tracheal stenosis.

2. **D.** A tracheal bronchus is not a risk factor for tracheal stenosis. Prolonged intubation, tracheostomy, and balloon cuff overdistention can all lead to tracheal stenosis.

3. **A.** Relapsing polychondritis involves only the cartilaginous portions of the trachea, sparing the posterior wall. Inflammatory bowel disease and granulomatosis with polyangiitis can result in diffuse or patchy tracheal wall thickening, including posterior membrane involvement. Amyloidosis typically involves the entire circumference and length of the trachea.

4. **D.** Hemoptysis is not a common sign of central airway stenosis. Many patients with central airway stenosis present with cough, stridor, and wheezing.

Comment

Differential Diagnosis

The axial computed tomography (CT) image (Fig. 100.1) shows narrowing of the lower cervical trachea. The coronal reformatted minimum intensity project (MinIP) (Fig. 100.2) demonstrates that the narrowing is focal and has an hour-glass shape. This is most typical of stenosis from tracheostomy or endotracheal intubation. Other causes of focal tracheal stenosis include granulomatosis with polyangiitis, inflammatory bowel disease, and other types of instrumentation.

Discussion

Tracheal stricture is the most common late complication of tracheal intubation and decannulation. In the illustrated case, the stenosis manifests as a characteristic focal, short-segment circumferential stenosis at the site of a previous intubation. Tracheal stenosis, tracheomalacia, or an ulcerative tracheoesophageal fistula can develop at the stomal site in the case of a tracheostomy, at the level of an endotracheal tube cuff, or at the site where the tip of a tracheal tube rests against the tracheal wall. Overdistention of an endotracheal tube cuff can produce pressure necrosis of the tracheal wall. Anterior angulation of an endotracheal tube can produce erosion of the tracheal wall and lead to perforation of the wall and rarely a fistula to the adjacent brachiocephalic artery; posterior angulation can result in a tracheoesophageal fistula.

Tracheal stenosis may be missed on conventional chest radiography, and a normal radiograph does not exclude the diagnosis. Multidetector CT is the imaging modality of choice and should include multiplanar and three-dimensional renderings when possible. Short-segment tracheal stenosis can be treated with resection and primary reanastomosis. Longer stenoses can require silicone stents.

REFERENCES
Lee KS, Yoon JH, Kim TK, et al. Evaluation of tracheobronchial disease with helical CT with multiplanar and three-dimensional reconstruction: correlation with bronchoscopy. *Radiographics.* 1997;17:555–567.
Thoracic Radiology: The Requisites, 3rd ed., pp. 137–158.

CASE 101

Thymic Hyperplasia

1. **A and C.** Thymoma most often has the appearance of a lobulated anterior mediastinal mass. Thymic hyperplasia can occasionally have a masslike appearance. Thymolipomas are generally quite large and contain large areas of fat

attenuation. The CT shows a heterogeneous intermediate-attenuation mass lesion, which is not typical of a thymic cyst.

2. **D**. Calcification is not a feature of normal thymus and but can be identified in thymomas or in treated lymphoma. Normal thymus has soft tissue attenuation. With aging, parts of the thymus undergo fatty replacement, and eventually the thymus is entirely replaced with fat which can be identified on CT.

3. **B**. Although myasthenia gravis is most commonly associated with thymoma, thymoma can also be seen in pure red cell aplasia. Thymic carcinomas are highly aggressive tumors and are less commonly associated with paraneoplastic syndromes than thymoma. Thymic carcinoids are most commonly associated with abnormal secretion of adrenocorticotropic hormone (ACTH) or antidiuretic hormone. Thymolipomas are generally not associated with paraneoplastic syndromes.

4. **B**. Magnetic resonance imaging (MRI) with chemical shift imaging is the most useful test for distinguishing thymic hyperplasia from thymic neoplasia because thymic hyperplasia has signal drop out on out-of-phase imaging because of fat content. FDG PET/CT and gallium scanning are not the most useful tests for distinguishing thymic hyperplasia from thymic neoplasia. Although CT is sensitive for detecting thymic mass lesions, distinguishing neoplasm from hyperplasia based on morphology alone can be difficult as illustrated in this case.

Comment

Differential Diagnosis

Contrast-enhanced CT image (Fig. 101.1) shows a homogeneous, ovoid soft tissue mass in the anterior mediastinum, most likely thymic hyperplasia, or thymic neoplasm. Further workup with axial T1 in-phase (Fig. 101.2) and out-of-phase (Fig. 101.3) MR images shows loss of signal from in-phase to out-of-phase, indicating the presence of fat in the mass, diagnostic of thymic hyperplasia.

Discussion

The normal thymus decreases in size with age as it undergoes fatty infiltration; it is visualized in less than 50% of patients older than 40 years on CT or MRI studies. The normal thymus manifests in the prevascular region of the anterior mediastinum as a bilobed homogeneous structure of soft tissue attenuation on CT. With progressive involution and fatty infiltration, it can appear speckled and lobular in configuration.

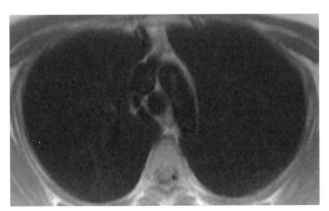

Fig. 101.2

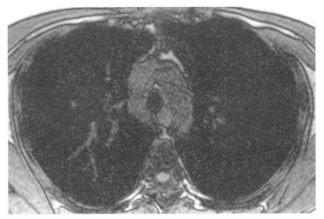

Fig. 101.3

Thymic enlargement can represent thymic hyperplasia or a thymic epithelial tumor. True thymic hyperplasia represents an increase in size and weight of the thymus with retention of its normal gross architecture and histologic appearance. Thymic hyperplasia can occur as a rebound phenomenon following chemotherapy, steroid therapy, or recovery from a severe systemic stress or insult (rebound thymic hyperplasia). Lymphoid (follicular) hyperplasia refers to a distinct entity characterized by an increased number of lymphoid follicles that is not usually associated with thymic enlargement. It is most commonly associated with myasthenia gravis, but it is also associated with autoimmune and systemic disorders including hyperthyroidism (Graves disease), acromegaly, systemic lupus erythematosus, scleroderma, rheumatoid arthritis, and cirrhosis.

Chemical shift MRI is often helpful in distinguishing thymic hyperplasia from thymoma and other thymic epithelial tumors. In this technique, comparison between in-phase and out-of-phase gradient-echo images reveal homogeneously decreased signal intensity in normal thymus and thymic hyperplasia on out-of-phase images due to diffuse fatty infiltration, as shown in this case. In contrast, thymic epithelial neoplasms usually do not exhibit this pattern. Whereas thymic hyperplasia generally requires no treatment (except for patients with myasthenia gravis, in which cases thymectomy can improve symptoms), thymic neoplasms are managed by surgical resection in most cases. Radiation therapy is often used in conjunction with surgery for invasive thymomas. Chemotherapy is typically reserved for recurrent or advanced disease.

REFERENCES

Inaoka T, Takahashi K, Mineta M, et al. Thymic hyperplasia and thymus gland tumors: differentiation with chemical shift MR imaging. *Radiology*. 2007;243:869–876.

Ackman JB, Wu CC. MRI of the thymus. *AJR Am J Roentgenol*. 2011 Jul;197(1):W15–20. https://doi.org/10.2214/AJR.10.4703.

Thoracic Radiology: The Requisites, 3rd ed., pp. 97–136.

CASE 102

Part-Solid Nodule (Lepidic Predominant Lung Adenocarcinoma)

1. **B and C**. Focal fibrosis can present as a ground-glass or mixed attenuation nodule. Additionally, lung adenocarcinoma can also present as a mixed attenuation (part solid) or ground-glass attenuation nodule. Respiratory bronchiolitis presents as multiple tiny, centrilobular ground-glass nodules in the

upper lobes. Histoplasmomas are usually large, solid nodules often with central calcification and do not have ground-glass attenuation.

2. **C.** Mixed attenuation nodules (solid and ground-glass components) are highly suggestive of lung adenocarcinoma. Most subcentimeter solid nodules are benign. Although a subcentimeter ground-glass nodule could represent a low-grade lung adenocarcinoma, other causes such as focal fibrosis, inflammation and atypical adenomatous hyperplasia are more frequent. Most calcified nodules represent the sequela of granulomatous infection, most commonly histoplasmosis and tuberculosis.

3. **A.** Lung adenocarcinoma is the most common primary type of lung cancer to manifest as ground-glass attenuation or part solid nodules. Squamous cell carcinomas are most commonly solid or cavitary, and large cell carcinomas are usually solid masses. Small cell carcinoma usually manifests with a central obstructing neoplasm, and bulky lymphadenopathy is usually present on diagnosis.

4. **B.** Current guidelines put forth by the the Fleischner Society recommend a 3 to 6 month follow up CT to see whether a part solid nodule persists and subsequent follow up CT on a yearly basis to determine if there is interval growth. The utility of FDG PET/CT for ground-glass or part-solid nodules is quite low with both poor sensitivity and specificity. Lobectomy, in general, should only be performed after the diagnosis of lung cancer is established. If the solid component exceeds 6 mm surgery may be warranted because of the likely development of invasive adenocarcinoma. Bronchoscopy is highly unlikely to provide any additional information at this time.

Comment

Differential Diagnosis

CT image (Fig. 102.1) shows a ground-glass attenuation nodule with small solid component in the left upper lobe. The differential diagnosis includes focal fibrosis, atypical adenomatous hyperplasia, low-grade lung adenocarcinoma (i.e., minimally invasive adenocarcinoma), focal organizing pneumonia, and infection.

On thin-section CT, a malignant solitary pulmonary nodule may be of soft-tissue or ground-glass attenuation, or it may be a combination of both ground-glass and solid components (part solid or mixed attenuation). Of those patterns, the mixed-attenuation solitary nodule is the most likely to be malignant, and the pure soft tissue nodule is the most likely to be benign.

A mixed-attenuation nodule with a halo of surrounding ground-glass opacity is also an imaging manifestation of invasive aspergillosis and mucormycosis, typically occurring in a severely neutropenic patient, and of cytomegalovirus, most commonly occurring 1 month or longer following organ transplantation.

Current guidelines put forth by the Fleischner Society recommend a 3 to 6 month follow up CT to assess for stability because many inflammatory nodules resolve while a low-grade malignancy will remain stable and eventually with longer term follow up manifest growth and increased solidity. Solitary solid pulmonary nodules are also variable in their border characteristics and can manifest as spiculated, ill-defined, or well-defined nodular opacities.

REFERENCES

Ko JP, Naidich DP. Current readings: radiologic interpretation of the part-solid nodule: clinical relevance and novel technologies. *Semin Thorac Cardiovasc Surg.* 2014;26(2):145–156.
MacMahon H, Naidich DP, Goo JM, Lee KS, Leung ANC, Mayo JR, Mehta AC, Ohno Y, Powell CA, Prokop M, Rubin GD, Schaefer-Prokop CM, Travis WD, Van Schil PE, Bankier AA. Guidelines for management of incidental pulmonary nodules detected on CT images: from the Fleischner Society 2017. *Radiology.* 2017 Jul;284(1):228–243.
Thoracic Radiology: The Requisites, 3rd ed., pp. 428–440.

Challenge

CASE 103

Pulmonary Alveolar Proteinosis

1. **A, B, C, D, and E.** The differential diagnosis for the imaging pattern includes acute and chronic conditions, all of which as listed.
2. **E.** The history indicated a chronic cough in this patient, implying the imaging abnormality may have existed for some time. Of the choices, most have acute presentations, whereas pulmonary alveolar proteinosis is most likely to have a protracted course.
3. **B.** The crazy-paving pattern indicates the presence of ground-glass opacity with superimposed interlobular septal thickening, giving the appearance of sidewalk or patio pavers. Signet ring sign is evoked in the setting of bronchiectasis. Comet tail sign is a manifestation of rounded atelectasis. CT halo refers to a ground-glass opacity ring surrounding a solid nodule, typically suggestive of perilesional hemorrhage in invasive infections. Reverse CT halo sign is also known as the "atoll sign" and may manifest in organizing pneumonia, pulmonary infarct, and some types of fungal infection.
4. **C.** An essential step in forming a differential diagnosis for ground-glass opacities and crazy-paving pattern is to determine its chronicity.

Comment

Differential Diagnosis

Crazy-paving pattern (acute): edema, infection (including atypical infection with *Pneumocystis* spp), acute lung injury, diffuse alveolar damage, diffuse alveolar hemorrhage, radiation pneumonitis.

Crazy-paving pattern (chronic): nonspecific interstitial pneumonitis, eosinophilic pneumonia, organizing pneumonia, lung adenocarcinoma, lymphangitic carcinomatosis, lipoid pneumonia.

Discussion

Pulmonary alveolar proteinosis (PAP) is characterized by filling of the alveolar spaces with periodic acid-Schiff positive proteinaceous material, with little or no associated tissue reaction. Causes include autoimmune, hereditary, and secondary causes, but all result in excessive production or impaired removal of surfactant. Although most cases are autoimmune, PAP has been reported to occur in association with acute large exposures to silica (silicoproteinosis). PAP typically affects men in the fourth and fifth decades of life and often have a history of smoking. Presenting symptoms might include non-productive cough and dyspnea. Patients may develop superimposed infection with fungi or *Nocardia*.

Chest radiographic findings include chronic, often symmetric perihilar or midlung zone distribution of hazy lung opacity and faint reticulation (Fig. 103.1), occasionally with areas of consolidation. CT findings include the classic "crazy-paving" pattern, a description of interlobular septal thickening superimposed on ground-glass opacity (Fig. 103.2), which are often lobular or geographic.

Treatment is with bronchioalveolar lavage and may be repeated in cases of relapsing disease. Other treatment options are targeted to the cause, including granulocyte-macrophage colony-stimulating factor (GM-CSF), rituximab, plasmapheresis, or even lung transplantation.

REFERENCES

Frazier AA, et al. From the archives of the AFIP: pulmonary alveolar proteinosis. *RadioGraphics.* 2008;28(3):883–899.

Suzuki T, et al. Pulmonary alveolar proteinosis syndrome. *Clin Chest Med.* 2016;37(3):431–440.

Thoracic Radiology: The Requisites, 3rd ed., pp. 310–322, 343–345.

CASE 104

Allergic Bronchopulmonary Aspergillosis (ABPA)

1. **C.** The so-called *finger-in-glove* pattern is typical of ABPA wherein the dilated, mucus-filled bronchus (mucocele) manifests as a branching pattern radiating from the hilum, like that of a gloved hand. Signet ring sign is evoked in the setting of bronchiectasis. The crazy-paving pattern indicates the presence of ground-glass opacity with superimposed interlobular septal thickening, giving the appearance of sidewalk or patio pavers. CT halo refers to a ground-glass opacity ring surrounding a solid nodule, typically suggestive of perilesional hemorrhage in invasive infections. Reverse CT halo sign is also known as the "atoll sign" and may manifest in organizing pneumonia, pulmonary infarct, and some types of fungal infection.
2. **D.** ABPA is a chronic hypersensitivity response to *Aspergillus* fungus colonization. Tracheobronchial papillomatosis is the result of HPV-6 infection. *Mycobacterium tuberculosis* and *Staphylococcus aureus* are implicated in atypical and typical community-acquired pneumonia, respectively.
3. **C.** Bronchiectasis is a risk factor for ABPA, such as in cystic fibrosis.
4. **B.** Patients with ABPA typically present with chronic cough and asthma-type symptoms owing to reactive airways.

Comment

Differential Diagnosis

Cystic fibrosis, bronchial atresia, post-obstructive mucoid impaction, primary ciliary dyskinesia, congenital immunodeficiency, postinfectious or aspiration bronchiectasis.

Discussion

ABPA represents a chronic hypersensitivity response of the airways to *Aspergillus* fungus colonization. Affected patients often have a protracted history of asthma, cystic fibrosis, or other atopic condition with positive cutaneous reactivity to *Aspergillus fumigatus* antigen. Chronic cough and asthma exacerbations in association with expectoration of thick mucus plugs or hemoptysis may occur. Elevated IgE antibodies and eosinophils in the airways, mucus, and serum are typical. Treatment includes oral corticosteroids and antifungals, which may be prescribed long-term to prevent recurrent symptoms.

Diagnostic criteria include chest imaging findings typical for ABPA, including most classically upper or mid-lung distribution of predominantly central, perihilar branching tubular opacities (*finger-in-glove* pattern) representing mucus-impacted bronchi (Fig. 104.1). CT offers detailed evaluation of additional airway findings such as cystic and varicoid bronchiectasis, mucoceles (Fig. 104.2), bronchial wall thickening, tree-in-bud nodules, and air-trapping. High attenuation of impacted mucus on CT (70-100 Hounsfield unit) is caused by fungal debris, mineral deposition (iron, manganese), and desiccated mucus, a feature present in 30% of cases and highly suggestive of ABPA.

REFERENCES
Jeong YJ, et al. Eosinophilic lung diseases: a clinical, radiologic, and pathologic overview. *RadioGraphics*. 2007;27:617–639.
Milliron B, et al. Bronchiectasis: mechanisms and imaging clues of associated common and uncommon diseases. *RadioGraphics*. 2015;35:1011–1030.
Thoracic Radiology: The Requisites, 3rd ed., pp. 155.

CASE 105

Mucoid Impaction (Endobronchial Hamartoma)

1. **C**
2. **A**
3. **E**

Comment

Differential Diagnosis

Neoplasm (endobronchial hamartoma, lipoma, papilloma, lung cancer, carcinoid tumor, metastases), broncholithiasis, foreign body, allergic bronchopulmonary aspergillosis, cystic fibrosis, bronchial atresia.

Discussion

Mucoid impaction refers to filling of bronchi with normal secretions and may affect large or small airways. Many causes of mucoid impaction are related to infection or inflammation, such as in cystic fibrosis wherein bronchiectatic airways become filled with bronchial secretions and often superinfected due to poor mucociliary clearance. Other causes may be a result of proximal bronchial obstruction the natural movement of mucus from the bronchi via the mucociliary elevator mechanism. Causes of obstruction include benign and malignant etiologies ranging from foreign body aspiration to lung cancer. Congenital causes of mucoid impaction include bronchial atresia. Endobronchial hamartoma is an uncommon benign tumor. Clinical features include cough, dyspnea, hemoptysis, and recurrent pneumonia.

In the acute setting, alveoli distal to the obstruction tend to become hyperinflated due to collateral ventilation through Pores of Kohn and Canals of Lambert. However, chronic obstruction will lead to resorptive (obstructive) atelectasis and, with more proximal obstruction, lobar or whole lung collapse. Endobronchial obstruction usually results in lobar collapse. Thus, when typical patterns of lobar atelectasis are encountered, especially in the outpatient setting, a centrally obstructing lesion must be assumed and further interrogated with CT and bronchoscopy.

Radiographic features include secondary signs such as the finger-in-glove sign, whereby occluded and mucus-filled bronchi become more radiopaque and manifest with tubular branching opacities radiating from the hilum. Alternatively, in lobar atelectasis, typical patterns of lobar collapse will be seen depending on which lobar bronchus is occluded (Fig. 105.1). CT features of mucoid impaction include branching tubular opacities representing the bronchi filled with mucus (Fig. 105.2). The collapsed lobe will typically enhance homogenously around the impacted bronchi differentiating the consolidation from pneumonia. The endobronchial tumor can be better characterized on CT, highlighting soft tissue, fat, and calcification in the setting of hamartomas. Malignant causes of bronchial obstruction must be excluded.

REFERENCES
Martínez-Jiménez S, et al. Mucoid impactions: finger-in-glove sign and other CT and radiographic features. *RadioGraphics*. 2008;28:1369–1382.
Thoracic Radiology: The Requisites, 3rd ed., pp. 50–59.

CASE 106

Solitary Fibrous Tumor of the Pleura

1. **B**. The axial contrast-enhanced computed tomography (CT) image (Fig. 106.1) shows an enhancing circumscribed mass arising from the pleura. Note the obtuse angles formed between the mass and the pleural interface. Also note some trace pleural fluid outlining the medial aspect of the lesion, confirming its pleural location. The extrapleural intercostal fat is not effaced.
2. **B**. Lesions that form an obtuse angle with the lung parenchyma are typically of pleural origin. Conversely, those that form acute angles with the lung interface are more likely to have arisen from the lung proper. Chest wall and rib invasion can be seen with any aggressive tumor, whether from lung, pleura, or chest wall structures.
3. **E**. Solitary fibrous tumors of the pleura can produce paraneoplastic syndromes that may include digital clubbing, hypertrophic osteoarthropathy, or hypoglycemia.
4. **D**. Typical MRI signal characteristics of solitary fibrous tumors include low-to-intermediate signal intensity on T1- and T2-weighted images with slow progressive enhancement curves, reflecting their fibrous histology (Fig. 106.2).

Comment

Differential Diagnosis

Pleural metastasis, primary pleural mesothelioma, chest wall lesion, thymoma with drop metastasis, neurogenic tumor, primary lung cancer.

Discussion

Solitary (localized) fibrous tumor of the pleura is an uncommon mesenchymal neoplasm of unknown etiology. Most are benign neoplasms comprised of low-grade spindle-shaped cells embedded in various amounts of collagen; 12% exhibit malignant histology. Up to 80% of tumors originate from the visceral pleura and up to 50% may arise from a stalk or pedicle, making them potentially mobile and at risk for torsion. Patients may present at any age, more than half with symptoms (dyspnea, cough, chest pain), especially with larger tumors. Less commonly, patients may present with paraneoplastic signs that may include digital clubbing, hypertrophic osteoarthropathy, or hypoglycemia that resolves after resection. Even tumors of benign histology may recur, often decades after resection, so long-term imaging surveillance is recommended.

Radiographic features depend on the size of the lesion, but typically include a peripheral nodule or mass. Given the pleural location, they may manifest the *incomplete border sign*, wherein a well-defined interface is formed by the part of the tumor in contact with lung and an indistinct margin is formed by the side of the tumor adjacent to the parietal pleura and chest wall. CT features typically include a well-defined intermediate-to-high attenuation, homogenous mass forming obtuse angles with the adjacent pleura. However, larger tumors may be more heterogeneous in attenuation depending on their degree of necrosis, hemorrhage, or calcification. Compressive atelectasis on the adjacent lung is typical.

Pleural effusions are associated in 30% of cases. Large lesion size, heterogeneity, and pleural effusions may be predictive of malignancy. MRI is a helpful tool to better characterize tissue properties, assess for local invasion, and differentiate pleural effusion from tumor. Typical MRI signal characteristics of benign solitary fibrous tumors include low-to-intermediate signal intensity on T1- and T2-weighted images reflecting the fibrous histology. Progressive dynamic contrast enhancement patterns are typical of fibrous tumors. In the absence of frank invasive features, MRI cannot reliably differentiate benign from malignant fibrous tumors, which must be determined after surgical resection.

REFERENCES

Ginat DT, et al. Imaging features of solitary fibrous tumors. *AJR Am J Roentgenol.* 2011;196(3):487–495.
Thoracic Radiology: The Requisites, 3rd ed., pp. 168–172.

CASE 107

Complete Lung Collapse Secondary to an Endobronchial Lesion (Lung Cancer)

1. **C**
2. **D**
3. **C**
4. **A, B, C, D, and E**

Comment

Differential Diagnosis

Neoplasm (endobronchial hamartoma, lipoma, papilloma, lung cancer, carcinoid tumor, metastases); broncholithiasis; foreign body; aspirated mucus plug; pneumonectomy; pneumonia; pleural disease (large pleural effusion, hemothorax, infusothorax, chylothorax, empyema, pleural metastases, malignant mesothelioma, large fibrous tumor of the pleura); large diaphragmatic hernia; pulmonary agenesis.

Discussion

Resorptive atelectasis occurs when communication between airways and alveoli is obstructed. Alveolar gas diffuses across the alveolar-capillary membrane but cannot be replaced by inspired air. Various patterns of segmental, lobar, or complete lung atelectasis depends on the level of obstruction along the tracheobronchial tree. Causes may be endoluminal or extrinsic compression of the bronchi (lymphadenopathy, masses, vasculature.) Lobar or complete lung collapse occurring in the outpatient setting should prompt suspicion for a centrally obstructing lesion and further interrogated with CT and bronchoscopy should be pursued.

Direct radiographic signs of atelectasis (fissural displacement and bronchovascular crowding) are less reliable in complete lung collapse (Fig. 107.1). Therefore indirect signs of increased lung opacity, ipsilateral tracheal and mediastinal shift, contralateral lung compensatory hyperinflation, and elevation of the ipsilateral hemidiaphragm must be sought. On CT (Fig. 107.2), the collapsed lung will typically enhance homogenously assuming the tumor has not compromised pulmonary arteries. Preservation of enhanced vessels in the atelectatic lung is known as the *CT angiogram sign* (Fig. 107.3). The endobronchial tumor can be better characterized on CT, highlighting soft tissue and mediastinal invasion.

The differential diagnosis for complete hemithorax opacification includes complete lung collapse; pneumonectomy; pneumonia; large pleural effusion, hemothorax, infusothorax, chylothorax or empyema; pleural metastases; malignant mesothelioma; large fibrous tumor of the pleura; large diaphragmatic hernia; and pulmonary agenesis. Pleural abnormalities should generally cause mass effect rather than volume loss. Lung volume is typically preserved in the setting of pneumonia. Clinical history and CT findings are valuable in distinguishing other potential etiologies.

REFERENCES

Detterbeck FC, et al. The eight edition lung cancer stage classification. *Chest.* 2017;151(1):193–203.
Carter BW, et al. Revisions to the TNM staging of lung cancer: rationale, significance, and clinical application. *RadioGraphics.* 2018;38:374–391.
Thoracic Radiology: The Requisites, 3rd ed., pp. 48–49, 453–455.

CASE 108

Mycobacterium avium complex (MAC) infection

1. **B**
2. **D**
3. **B**

Comment

Differential Diagnosis

Tuberculosis, other cavitary or airway-centric infection (fungal, nocardia, etc.), aspiration, cystic fibrosis, lung cancer.

Discussion

Nontuberculous mycobacteria (NTM) represent a ubiquitous species which comprise more than 100 organisms. MAC and *Mycobacterium kansasii* are the most commonly encountered human pathogens of this species, often colonizing airways. Careful synthesis of clinical, radiographic, and microbiologic findings is required for diagnosis, which would ultimately prompt a prolonged course of empirical antibiotics which may carry serious side effects. Therefore, accurate diagnosis and appropriate selection of patients for treatment (symptomatic or progressive disease) is paramount.

NTM infection is divided into cavitary (classic) and bronchiectatic (non-classic) forms. However, nodular (deglutition), hypersensitivity (hot tub lung), and immunocompromised host forms may also be encountered. Classic NTM pattern tends to affect older men with preexisting lung disease (e.g., emphysema) and may mimic cavitary tuberculosis. Non-classic NTM pattern typically affects thin, older women without preexisting lung disease. The term *Lady Windermere syndrome* has been applied historically to refer to non-classic NTM pattern in elderly women who might have suppressed their cough.

Imaging manifestations depend on the NTM form. Classic NTM pattern manifests radiographically as upper lung zone cavities with volume loss and surrounding nodular opacities indicating endobronchial disease. Fibrothorax may manifest as pleural thickening. Radiographic findings may be subtle in patients with early disease. In the non-classic form, radiographs may show cylindrical or cystic bronchiectasis with nodules, most commonly affecting the lingula and right middle lobe. Radiographically occult cavities are better demonstrated with CT as is airway involvement. Bronchiectasis may or may not be present in the classic form but is a predominant feature of non-classic NTM pattern. Nodules suggested on radiographs are more clearly defined with CT including centrilobular nodules and tree-in-bud opacities (Fig. 108.1). Multifocal consolidations may occasionally be present.

REFERENCES
Martínez-Jiménez S, et al. The many faces of pulmonary nontuberculous mycobacterial infection. *AJR Am J Roentgenol.* 2007;189(1):177–186.
Thoracic Radiology: The Requisites, 3rd ed., p. 333.

CASE 109

Sarcoidosis (Perilymphatic Nodules)

1. **D**. Perilymphatic distribution of nodules includes involvement of the peripheral (subpleural/interlobular septal) and axial (peribronchovascular) lymphatics. Note the beaded appearance of several vascular structures in the right upper lobe on the coronal CT image. The sagittal CT image shows well the nodular studding of the subpleural lymphatics, including along the right major fissure.
2. **A, B, C, and D**. All of the choices *except* E may manifest with perilymphatic nodules. Miliary tuberculosis manifests as innumerable randomly distributed micronodules.
3. **D**. The galaxy sign refers to the CT appearance of coalescent nodules to form a more discrete nodule or mass with nodular radiating lines and surrounding smaller nodules, like images of galaxies in space. Comet tail sign is associated with rounded atelectasis. Mosaic attenuation refers to geographic areas of lucent and ground-glass lung attenuation. Reverse CT halo sign is associated with organizing pneumonia and occasionally pulmonary infarct.
4. **A**. Most patients with sarcoidosis have no symptoms. Whereas others may present with dry cough, weight loss, neurologic symptoms, or other systemic manifestations in the setting of Lofgren syndrome (erythema nodosum, polyarthritis, and fever) or Heerfordt syndrome (fever, parotid enlargement, facial palsy, and uveitis).

Comment

Differential Diagnosis

Pneumoconiosis (silicosis, coal worker's pneumoconiosis, berylliosis), lymphangitic carcinomatosis, immunoglobulin G4 (IgG4)-related lung disease, alveoloseptal amyloidosis, lymphoma, Kaposi sarcoma.

Discussion

Sarcoidosis is an idiopathic multisystem disorder characterized by non-caseating granulomas, which typically affects younger adults (age <40) and women twice as often as men. Over 50% of patients are asymptomatic despite more than 90% having chest radiographic abnormalities.

Pulmonary abnormalities are present radiographically in about 60% of patients whether in conjunction with hilar disease (Stage II), isolated to the parenchyma (Stage III), or in the setting of end-stage fibrosis (Stage IV). Parenchymal involvement manifests as a reticulonodular pattern in an upper lung zone distribution. *Perilymphatic* distribution of nodules is characteristic of sarcoidosis and refers to simultaneous localization of non-caseating granulomas within the axial (peribronchovascular/centrilobular) and peripheral (interlobular septal/subpleural) interstitium (Figs. 109.1 and 109.2). Nodules tend to radiate peripherally from the hila in the axial distribution and stud along pleural or fissural surfaces in the peripheral distribution. However, nodular septal thickening is typically to a lesser degree than that seen in lymphangitic carcinomatosis. Micronodules may coalesce to form larger discrete nodules or masses

with or without air bronchograms (alveolar sarcoid) and may exhibit radiating lines and smaller nodules (CT galaxy sign). Conglomeration of granulomas along the subpleural interstitium may produce *pseudoplaques* and mimic pleural plaques of asbestos-related pleural disease.

REFERENCES
Nakatsu M, et al. Large coalescent parenchymal nodules in pulmonary sarcoidosis "sarcoid galaxy" sign. *AJR Am J Roentgenol.* 2002;178:1389–1393.
Criado E, et al. Pulmonary sarcoidosis: typical and atypical manifestations at high-resolution CT with pathologic correlation. *RadioGraphics.* 2010;30(6):1567–1586.
Little BP. Sarcoidosis: overview of pulmonary manifestations and imaging. *Semin Roentgenol.* 2015 Jan;50(1):52–64.
Thoracic Radiology: The Requisites, 3rd ed., pp. 335–350, 365–366.

CASE 110

Small Airways Disease (Infectious Bronchiolitis)

1. **C**
2. **C and D**
3. **A**

Comment

Differential Diagnosis

Infectious bronchiolitis (bacterial, mycobacterial, fungal, viral), aspiration bronchiolitis, follicular bronchiolitis, diffuse panbronchiolitis, sarcoidosis, bronchiectasis (cystic fibrosis, allergic bronchopulmonary aspergillosis, immotile cilia syndrome), vascular tree-in-bud pattern (e.g., excipient lung disease, intravascular metastases).

Discussion

Infectious bronchiolitis is the most common cause of bronchiolitis because of a wide variety of pathogens, including bacteria (typical and atypical), viruses (respiratory syncytial virus, adenovirus), and fungi. Immunocompromised patients are at particular risk for atypical infections by viruses, fungi, and other atypical bacteria such as *Chlamydia* and mycobacteria. The most common manifestations of infectious bronchiolitis on CT are centrilobular nonbranching and branching (tree-in-bud) nodules (Fig. 110.1).

Normal bronchioles are usually invisible on radiography and CT given their small diameter (2 mm) and lack of a cartilaginous wall. The *tree-in-bud sign* describes the CT appearance of peripheral centrilobular bronchioles which may be impacted with cellular material or fluid (e.g., mucus, fluid, pus, aspirated material, or tumor). The tree-in-bud pattern appears as centrilobular branching V- or Y-shaped opacities, outlining the microanatomy of the secondary pulmonary lobule (bronchiole or arteriole). Tree-in-bud opacities caused by infection or aspiration are often clustered as opposed to diffuse. Whereas infectious bronchiolitis may occur in any craniocaudal or ventral-dorsal distribution, aspiration bronchiolitis tends to occur in dependent aspects of the lung. Associated bronchiolar dilation, mural and peribronchial inflammation can increase the conspicuity of this pattern on imaging. Bronchiolectasis may be a clue to the chronicity of small airway inflammation.

REFERENCES
Eisenhuber E. The tree-in-bud sign. *Radiology.* 2002;222:771–772.
Winningham PJ, et al. Bronchiolitis: a practical approach for the general radiologist. *RadioGraphics.* 2017;37:777–794.
Thoracic Radiology: The Requisites, 3rd ed., pp. 155–157, 340–343.

CASE 111

Mosaic Attenuation (Small Airway Disease)

1. **B and C**
2. **C and D**
3. **A**

Comment

Differential Diagnosis

Small airways disease (cellular or constrictive bronchiolitis), diffuse idiopathic pulmonary neuroendocrine cell hyperplasia (DIPNECH), pulmonary vascular disease, groundglass opacity (edema, hemorrhage, infection, diffuse alveolar damage, organizing pneumonia, hypersensitivity pneumonitis, non-specific interstitial pneumonia).

Discussion

Mosaic attenuation refers variable areas of both increased and decreased parenchymal attenuation on CT. *Air trapping* is not synonymous and instead refers to areas of lung which do not increase in attenuation as would be expected with physiologic microatelectasis during exhalation phase imaging. The transition between these areas is usually well-defined and geographic following the boundaries of secondary pulmonary lobules. Causes of mosaic attenuation pattern can include problems with the small airways (most commonly infectious bronchiolitis), pulmonary vascular disease, or parenchymal diseases associated with increased lung attenuation.

It can be difficult to determine which parts of the lung are normal and diseased, especially without the exhalation phase data. Abnormal lung can be identified when a lobe or lobule becomes more lucent and slightly expanded on exhalation phase images (air trapping) in the setting of small airways diseases. Mosaic attenuation occurring in the setting of pulmonary vascular disease (e.g., thromboembolism), areas lung may appear lucent as a result of diminished vascular perfusion. Because the airway supplying the affected segment is typically normal in these regions, exhalation should lead to microatelectasis of the alveoli, decrease in volume, and increase in relative lung attenuation. Vessel caliber within the abnormal lung segments in both airway- and vascular causes of mosaic attenuation may be altered by vasoconstriction and alone is not helpful in distinguishing between the two etiologies. Ancillary CT clues to small airways disease include bronchial wall thickening, bronchiectasis, centrilobular nodules and mucus plugging in airways supplying the lucent lung segments. Clues to vascular causes of mosaic attenuation include pulmonary arterial dilation, abrupt tapering, or corkscrew configuration (suggesting pulmonary hypertension); endovascular webs and eccentric thrombi; dilated bronchial arteries; and right ventricular hypertrophy or dilation.

REFERENCES
Kligerman SJ, et al. Mosaic attenuation: etiology, methods of differentiation, and pitfalls. *RadioGraphics*. 2015;35:1360–1380.
Thoracic Radiology: The Requisites, 3rd ed., p. 354.

CASE 112

Chronic Beryllium Disease

1. **A and C**
2. **A**
3. **A, B, C, D, and E**
4. **E**

Comment

Differential Diagnosis

Sarcoidosis, silicosis, coal worker's pneumoconiosis, chronic tuberculosis, chronic hypersensitivity pneumonitis, post-radiation change, lung cancer (progressive massive fibrosis).

Discussion

Chronic beryllium disease is a systemic granulomatous disorder that develops as a cell-mediated (type IV) hypersensitivity reaction to beryllium metal salt fumes, dust, or aerosol. The lung is the most commonly affected organ. Primary sources of occupational exposure include those working in ceramics, dentistry, aerospace, and electronics manufacturing industries (e.g., telecommunication, computers, electronics). The disorder was first described among fluorescent lamp workers in 1946. Unlike other pneumoconioses, the incidence and severity of disease are not necessarily dose-related, and extensive disease may occur with minimal exposure. Diagnosis of chronic beryllium disease requires evidence of beryllium sensitization and lung histology showing noncaseating granulomas. Beryllium sensitization occurs in 2% to 10% of patients within a few weeks of exposure and can be detected using the beryllium lymphocyte proliferation test (BeLPT), even before workers experience symptoms or have radiographic abnormalities.

The imaging features of chronic beryllium disease are indistinguishable from those found in sarcoidosis, including reticulonodular opacities, perilymphatic nodules, ground-glass opacities (early), bronchial wall thickening, and interlobular septal thickening. In advanced disease, fibrosis may develop and manifests as reticulation, honeycombing, upper lobe volume loss, architectural distortion, and paracicatricial emphysematous bullae. The fibrosis may become confluent forming consolidations and marked distortion, often retracted posteriorly and cranially, a term called *progressive massive fibrosis*. Mediastinal and hilar lymphadenopathy are seen, but less commonly than in sarcoidosis, occurring in only 25% of patients. Amorphous or egg shell patterns of lymph node calcification are characteristic, as in sarcoidosis and other pneumoconioses. Patients with rare acute beryllium disease may present with a diffuse pulmonary edema pattern suggestive of acute chemical pneumonitis that is associated with 10% mortality and risk for developing lung cancer.

REFERENCES
Cox CW, et al. State of the art: imaging of occupational lung disease. *Radiology*. 2014;270(3):681–696.
Thoracic Radiology: The Requisites, 3rd ed., pp. 386–388.

CASE 113

Chronic Eosinophilic Pneumonia

1. **A, B, C, D, and E**
2. **D**
3. **C**
4. **C**

Comment

Differential Diagnosis

Pneumonia, aspiration, simple pulmonary eosinophilia (Löffler syndrome), vasculitis (Churg-Strauss syndrome), cryptogenic organizing pneumonia, pulmonary infarcts, sarcoidosis, pulmonary alveolar proteinosis, lung adenocarcinoma.

Discussion

Chronic eosinophilic pneumonia (CEP) is an idiopathic chronic respiratory condition characterized on histopathology by infiltration of packing of alveoli with eosinophils. Patients typically present with weeks to months of smoldering dyspnea, fever, chills, night sweats, and weight loss. CEP affects women more commonly than men, occurring around the fifth decade. In 53% of patients, an association with asthma and atopy is found. Mild to moderate peripheral blood eosinophilia of at least 6% of total white cell count is typical, or bronchioalveolar lavage showing greater than 25% eosinophils. If treated, the prognosis for patients with CEP is favorable with an often dramatic clinical and radiographic response to corticosteroid treatment occurring over hours to days, respectively. However, if untreated the disease may progress to irreversible fibrosis and may be fatal.

Radiographic features include migratory peripheral consolidations characteristically distributed in apical and axillary regions (Fig. 113.1), unlike in cryptogenic organizing pneumonia which has a basal predilection. When the opacities frame the lung, the pattern may be described as *photographic negative of pulmonary edema*. Pleural effusions are less common than in acute eosinophilic lung conditions. CT shows peripheral consolidation often with areas of ground-glass opacity (Figs. 113.2 and 113.3). In some cases, the opacities in CEP may wax and wane in the exact location with identical configuration. Imaging abnormalities tend to resolve in a lateral to medial pattern, leaving bands of consolidation in parallel to the lung edge. Findings which may manifest in later stages of the disease include ground-glass opacities, crazy-paving, nodules, atelectasis, bandlike opacities, and reticulation. Half of patients will have mediastinal lymphadenopathy.

REFERENCES

Price M, et al. Imaging of eosinophilic lung disease. *Radiol Clin North Am*. 2016;54(6):1151–1161.
Thoracic Radiology: The Requisites, 3rd ed., p. 371.

CASE 114

Tracheal Diverticulum

1. **A**
2. **C**
3. **B**

Comment

Differential Diagnosis

Pneumomediastinum, apical paraseptal bullae, iatrogenic tracheal injury (intubation, endoscopy, surgery, radiation, caustic injury), tracheobronchomegaly (Mournier Kuhn Syndrome), traction diverticulum (upper lobe fibrosis), tracheal fistula, laryngocele, pharyngocele, Zenker diverticulum.

Discussion

Tracheal diverticula represent congenital or acquired foci of protruded ciliated respiratory mucosa laterally through a weakened area in the tracheal wall. Tracheal diverticulae occur on the right side in 98% of cases, most often at the T1-T2 level (4-5 cm below the vocal cords). Prevalence has been reported in up to 8% of CTs. Congenital diverticulae are more common in men, have smaller diameters and narrow connections with the tracheal lumen. They represent developmental defects in the posterior tracheal membrane or a primary defect in tracheal cartilage. Conversely, acquired diverticulae represent pseudo-diverticulae with walls lined only by respiratory mucosa (no muscle or cartilage), often larger, and have wider connection to the trachea. Most diverticulae are discovered incidentally in asymptomatic patients. However, some individuals may report signs and symptoms related to recurrent airway infections and chronic cough. Clinical history of recent iatrogenic intervention should lead the imager to consider more acute etiologies for paratracheal air, especially pneumomediastinum and tracheal rupture.

An association between tracheal diverticulae and reduced expiratory flow rates and FEV1/FVC has been described, and the presence of a tracheal diverticulum may represent an indirect sign of obstructive lung disease.

Small tracheal diverticula are often not visible on chest radiographs and are more easily identified on CT. Characteristics of tracheal diverticulae on CT include thin-walled air-containing paratracheal air sacs, with luminal connection variably seen. CT also can distinguish tracheal diverticula from other paratracheal air collections, including laryngocele, pharyngocele, Zenker diverticulum, and apical bullae.

REFERENCES

Bae HJ, et al. Paratracheal air cysts on thoracic multidetector CT: incidence, morphological characteristics and relevance to pulmonary emphysema. *Br J Radiol*. 2013;86(1021):2012–2018.
Sayit AT, et al. The diseases of airway-tracheal diverticulum: a review of the literature. *J Thorac Dis*. 2016;8(10):E1163–E1167.
Thoracic Radiology: The Requisites, 3rd ed., p. 138.

CASE 115

Sternal Dehiscence After Median Sternotomy

1. **C**
2. **C**
3. **E**
4. **E**

Comment

Discussion

Sternotomy access procedures are often required to treat cardiovascular and pulmonary pathology and have become a mainstay in thoracic surgery. Several variations on the standard alternating transsternal-peristernal wire technique include bilateral pericostal and peristernal wires (Robicsek closure), plate and screw fixation, and transverse thoracosternotomy (clam-shell), the latter preferred for lung transplantation. Complications of standard sternotomy techniques include wire fracture (2%–3%) and displacement (wire migration and sternal dehiscence), osseous non-union and fracture, infection, and hematoma. Clinical evidence for sternotomy complications are often non-specific, including no symptoms, pain, fever, sternal clicking, and wire protrusion. Risk factors for sternal dehiscence include both patient and operative factors such as obesity, diabetes, chronic obstructive pulmonary disease (COPD), osteoporosis, prolonged bypass time, sacrifice of the internal mammary artery, and reoperation.

As clinical signs and symptoms of sternal dehiscence are nonspecific, imaging plays a critical role in early detection and characterization of sternotomy complications. High mortality associated with sternotomy complications is reduced if findings are detected early, which is possible by imaging even before clinical suspicion arises. Wire fracture alone should not imply dehiscence. Wire displacement describes offset of the vertical alignment of adjacent wires. When wires pull out or cut through the sternum but remain intact, they are described as "wandering." Wires may also rotate, with alteration of the axis of orientation relative to the baseline chest radiograph. Disrupted wires appear unraveled or fractured. Rotation and unraveling of sternal wires are specific signs of dehiscence and are seen in nearly 90% of cases. Computed tomography (CT) better characterizes the sternal gap of the sternal incision and can detect early changes of osteomyelitis as well as soft tissue inflammation and fluid collections.

REFERENCES

Boiselle PM, et al. Wandering wires: frequency of sternal wire abnormalities in patients with sternal dehiscence. *AJR Am J Roentgenol.* 1999;173:777–780.

Hota P, et al. Poststernotomy complications: a multimodality review of normal and abnormal postoperative imaging findings. *AJR Am J Roentgenol.* 2018;211:1194–1205.

Thoracic Radiology: The Requisites, 3rd ed., p. 277.

CASE 116

Mediastinitis

1. **C**
2. **A, B, C, D, and E**
3. **C**

Comment

Differential Diagnosis

Mediastinal hemorrhage, postoperative seroma, fibrosing mediastinitis, diffuse lymphangiomatosis.

Discussion

Acute mediastinitis is a potentially life-threatening condition resulting from acute inflammation of mediastinal structures and the surrounding fat. Although most commonly associated with esophageal perforation, other causes may be postoperative (especially sternotomy), posttraumatic, or infectious. The latter may be from primary mediastinal inoculation or from inferior extension of head and neck disease (acute descending necrotizing mediastinitis). Patients present with high fevers, chest pain, dyspnea, and leukocytosis. Regardless of the cause, acute mediastinitis is associated with high mortality, up to 50% in some series, and requires urgent treatment.

Chest radiography may show mediastinal widening and obscuration of normal mediastinal landmarks. Mediastinal gas or air-fluid levels may be seen in the setting of abscess or gas-forming infection. Despite findings detected on radiography, contrast-enhanced CT is required for evaluation of any suspected acute mediastinal condition. Positive oral contrast material is recommended for evaluation of suspected esophageal injury. CT findings of increased mediastinal fat attenuation, loculated fluid or air collections, lymphadenopathy, pleural effusions and empyema may be seen. Similar findings may be found on magnetic resonance imaging (MRI) with increased signal in mediastinal fat on post-contrast T1- and T2 fat-suppressed sequences. Gas on MRI manifests as bubbles of signal void on all pulse sequences.

REFERENCES

Akman C, et al. Imaging in mediastinitis: a systematic review based on aetiology. *Clin Radiol.* 2004;59:573–585.

Katabathina VS, et al. Nonvascular, nontraumatic mediastinal emergencies in adults: a comprehensive review of imaging findings. *RadioGraphics.* 2011;31:1141–1160.

Thoracic Radiology: The Requisites, 3rd ed., pp. 131–132.

CASE 117

Cryptogenic Organizing Pneumonia

1. **D**. The axial CT image (lung windows) shows peripheral (subpleural) distribution of involvement. Note the irregular consolidation primarily distributed in the immediate subpleural lung.
2. **B**. The axial CT image (lung windows) shows peripherally distributed crescent rings of consolidation surrounding central regions of ground-glass opacity, compatible with the "reverse CT halo sign" or so-called "atoll" sign. The opposite pattern is found in the CT halo sign, wherein there is a central consolidation surrounded by ground-glass opacities.
3. **A**. This is a classic presentation of organizing pneumonia, a nonspecific pattern of lung injury from a variety of causes. Occasionally, the cause cannot be elicited after clinical investigation leaving the diagnosis of cryptogenic (or idiopathic) organizing pneumonia. Corticosteroids are the treatment of choice for organizing pneumonia after other etiologies are excluded.
4. **A, B, C, D, and E**. Lung involvement of the listed entities can manifest with an organizing pneumonia pattern.

Comment

Differential Diagnosis

Pneumonia, aspiration, chronic eosinophilic pneumonia, pulmonary hemorrhage, infarct, vasculitis (e.g., granulomatosis with polyangiitis), primary pulmonary lymphoma, primary lung cancer.

Discussion

Organizing pneumonia (OP) is a histologic pattern of lung injury in response to a wide variety of insults with protean imaging manifestations. Most cases are associated with an identifiable cause such as collagen vascular disease, radiation therapy, medication, aspiration, pneumonia, or organ and stem cell transplantation. In up to 70% of cases, no specific etiology can be determined, and the term *cryptogenic* OP (formerly bronchiolitis obliterans with OP) is applied. Cryptogenic OP is considered a distinct entity among the idiopathic interstitial pneumonias, albeit a predominantly airspace process with some component of interstitial inflammation. Histologically, OP is characterized by peribronchiolar and intra-alveolar plugs composed of fibroblasts and myofibroblasts embedded in a matrix of type III collagen and other glycoproteins. Importantly, the underlying alveolar septal architecture is preserved. Cryptogenic OP has a good response to corticosteroid therapy, although relapses are common. A subset of patients may progress from OP to lung fibrosis despite treatment (often a non-specific interstitial pneumonia pattern), portending a poorer prognosis.

No histopathologic or imaging features can distinguish cryptogenic from secondary forms of OP. Focal or multifocal consolidation with or without air bronchograms are the most common findings on radiography and CT. Air bronchograms represent transient dilation of small airways within the consolidations. Most patients (60%–90%) present with diffuse parenchymal abnormality, usually in a peripheral or bronchocentric distribution, often affecting the lower lung zones. Temporally, opacities may be migratory or spontaneously regress. A perilobular pattern may be seen in up to 57% of cases, consisting of polygonal opacities that border the secondary pulmonary lobule, with or without septal thickening that correspond histologically to dilated lymphatics and accumulation of organizing tissue and fibrosis along the periphery of the pulmonary lobule. Although non-specific, a classic CT finding associated with OP is the *reversed CT halo (atoll) sign*, described as a crescent or ring of consolidation that surrounds a central region of ground-glass opacity.

REFERENCES

Kligerman SJ, et al. Organizing and fibrosis as a response to lung injury in diffuse alveolar damage, organizing pneumonia, and acute fibrinous and organizing pneumonia. *RadioGraphics.* 2013;33:1951–1975.
Torreaba JR, et al. Pathology-radiology correlation of common and uncommon computed tomographic patterns of organizing pneumonia. *Hum Pathol.* 2018;71:30–40.
Thoracic Radiology: The Requisites, 3rd ed., pp. 357–358.

CASE 118

Tracheobronchial Amyloidosis

1. **A, B, and D**
2. **A**
3. **A**
4. **A**

Comment

Differential Diagnosis

Acquired tracheal stenosis, broncholith, foreign body, tracheobronchopathia osteochondroplastica, granulomatosis with polyangiitis, sarcoidosis, relapsing polychondritis, tracheal neoplasm (hamartoma, carcinoid, adenoid cystic carcinoma, mucoepidermoid carcinoma, squamous cell carcinoma, primary lung carcinoma, metastasis), tracheobronchial papillomatosis, infection (tuberculosis [TB], Histoplasma, Aspergillus, Klebsiella rhinoscleromatis).

Discussion

Amyloidosis is a systemic disorder characterized by deposition of insoluble amyloid fibrils in tissues. Accumulation of these fibrils within the submucosal of the airway disrupt its normal architecture forming endoluminal calcified or ossified masses. Diffuse or multifocal airway involvement is common in systemic amyloidosis, but usually does not cause symptoms. Any portion of the tracheobronchial tract may be involved. Amyloid nodules may lead to airway obstruction and air-trapping, which can progress to respiratory distress and post-obstructive pneumonia. Chronic irritation and damage to the submucosa over time may predispose to hemoptysis.

CT features of the affected airways demonstrate focal and nodular or diffuse contiguous narrowing of the central airways. Unlike in relapsing polychondritis and tracheobronchopathia osteochondroplastica, the posterior membrane of the airway is typically involved. Focal amyloid deposits may enhance after intravenous contrast administration. Treatment options include debridement, laser ablation, balloon dilation, stent placement, and resection.

REFERENCES

Aylwin AC, et al. Imaging appearance of thoracic amyloidosis. *J Thorac Imaging.* 2005;20(1):41–46.
Ngo AH, et al. Tumors and tumorlike conditions of the large airways. *AJR Am J Roentgenol.* 2013;201:301–313.
Thoracic Radiology: The Requisites, 3rd ed., pp. 142–143.

CASE 119

Constrictive Bronchiolitis (Swyer-James-MacLeod Syndrome)

1. **A, B, C, D, and E**
2. **C**
3. **B**
4. **B**

Comment

Differential Diagnosis

Technical (rotated patient position), chest wall abnormalities (mastectomy, Poland syndrome), compensatory overinflation (lobectomy), pneumothorax, bullae, asthma, bronchiectasis (cystic fibrosis, primary ciliary dyskinesia, immunodeficiency syndromes), endobronchial obstruction (aspirated material, foreign body, broncholith, tumor), congenital (pulmonary underdevelopment spectrum, congenital lobar emphysema, bronchial atresia, hypogenetic lung syndrome), pulmonary vascular disorders (proximal interruption of pulmonary artery, chronic thromboembolic disease, fibrosing mediastinitis).

Discussion

Constrictive bronchiolitis is characterized by bronchiolar submucosal fibrosis as a result of damage to the respiratory epithelium leading to concentric luminal narrowing and occlusion. Causes include previous infection, toxic inhalation, lung transplant rejection, graft-versus-host disease in stem cell transplant recipients, connective tissue disease, and diffuse idiopathic neuroendocrine cell hyperplasia (DIPNECH).

Swyer-James-MacLeod syndrome is a variant of post-infectious constrictive bronchiolitis as sequela of a remote childhood viral respiratory infection. Infection before the age of alveolar maturation (around 8 years) impairs development of alveoli and pulmonary vessels. Most patients are asymptomatic but may present with progressive dyspnea and cough, with non-reversible obstructive ventilatory defects.

Chest radiographs classically demonstrate a hyperlucent lung because of decreased vascularity with normal to slightly decreased volume. On computed tomography (CT), typical findings include bronchiectasis and mosaic attenuation, with areas of diminished vascularity within areas of lucent lung and accentuation of the lucency on expiratory images (air trapping). Although radiographic findings of Swyer-James-MacLeod syndrome tend to be unilateral, CT will often reveal asymmetric bilateral lung involvement.

REFERENCES

Nemec SF, et al. Pulmonary hyperlucency in adults. *AJR Am J Roentgenol.* 2013;200:W101–113.
Mosquera RA, et al. Dysanaptic growth of lung and airway in children with post-infectious bronchiolitis. *Clin Respir J.* 2014;8(1):63–71.
Thoracic Radiology: The Requisites, 3rd ed., pp. 391–404.

CASE 120

Metastasizing Leiomyomatosis

1. **C**
2. **D**
3. **A**

Comment

Differential Diagnosis

Hematogenous metastases, miliary infection (tuberculosis [TB], fungal, bacille Calmette-Guerin [BCG] *Mycobacterium bovis*), Langerhans cell histiocytosis, sarcoidosis.

Discussion

The anatomic distribution of multiple pulmonary nodules on chest radiography and CT provides an important clue to the differential diagnosis. A diffuse random distribution of nodules implies that nodules involve all parts of the secondary pulmonary lobule (centrilobular and acinar) and interstitium (peribronchovascular, septal, subpleural). Random nodules are typically bilateral and symmetric, and may have upper, lower, or diffuse craniocaudal distribution. Generally, this pattern should evoke the possibility of hematogenous metastases or disseminated (miliary) tuberculosis or fungal infection. Occasionally, a pulmonary vessel may be found coursing to the nodule (*feeding vessel sign*), implying its vascular route of distribution.

Metastasizing leiomyomatosis is a rare entity that may occur in women with a remote history of uterine leiomyoma and hysterectomy. The lung is the most common site of extrauterine involvement. Most patients are asymptomatic, often being diagnosed decades after hysterectomy when diffuse pulmonary nodules are revealed on imaging studies. Pulmonary lesions represent well-differentiated leiomyomas, ranging in size from subcentimeter nodules to masses (≥3 cm). Less common patterns include miliary and cavitary nodules. Nodules typically show enhancement and slow growth, while those with aggressive features such as vascular invasion or rapid growth may suggest a higher-grade histology. These tumors are responsive to hormonal stimuli (progesterone and estrogen).

REFERENCES
Abrahamson S, et al. Benign metastasizing leiomyoma: clinical, imaging, and pathologic correlation. *AJR Am J Roentgenol.* 2001;176:1409–1413.
Fasih N, et al. Leiomyoma beyond the uterus: unusual locations, rare manifestations. *RadioGraphics.* 2008;28(7):1931–1948.
Thoracic Radiology: The Requisites, 3rd ed., pp. 340–343, 434–439.

CASE 121

Asbestosis

1. **B.** CT images show mild peripheral lung fibrosis with bilateral pleural plaques. The constellation of findings is essentially diagnostic of asbestosis. There are no specific findings to suggest hypersensitivity pneumonitis (ground-glass opacity, mosaic pattern due to air trapping, head-cheese sign) or sarcoidosis (nodularity, symmetric mediastinal lymphadenopathy). Idiopathic pulmonary fibrosis (UIP) could have this appearance on the lung windows; however, the presence of pleural plaques is strongly suggestive of asbestos exposure as the cause of fibrosis rather than idiopathic disease.
2. **C.** In approximately half of the cases of UIP the diagnosis can be established solely based on chest CT findings using current guidelines.
3. **B.** A substantial majority of fibrotic HP cases show relative sparing of the lung bases. This contrasts with UIP and NSIP which are most often basilar predominant; basilar predominance is seen with high frequency in NSIP cases though UIP can have a more heterogeneous zonal distribution.

4. **B.** Sarcoidosis and chronic beryllium disease look identical histologically and share many imaging characteristics. However, isolated lymphadenopathy, fibrosis, and airway involvement is much more common in sarcoidosis than chronic beryllium disease; and should point away from this diagnostic consideration unless there is a strong occupational or exposure history.

Comment

Asbestosis refers to pulmonary fibrosis that occurs in asbestos workers. It usually occurs in individuals who have been exposed to high concentrations over a prolonged period. Affected patients typically present with symptoms of a dry cough and dyspnea. Pulmonary function tests reveal a progressive reduction in vital capacity and diffusing capacity.

On conventional radiographs, you may observe a linear or reticular pattern of parenchymal opacities in the lower lung zones, which may progress to honeycombing. The identification of pleural plaques or pleural thickening supports the diagnosis. However, pleural abnormalities may be absent. It is important to recognize that normal conventional radiographs do not exclude a diagnosis of asbestosis. Occasionally the histologic findings in asbestosis are consistent with NSIP rather than UIP.

CT, particularly high-resolution CT (HRCT), is superior to radiography in the detection, quantification, and characterization of asbestosis. HRCT findings include reticulation, subpleural curvilinear lines, subpleural dependent density, parenchymal bands, and honeycombing. In an asbestos-exposed individual, these HRCT findings are suggestive of asbestosis; however, they are not specific for this process. An occupational history, pleural plaques and a characteristic interstitial pattern on CT are usually sufficient to support the diagnosis. Lung biopsy is seldom required for a worker to obtain compensation.

REFERENCES
Cox CW, Rose CS, Lynch DA. State of the art: imaging of occupational lung disease. *Radiology.* 2014 Mar;270(3):681–696.
Thoracic Radiology: The Requisites, 3rd ed., pp. 377–390.

CASE 122

Mounier-Kuhn Syndrome

1. **A.** Axial chest computed tomography (CT) image (Fig. 122.1) in lung window shows marked dilation of the trachea. Sagittal reconstructed image (Fig. 122.2) shows multiple diverticula (arrows) projecting posteriorly from the enlarged trachea, essentially diagnostic of Mounier-Kuhn syndrome. None of the other answer choices would present with this constellation of findings. In fact, the other three choices could all cause tracheal narrowing. Other causes of diffuse tracheal dilation include chronic obstructive pulmonary disease (COPD) (mild) and upper lung pulmonary fibrosis.
2. **D.** Nodules are not a common finding in Mounier-Kuhn syndrome. The other listed imaging findings are quite common in this condition.
3. **D.** Tracheobronchopathia osteochondroplastica (TBO) is an under-diagnosed condition, which is usually incidentally detected on imaging for another indication. No specific treatment is mandated for TBO.
4. **C.** The posterior wall of the trachea is free of any cartilaginous support. The cartilage in the anterior and lateral walls of the trachea is the main framework, which gives the trachea its unique arch-shaped appearance on axial chest CT.

Comment

Mounier-Kuhn syndrome, also referred to as *congenital tracheobronchomegaly*, is characterized pathologically by atrophy or absence of elastic fibers and thinning of the muscular mucosa of the trachea and main bronchi. This results in a flaccid airway that abnormally dilates during inspiration and excessively collapses on expiration. An ineffective coughing mechanism and pooling of secretions within outpouchings of the mucosa predispose affected patients to recurrent bouts of respiratory infections. Pulmonary complications include bronchiectasis most frequently, but emphysema and pulmonary fibrosis may also occur.

The second figure reveals an enlarged trachea and a wide-mouthed tracheal diverticulum (arrows). The posterolateral wall of the trachea is the most common location for a diverticulum in patients with Mounier-Kuhn syndrome. This site represents the junction of the posterior membranous and the anterior cartilaginous portions of the trachea. A minority of patients with Mounier-Kuhn syndrome demonstrate widespread tracheal and bronchial diverticula.

Other associations with primary tracheomegaly include Ehlers-Danlos syndrome, Marfan syndrome, and cutis laxa. Secondary tracheomegaly may develop in patients with long-standing pulmonary fibrosis, possibly secondary to chronic coughing and recurrent infections.

REFERENCES
Chung JH, Kanne JP, Gilman MD. CT of diffuse tracheal diseases. *AJR Am J Roentgenol.* 2011 Mar;196(3):W240–246.
Thoracic Radiology: The Requisites, 3rd ed., pp. 137–158.

CASE 123

Tracheomalacia

1. **B.** An inspiratory computed tomography (CT) image demonstrates a normal appearing trachea (Fig. 123.1). However, during dynamic expiration (Fig. 123.2), there is severe anterior bowing of the posterior wall of the trachea resulting in severe narrowing of the tracheal lumen. The findings are highly consistent with the diagnosis of tracheomalacia.
2. **B.** Tracheomalacia is best detected during the dynamic expiratory phase of the respiratory cycle. It may also be visible on end-expiratory images but not consistently.
3. **D.** Tracheobronchopathia osteochondroplastica, like relapsing polychondritis, preferentially affects the cartilaginous portions of the trachea with sparing of the posterior wall of the trachea. The other listed conditions typically affect the trachea wall diffusely.
4. **C.** The imaging description is that of the lunate trachea. This is a finding on inspiratory imaging, which is associated with tracheomalacia. Patients with a lunate trachea should be further evaluated with dynamic expiratory imaging to assess for tracheal collapse.

Comment

Tracheomalacia refers to excessive collapsibility of the airway. Such collapsibility is usually most apparent during coughing and during forced expiration. The abnormally flaccid airway is associated with physiologic alterations, including an inefficient coughing mechanism, and retained secretions. This may lead to recurrent infections and bronchiectasis. Rarely, it may be complicated by respiratory failure.

Tracheomalacia occurs rarely as a congenital abnormality due to a deficiency of cartilage formation. Acquired causes include prior intubation, chronic obstructive pulmonary disease (COPD), obesity, trauma, infection, relapsing polychondritis, and extrinsic compression (e.g., from a thyroid goiter).

Patients with severely symptomatic tracheomalacia may potentially benefit from surgery such as tracheoplasty, a technique that involves reinforcement of the posterior membranous wall of the trachea with a graft. This procedure has shown promising results in patients with acquired tracheomalacia in whom excessive tracheal collapsibility is mostly because of an abnormally flaccid posterior tracheal wall rather than a cartilage deficiency.

REFERENCES
Javidan-Nejad C. MDCT of trachea and main bronchi. *Radiol Clin North Am.* 2010 Jan;48(1):157–176.
Thoracic Radiology: The Requisites, 3rd ed., pp. 137–158.

CASE 124

Adenoid Cystic Carcinoma

1. **A, B, C, and D**. All of the listed conditions may present as a focal tracheal mass. The two most common primary neoplasms of the trachea are squamous carcinoma and adenoid cystic carcinoma.
2. **C.** Typically, the trachea must be narrowed by greater than 75% for patients to become symptomatic.
3. **A.** The most common distant primary malignancies to metastasize to the trachea are melanoma, breast cancer, renal cell carcinoma, and colon cancer.
4. **B.** Large airway hamartomas often contain a substantial amount of fat. This is a helpful finding in the setting of an airway tumor because such fat containing lesions are almost invariably benign (lipoma or hamartoma). Hamartomas may also demonstrate a popcorn pattern of calcification, which is highly suggestive of the diagnosis. Although hamartomas are the most common benign tumor of the lung, they rarely involve the large airways.

Comment

Primary tracheal neoplasms are quite rare. In adult patients, the majority of tracheal neoplasms are malignant. Presenting symptoms include shortness of breath and wheezing. Affected patients may initially be misdiagnosed as having adult-onset asthma.

Squamous cell carcinoma has a male predilection, and it is strongly associated with cigarette smoking. Squamous cell carcinoma carries a poor prognosis. Therapy consists of surgery and radiation for localized disease and radiation alone for surgically unresectable cases.

Adenoid cystic carcinoma is a low-grade malignancy that has no gender predilection and no relationship to cigarette smoking. Adenoid cystic carcinoma has a significantly better prognosis than squamous cell carcinoma, and surgical resection is potentially curative for patients with localized disease. Adjuvant radiation therapy is often required because of the predilection for these tumors to spread perineurally and submucosally. Late recurrences and metastases have been reported, however, especially among patients treated only with radiation therapy.

Axial image from contrast enhanced chest computed tomography (CT) demonstrates a focal bulky mass which appears to emanate from the right lateral aspect of the trachea causing moderate narrowing of the tracheal lumen (Fig. 124.1). Coronal CT minIP reformatted image demonstrates extension of the mass into the right main stem bronchus; there is complete obstruction of the right main stem bronchus (Fig. 124.2). There is relative hypoattenuation of the right lung relative to the left due to air-trapping.

CT plays an important role in preoperative planning of tracheal neoplasms by determining the amenability of a lesion to complete resection and by guiding the surgeon with respect to the approach, type, and extent of resection. Multiplanar reformation and three-dimensional reconstruction images play a complementary role to axial images by enhancing the accurate assessment of the craniocaudal extent of a neoplasm and its relationship to adjacent mediastinal structures.

REFERENCES

Javidan-Nejad C. MDCT of trachea and main bronchi. *Radiol Clin North Am.* 2010 Jan;48(1):157–176.

Thoracic Radiology: The Requisites, 3rd ed., pp. 137–158.

CASE 125

Nocardia

1. **B and D**. Nocardia and Aspergillus species are the most common infections to present as a solitary pulmonary nodule in the setting of organ transplantation.
2. **A**. Primary graft failure is the major cause of mortality within the first 30 days after cardiac transplantation. Infections are the leading cause of mortality between 6 months and 1 year after cardiac transplantation. Acute allograft rejection accounts for 10% of all deaths in the first 3 years after cardiac transplantation. Allograft vasculopathy is an important cause of mortality after the first year, ranking among the top three causes of death in this time range.
3. **B**. It would be unusual for invasive aspergillosis to present with a tree in bud pattern. All other listed entities commonly demonstrate a tree in bud pattern on CT which is caused by small airway impaction with pus or inflammatory debris.

Comment

Cardiac transplantation is currently a widely accepted treatment for end-stage heart disease. The most common causes of morbidity and mortality following heart transplantation are infection and rejection.

Most heart transplant patients undergo annual surveillance with chest radiography. Infectious complications manifest as pulmonary nodules, masses, ground-glass opacities and/or consolidations and should prompt further evaluation with chest CT (Fig. 125.1). When single or multiple lung nodules or masses occur in the lungs of a patient who is status post heart transplantation, one should first consider infectious etiologies such as *Aspergillus* and *Nocardia* species. In a series of 257 patients who underwent heart transplantation, single or multiple lung nodules or masses were detected on chest radiographs in approximately 10% of patients. Infections were the most common etiology, with *Aspergillus* encountered slightly more frequently than *Nocardia*. *Aspergillus* infection developed within a median of 2 months following transplantation. The median time to development of *Nocardia* infection was 5 months.

The time course for susceptibility to specific organisms is similar among patients following heart and other solid organ transplants. In the first month after transplantation, bacterial nosocomial infections are most common. Between 2 and 6 months, viral and opportunistic fungal infections are most common. After 6 months posttransplantation, bacterial community-acquired pneumonias are most common.

Posttransplant lymphoproliferative disorder is an important noninfectious cause of lung nodules and masses that is closely associated with the Epstein-Barr virus. The incidence of this disorder is highest during the first year following transplantation, corresponding to the time of most severe immunosuppression.

Lung parenchymal abnormalities are frequently accompanied by mediastinal and/or hilar lymph node enlargement, a finding that is not typically associated with *Aspergillus* and *Nocardia* infections.

REFERENCES

Knollmann FD, Hummel M, Hetzer R, Felix R. CT of heart transplant recipients: spectrum of disease. *Radiographics.* 2000 Nov–Dec;20(6): 1637–1648.

Smith JD, Stowell JT, Martínez-Jiménez S, Desouches SL, Rosa-do-de-Christenson ML, Jain KK, Magalski A. Evaluation after orthotopic heart transplant: what the radiologist should know. *Radiographics.* 2019 Mar–Apr;39(2):321–343.

Thoracic Radiology: The Requisites, 3rd ed., pp. 310–322.

CASE 126

Chronic Thromboembolic Disease

1. D. Axial image from contrast enhanced chest CT demonstrates eccentric feeling defects within the central pulmonary arteries essentially diagnostic of chronic thromboembolic disease (Fig. 126.1).
2. A. Although mosaic attenuation may be due to small airways disease, small vessel disease, or lobular infiltration of the lung; the most common cause of mosaic attenuation is constrictive small airway disease(air-trapping).
3. D. Mosaic attenuation, ground-glass opacity, and central arterial filling defects can be seen in both acute and chronic thromboembolic disease. However, decreased caliber of a pulmonary arterial branch (when associated with an internal filling effect) is diagnostic of chronic thromboembolic disease. This finding contrasts with acute pulmonary embolism which is characterized by dilation of the affected pulmonary arterial branch.
4. D. Proximal interruption of pulmonary artery is almost always associated with ipsilateral diffuse pulmonary scarring/fibrosis. Other associated findings include large ipsilateral bronchial arteries and a corrugated appearance to the subpleural lung due to peripheral collateral arteries. The aortic arch is almost always contralateral to the interrupted pulmonary artery.

Comment

Chronic pulmonary thromboembolism is a relatively uncommon but treatable cause of pulmonary artery hypertension. Because many affected patients do not present with a history of prior embolic episodes, the diagnosis may be difficult.

CT is playing an increasingly prominent role in the diagnosis of chronic pulmonary thromboembolism. Characteristic findings have been described in the lung parenchyma and pulmonary vessels. Regarding the lung parenchyma, you may observe variable areas of lung attenuation, with a lobular or multilobular distribution, referred to as a mosaic attenuation pattern. The low-attenuation areas of the lung often exhibit both a diminished number and decreased size of vessels compared with adjacent areas of higher attenuation (Fig. 126.2). In patients with chronic pulmonary thromboembolism, this pattern reflects diminished blood flow to areas of the lung distal to chronic emboli.

The vascular hallmark of chronic pulmonary thromboembolism is the presence of a mural thrombus. Chronic thrombus is typically adherent to the vascular wall, and it may contain foci of calcification. In patients with chronic pulmonary thromboembolism, you may also observe complete occlusion of a vessel that is diminished in size; a peripheral intraluminal defect; contrast flowing through a thickened, often smaller artery because of recanalization; and a web or flap within a contrast-filled artery. In addition, extensive bronchial collateral vessels may also be observed.

REFERENCES

Castañer E, Gallardo X, Ballesteros E, Andreu M, Pallardó Y, Mata JM, Riera L. CT diagnosis of chronic pulmonary thromboembolism. *Radiographics.* 2009 Jan–Feb;29(1):31–50; discussion 50–53.

Thoracic Radiology: The Requisites, 3rd ed., pp. 238–258.

CASE 127

Metastatic Thyroid Cancer

1. **D.** Frontal chest radiograph (Fig. 127.1) and chest CT image (Fig. 127.2) demonstrate innumerable pulmonary nodules throughout the lungs. The pattern of nodular lung disease on CT is most consistent with a random pattern. Of the listed conditions, metastatic cancer is most likely. The pattern of nodularity in sarcoidosis is typically perilymphatic. Silicosis tends to favor the subpleural and centrilobular portions of the lungs, often mimicking the perilymphatic pattern common in sarcoidosis. A combination of centrilobular nodules and cysts occurs in Langerhans cell histiocytosis.
2. **A.** In addition to metastatic disease, hematologic spread of certain granulomatous infections (tuberculosis [TB]) can also present with a random pattern of diffuse nodular lung disease. Hypersensitivity pneumonitis, when it is characterized by centrilobular ground-glass opacities is usually predominant in the upper lobes. Chronic beryllium disease mimics the perilymphatic pattern of sarcoidosis.
3. **A.** Silicosis is characterized by upper zone predominant solid nodules. Sarcoidosis and Langerhans cell histiocytosis may also present with upper lung predominant nodules.
4. **C.** The presented clinical scenario is suggestive of chronic beryllium disease. At risk individuals are typically those involved directly in the manufacturing of certain materials such as thermal coating, nuclear reactors, rocket heat shields, ceramics, electronics, and x-ray tubes. Beryllium lymphocyte proliferation test (BeLPT) is the first step in determining whether someone is sensitized to beryllium. Confirmed abnormal BeLPT is highly suggestive of the diagnosis if clinical and imaging findings are supportive. Imaging findings most commonly mimic sarcoidosis although progression to frank fibrosis or significant airway involvement is unusual in chronic beryllium disease.

Comment

The radiograph and CT image demonstrate a diffuse, nodular pattern of parenchymal opacities. Most nodules are 2 to 3 mm in diameter, although a few are slightly larger. Characterization of diffuse nodular lung disease on radiography is challenging and is better performed on chest CT.

The random pattern of diffuse nodules in this case is most consistent with hematogenous spread of infection or metastases. One of the most helpful findings in differentiating the different patterns of nodular lung disease is presence or absence of subpleural sparing. Perilymphatic nodules typically are subpleural and perifissural in contradistinction to centrilobular nodules which will spare these areas. Random nodules are often basilar predominant because of their hematogenous mode of spread; the lung bases receive a substantial higher proportion of pulmonary blood flow as compared to the lung apices.

REFERENCES

Boitsios G, Bankier AA, Eisenberg RL. Diffuse pulmonary nodules. *AJR Am J Roentgenol.* 2010 May;194(5):W354–366.

Thoracic Radiology: The Requisites, 3rd ed., pp. 405–427.

CASE 128

Castleman Disease (Benign Lymph Node Hyperplasia)

(Case courtesy of Travis Henry, MD)

1. **C and D.** Axial image from contrast enhanced chest CT (Fig. 128.1) shows an avidly enhancing mediastinal lymph node in the low paratracheal region. Differential diagnosis includes Castleman's disease and hypervascular metastases. Sarcoidosis could be considered but is less likely because it typically does not demonstrate this degree of focal isolated mediastinal lymphadenopathy. Tuberculosis more typically causes necrosis within lymph nodes.
2. **C.** All of the listed primary malignancies are associated with hypervascular nodal metastases except for colon cancer.
3. **A.** Avid nodal enhancement after intravenous contrast administration is typical of the hyaline vascular subtype of Castleman's disease and is less common in the plasma cell variant. The other listed answer options are all much more common in the plasma cell variant.
4. **B.** HIV is highly associated with human herpesvirus 8 (HHV-8) associated Castleman's disease variant.

Comment

The identification of enhancing lymph nodes significantly narrows the wide differential diagnosis of mediastinal adenopathy. In most cases, enhancing nodes are due to metastatic disease from hypervascular neoplasms such as renal cell carcinoma, thyroid carcinoma, melanoma, and carcinoid neoplasms. The most common benign etiology is Castleman's disease, the diagnosis in this case, which is an additional important diagnosis to consider when you identify markedly enhancing lymph nodes.

Castleman's disease, also referred to as *angiofollicular benign lymph node hyperplasia*, is an uncommon lymphoproliferative disorder. This disorder has been divided into two major histologic subtypes: hyaline vascular and plasma cell. The hyaline vascular subtype is present in the vast majority (90%) of cases. This subtype is characterized by hyperplasia of lymphoid follicles with germinal center formation and the presence of numerous capillaries with hyalinized walls. It usually manifests as a solitary hilar or mediastinal enhancing nodal mass in asymptomatic patients and is generally curable with surgical resection.

The plasma cell subtype is characterized by the presence of mature plasma cells located between the hyperplastic germinal centers and relatively few capillaries. This form is frequently associated with clinical symptoms, including fever, fatigue, anemia, polyclonal hypergammaglobulinemia, and bone marrow plasmacytosis. In contrast to the hyaline vascular sub-type, bilateral hilar and multifocal mediastinal lymph node enlargement is commonly observed. Another differentiating feature is the relatively low level of enhancement of nodes observed in the plasma cell subtype compared with the marked enhancement of nodes in the hyaline vascular subtype.

Castleman's disease may also be categorized as either unicentric or multicentric in distribution. The former is usually due to the hyaline vascular subtype and the latter is usually secondary to the plasma cell variety. Multicentric Castleman's disease is associated with a worse prognosis than the unicentric variety. Although both varieties may be complicated by development of lymphoma, malignancy is much more common in the multicentric form.

HHV-8–associated Castleman disease is rare and has a worse prognosis than the plasma cell and hyaline vascular variants. Average survival times are usually within a few months. This subtype occurs almost exclusively in those who are immunosuppressed patients and in those who are HIV-positive. Typically, patients will present with lymphadenopathy, immunological conditions, or systemic complaints.

REFERENCES

Bonekamp D, Horton KM, Hruban RH, Fishman EK. Castleman disease: the great mimic. *Radiographics.* 2011 Oct;31(6):1793–1807.
Thoracic Radiology: The Requisites, 3rd ed., pp. 61–87, 97–136.

CASE 129

Aortic dissection

1. **C.** Axial and sagittal images from contrast enhanced chest computed tomography (CT) (Fig. 129.1) demonstrate a dissection flap in the descending thoracic aorta, distal to the left subclavian artery consistent with a type B aortic dissection.
2. **C.** Blood pressure control (along with decreasing heart rate and pain) is a mainstay of medical therapy for type B aortic dissections. Surgery is usually not pursued unless the patient has recurrent or persistent pain despite analgesia, imaging demonstrates an acute increase in the size of the false lumen or a contained rupture, or if there are signs of organ or limb hypoperfusion
3. **D.** Penetrating aortic ulcerations most commonly affect the descending thoracic aorta.
4. **A.** The right pulmonary artery and the ascending aorta share adventitia. Therefore hematoma in the wall of the ascending aorta may extend into the right pulmonary artery and extend to other portions of the pulmonary arterial system.

Comment

This case demonstrates an aortic dissection. Note the presence of an intimal flap, which manifests as a linear soft tissue density within the contrast-opacified vessel. Aortic dissection is characterized by a tear in the intima of the aortic wall, followed by separation of the tunica media. This process results in the creation of two channels for the passage of blood: a true and a false lumen.

Once an aortic dissection has been identified, it is important to determine its precise extent. Stanford type A dissections require surgical therapy. Extension of the dissection into the great vessels is an important preoperative finding. In contrast, Stanford type B are generally managed medically. Radiologists and surgeons may define these types differently. Radiologists typically define the Stanford type A dissections as those that involve the aorta proximal to the left subclavian artery; surgeons instead use the innominate artery as the anatomical marker. Some have proposed a refinement to the classification addressing those dissections which originate between the innominate and left subclavian arteries but do not involve the aorta proximal to the innominate artery as "type B dissections with aortic arch involvement." The most important advice for the radiologist is to provide a clear definition in the report of the origin of the dissection.

REFERENCES

Lempel JK, Frazier AA, Jeudy J, Kligerman SJ, Schultz R, Ninalowo HA, Gozansky EK, Griffith B, White CS. Aortic arch dissection: a controversy of classification. *Radiology.* 2014 Jun;271(3):848–855.
Gutschow SE, Walker CM, Martínez-Jiménez S, Rosado-de-Christenson ML, Stowell J, Kunin JR. Emerging concepts in intramural hematoma imaging. *Radiographics.* 2016 May–Jun;36(3):660–674.
Thoracic Radiology: The Requisites, 3rd ed., pp. 97–136, 279–288.

CASE 130

Relapsing Polychondritis

1. **B.** Computed tomography (CT) image (Fig. 130.1) shows thickening of the anterior and lateral tracheal walls with sparing of the posterior tracheal membrane. Of the listed answer choices, the only disease entity which typically spares the posterior aspect of the trachea is relapsing polychondritis. There is no cartilage within the posterior wall of the trachea.
2. **A.** The subglottic trachea is most commonly affected in the setting of granulomatosis with polyangiitis.
3. **C.** Amyloidosis and tracheobronchopathia osteochondroplastica (TBO) can both lead to hyperdense nodular lesions within the tracheal wall. Differentiating between these two entities can usually be achieved by assessing the posterior tracheal wall ie. amyloidosis involves the trachea circumferentially as opposed to TBO which spares the posterior aspect of the trachea. TBO is a benign condition which only involves the cartilaginous portion of tracheal wall.
4. **C.** Upper lung predominant pulmonary fibrosis can lead to tracheal dilation likely due to traction effect. Tracheobronchomegaly (Mounier-Kuhn syndrome) is a rare condition which may also manifest with diffuse central airway dilation and is thought to be caused by inherent atrophy or absence of the elastic fibers of the trachea and main bronchi.

Comment

Relapsing polychondritis is a rare inflammatory disease that affects the cartilages of the ears, nose, upper respiratory tract, and joints. The etiology of this condition is uncertain, but it is likely an autoimmune disorder. Recurrent bouts of inflammation result in fragmentation and subsequent fibrosis of cartilaginous structures. Auricular chondritis is the most common manifestation of this disorder, occurring in approximately 90% of patients. Respiratory tract involvement is seen in approximately 50% of patients and is the major cause of morbidity associated with this condition.

Regarding airway involvement, the larynx, trachea, and mainstem bronchi are most commonly affected. Segmental and subsegmental bronchi are affected less frequently. Initially, airway narrowing results from mucosal edema. Later in the course of this condition, edema is replaced by granulation tissue and fibrosis. Airway involvement results in impaired clearance of secretions that may be complicated by recurrent respiratory infections and bronchiectasis. Recently, there has been increasing recognition of the presence of tracheobronchomalacia in patients with relapsing polychondritis. This may occur prior to development of morphologic abnormalities in some patients. Thus imaging evaluation of patients with suspected airway involvement from relapsing polychondritis should include both end-inspiratory and dynamic expiratory sequences. Dynamic expiratory CT imaging refers to the acquisition of a volumetric CT dataset during forced exhalation and has been shown to be more sensitive for detecting abnormal airway collapse than the less physiologic method of end-expiratory imaging.

REFERENCES

Chung JH, Kanne JP, Gilman MD. CT of diffuse tracheal diseases. *AJR Am J Roentgenol.* 2011 Mar;196(3):W240–246.
Thoracic Radiology: The Requisites, 3rd ed., pp. 137–158.

CASE 131

Swyer-James-Macleod Syndrome

1. **B and D.** The posteroanterior (PA) chest radiograph shows a small left lung with shift of the heart to the left. There is

a paucity of vasculature in the left lung (Fig. 131.1). Chest CT images show severe air-trapping affecting the left lung more than the right lung. The right upper lobe is normal and does not air trap on expiration (attenuation of the right upper lobe increases because of the decreased amount of air) (Fig. 131.2). Combined with history of childhood pneumonia, the findings are typical of Swyer-James-MacLeod syndrome, which is a subtype of obliterative bronchiolitis. The findings would be atypical for bronchial atresia or lobar emphysema.

2. **D**. Hyperdense mucus plugging of bronchi is essentially diagnostic of allergic bronchopulmonary aspergillosis. This condition leads to precipitation of salts in areas of mucus plugging. Elevated IgE and eosinophil levels are typical. Patients almost always have an underlying diagnosis of asthma and/or cystic fibrosis.

3. **A**. During expiration, the posterior wall of the trachea bows forward. The other portions of the trachea are reinforced by cartilage and generally maintain their convex morphology. Bronchi, on the other hand, have complete cartilaginous rings and tend to decrease in size more uniformly with expiration.

4. **D**. Diffuse idiopathic pulmonary neuroendocrine cell hyperplasia is a rare lung condition which occurs almost exclusively in women, most commonly in those who are middle-aged or elderly. The most significant manifestations of this condition are severe air-trapping from obliterative bronchiolitis and intraluminal proliferation of neuroendocrine cells. As these cells increase in size, they form multiple pulmonary nodules which pathologically are carcinoid tumorlets (smaller than 5 mm) and tumors (larger than 5 mm).

Comment

The imaging findings are characteristic of Swyer-James-Macleod syndrome, a variant of postinfectious bronchiolitis obliterans. This syndrome occurs secondary to an acute viral bronchiolitis in early infancy or early childhood that prevents the normal development of the affected lung. As shown in this case, the typical inspiratory radiograph findings include a unilateral hyperlucent lung or lobe with normal or reduced volume and reduced pulmonary vascularity.

CT imaging features of Swyer-James-Macleod syndrome include (1) areas of decreased lung attenuation with associated reduction in the number and size of vessels; (2) bronchiectasis; and (3) air trapping on expiratory images. Interestingly, although radiographic findings in patients with Swyer-James-Macleod syndrome are typically unilateral, CT often shows patchy areas of abnormality within the opposite lung as well.

Most patients are asymptomatic adults at the time of diagnosis, and the condition is often detected incidentally on a radiograph or CT performed for other reasons. Less commonly, patients present with recurrent infections or dyspnea.

REFERENCES
Dillman JR, Sanchez R, Ladino-Torres MF, Yarram SG, Strouse PJ, Lucaya J. Expanding upon the unilateral hyperlucent hemithorax in children. *Radiographics*. 2011 May–Jun;31(3):723–741.
Thoracic Radiology: The Requisites, 3rd ed., pp. 391–404.

CASE 132

Accessory Cardiac Bronchus

1. **D**. Axial (Fig. 132.1) and coronal minIP (Fig. 132.2) chest computed tomography (CT) images in this case demonstrate an anomalous blind-ending diverticulum arising from the medial wall of the bronchus intermedius. This anatomic variant is described as a cardiac bronchus.

2. **C**. Pulmonary artery sling (anomalous origin of the left pulmonary artery from the right artery) is associated with a bridging bronchus. The bridging bronchus is a large bronchus which ventilates a large proportion of the right lung (typically the right middle and right lower lobes) with an anomalous origin from the left main stem bronchus.

3. **A**. Bronchial atresia most commonly affects the left upper lobe. The right upper lobe accounts for most of the remaining cases.

4. **B**. A tracheal bronchus usually ventilates a portion of the right upper lobe. The inflated balloon of an endotracheal tube terminating near the carina could obstruct the tracheal bronchus proximally causing right upper lobe atelectasis.

Comment

This structure represents a cardiac bronchus, the only known true supernumerary anomalous bronchus. Other anomalies of the airway involve either a normal number of bronchi associated with ectopic locations (e.g., aberrant tracheal bronchus) or an absence of bronchi (e.g., bronchial atresia).

The cardiac bronchus always arises from the same location: the medial wall of the bronchus intermedius, above the origin of the superior segmental bronchus. It is directed caudally toward the mediastinum. For this reason, it has been designated as the *cardiac* bronchus.

Its length varies from a small, blind-ending pouch to a longer branching structure. The longer configuration may be associated with rudimentary alveolar tissue in some cases. The cardiac bronchus is lined by endobronchial mucosa and contains cartilaginous rings within its walls.

This anomaly is usually incidentally discovered in asymptomatic patients. However, occasionally a cardiac bronchus may serve as a reservoir for infected secretions resulting in recurrent respiratory infections. Associated inflammation and hypervascularity may also result in hemoptysis. Surgical excision is recommended for symptomatic patients.

REFERENCES
Unlu EN, Yilmaz Aydin L, Bakirci S, Onbas O. Prevalence of the accessory cardiac bronchus on multidetector computed tomography: evaluation and proposed classification. *J Thorac Imaging*. 2016 Jul 20
Chassagnon G, Morel B, Carpentier E, Ducou Le Pointe H, Sirinelli D. Tracheobronchial branching abnormalities: lobe-based classification scheme. *Radiographics*. 2016 Mar–Apr;36(2):358–373.
Ghaye B, Szapiro D, Fanchamps JM, et al. Congenital bronchial abnormalities revisited. *Radiographics*. 2001;21:105–119.
Thoracic Radiology: The Requisites, 3rd ed., pp. 193–209.

CASE 133

Intralobar Sequestration

1. **A**. The chest radiograph demonstrates a focal opacity in the retrocardiac portion of the left lower lobe (Fig. 133.1). Computed tomography (CT) image shows a multicystic lesion in the left lower lobe with a single artery extending from the descending thoracic aorta into this lesion (Fig. 133.2), this combination of findings is essentially diagnostic of a pulmonary sequestration.

2. **A**. Pulmonary extralobar sequestrations typically present during infancy. Intralobar sequestrations typically present later in life with recurrent infections.

3. **B**. Symptomatic congenital pulmonary airway malformations are usually surgically resected. There is some controversy regarding this approach and conservative management can be an option.

4. **C.** Pulmonary bronchogenic cysts are relatively rare compared to their mediastinal counterparts. When they do occur, they most commonly affect the lower lobes.

Comment

The imaging findings are essentially diagnostic of a *sequestration*, which refers to an area of aberrant lung tissue that has no normal connection with the bronchial tree or pulmonary arteries and is supplied by a systemic artery.

Sequestrations are classified as either *intralobar* (contained within the substance of the lung) or *extralobar* (contained within its own pleural envelope). Intralobar sequestration is the most common type. Affected patients may be asymptomatic or may present with a history of recurrent pulmonary infections. The posterior basal segment of the lower lobe is the most common location, and the left lung is affected twice as often as the right lung. Intralobar sequestrations may appear radiographically as a solid mass, a focal area of consolidation, or a cystic or multicystic lesion. The identification of a systemic arterial supply (usually a single artery from the aorta) confirms the diagnosis. A systemic artery is usually visible on either contrast-enhanced CT or magnetic resonance imaging (MRI). Failure to detect such a vessel does not exclude the diagnosis, however, and angiography may rarely be required for definitive diagnosis. Venous drainage typically occurs via the pulmonary veins although systemic drainage is occasionally identified.

In contrast with intralobar sequestration, the extralobar variety usually presents during infancy. The typical radiographic appearance is a well-defined, solitary mass near the posteromedial aspect of the hemidiaphragm. Less frequent sites of involvement include mediastinal and subdiaphragmatic locations. Approximately 90% of cases are in the left hemithorax. The arterial supply may arise from single or multiple systemic arteries. Extralobar sequestration is associated with systemic venous drainage, usually to the azygos system and less commonly into the portal vein, subclavian vein, or internal mammary vein.

Extra sequestration is widely recognized as a congenital anomaly. There is emerging consensus that intralobar sequestration may be acquired secondary to chronic infection.

REFERENCES
Lee EY, Boiselle PM, Cleveland RH. Multidetector CT evaluation of congenital lung anomalies. *Radiology.* 2008 Jun;247(3):632–648.
Walker CM, Wu CC, Gilman MD, et al. The imaging spectrum of bronchopulmonary sequestration. *Curr Probl Diagn Radiol.* 2014;43:100–114.
Thoracic Radiology: The Requisites, 3rd ed., pp. 193–209.

CASE 134

Acute Pulmonary Emboli With Right Heart Strain

1. **A.** The presence of endoluminal filling defects is the most important finding in acute pulmonary embolism. The filling defects are too large and well defined in this case to the result of flow artifacts. Pulmonary artery sarcoma is a rare neoplasm and can mimic pulmonary embolism; however, the bilateral and non-continuous location of these filling defects excludes that diagnosis. There are no findings of a pseudoaneurysm in this patient.
2. **C.** The right ventricle is enlarged but not hypertrophied and there is bowing of the interventricular septum, suggesting acute right heart strain. No findings of pulmonary infarct or hemorrhage or aortic dissection are present.
3. **D.** The Westermark sign describes oligemia on a chest radiograph distal to a centrally obstructing thrombus. This appearance is extremely uncommon and may be encountered more often in the setting of chronic pulmonary thromboembolic disease. It is often apparent only in retrospect. The S sign of Golden describes the appearance of an opaque atelectatic right upper lobe caused by an obstructing hilar mass, resulting in an S-like configuration of the pulmonary fissure. Hampton hump describes a peripheral wedge-shaped opacity on the chest radiograph that abuts the pleura and represents a pulmonary infarct. The Fleischner sign describes dilation of a central pulmonary artery on the chest radiograph resulting from an obstructing embolus.
4. **B.** On MRI bland thrombus does not enhance with gadolinium. In contrast, a pulmonary artery sarcoma does. Both a sarcoma and bland thrombus can have high T2 signal intensity. Although the shape of the filling defect might suggest a tumor rather than a bland thrombus, the finding is not reliable. The appearance of thrombus on T1-weighted imaging depends on its age. However, some pulmonary artery sarcomas can have foci of high T1 signal intensity.

Comment

Differential Diagnosis

Contrast-enhanced computed tomography (CT) shows bilateral filling defects in the pulmonary arteries (Fig. 134.1) in addition to dilation of the right ventricle (Fig. 134.2), consistent with acute pulmonary embolism and acute right heart strain. Other causes of pulmonary artery filling defects include tumor emboli, pulmonary artery sarcoma, and flow artifacts. Tumor emboli can be indistinguishable from bland thrombus and usually result when tumor elsewhere (e.g., kidney, IVC, liver) invades a large systemic vein such as the inferior vena cava. Pulmonary artery sarcomas are very rare and typically arise in one of the central pulmonary arteries as a single mass. Flow artifacts can occur with severe pulmonary hypertension or surgical shunts such as a Fontan shunt.

Comment

CT angiography is the reference standard examination for the detection of acute pulmonary embolism (PE). Findings of acute pulmonary embolism on CT include one or more filling defects in the pulmonary arteries which produce acute angles with the arterial wall with distension of the affected artery. Areas of ground-glass opacity or consolidation may be present distal to emboli, reflecting areas of pulmonary hemorrhage. Occasionally, a well-defined wedge-shaped focus of opacification often with a with a ground-glass center which abuts the pleura may be present. This finding represents a pulmonary infarct. Small ipsilateral pleural effusions are common.

Treatment for most patients with acute PE is with anticoagulation. Thrombolysis, either peripheral or catheter directed may be used in cases of severe right heart strain or cardiogenic shock.

REFERENCES
Devaraj A, Sayer C, Sheard S, et al. Diagnosing acute pulmonary embolism with computed tomography: imaging update. *J Thorac Imaging.* 2015;30:176–192.
Ohno Y, Yoshikawa T, Kishida Y, et al. Unenhanced and contrast-enhanced MR angiography and perfusion imaging for suspected pulmonary thromboembolism. *AJR Am J Roentgenol.* 2017:1–14.
Saad N. Aggressive management of pulmonary embolism. *Semin Intervent Radiol.* 2012;29:52–56.
Thoracic Radiology: The Requisites, 3rd ed., pp. 238–258.

CASE 135

Panlobular Emphysema (Alpha-1 Antitrypsin Deficiency)

1. **B and C**. Alpha-1 antitrypsin deficiency can lead to panlobular emphysema, which typically has a basal predominance. Additionally, intravenous injection of methylphenidate can also result in panlobular emphysema indistinguishable from alpha-1 antitrypsin deficiency. Although emphysema is a component of silicosis and coal-worker's pneumoconiosis, it is usually of the paracicatricial variety i.e., related to the areas of progressive massive fibrosis which occur in the upper lobes. It may also be of the centrilobular type of emphysema in workers who smoke. Nontuberculous mycobacterial infection is typically characterized by nodules, bronchiectasis, and consolidation.
2. **C**. Panlobular emphysema is the predominant type of emphysema in this patient. Centrilobular, paraseptal, and paracicatricial emphysema do not predominate in this patient.
3. **B**. Alpha-1 antitrypsin deficiency is inherited as an autosomal recessive trait. It is not inherited as an autosomal dominant, X-linked dominant, or X-linked recessive trait.
4. Liver cirrhosis is another complication of alpha-1 antitrypsin deficiency. Pancreatitis, renal cell carcinoma, and aortic aneurysm are not known complications of alpha-1 antitrypsin deficiency.

Comment

Differential Diagnosis

Posteroanterior (PA) and lateral radiographs (Figs. 135.1 and 135.2) show hyperinflated lungs with basal lucency and coronal CT shows attenuation of the vasculature in the lower lungs (Fig. 135.3), suggestive of panlobular emphysema. The differential diagnosis for basal predominant panlobular emphysema includes alpha-1 antitrypsin deficiency, IV drug abuse (especially methylphenidate), and occasionally cigarette smoking.

Discussion

Panlobular emphysema is characterized by hyperlucency, hyperinflation, and fewer and smaller-than-normal pulmonary vessels. This appearance has been described as a "simplification of normal lung architecture." Alpha-1 antitrypsin (AAT) deficiency, the diagnosis in this case, is characterized by a basilar distribution of panlobular emphysema.

AAT deficiency is an inherited autosomal recessive disorder that is characterized by abnormally low levels of α_1-protease inhibitor. This protein inhibits several lysosomal proteases and prevents the damaging effects of elastases released by macrophages and neutrophils. Because the administration of elastase has been shown to produce emphysema in animal models, it is not surprising that patients with reduced levels of protease inhibitors are at risk for developing this complication. Patients who are homozygous for this disorder have a very low level (roughly 20% of normal) of α_1-protease inhibitor and are at high risk for developing emphysema. Cigarette smoking increases this risk.

Interestingly, patients with AAT deficiency have a high prevalence of bronchiectasis, which has been reported in approximately 40% of cases. The mechanism by which bronchiectasis develops in these patients is uncertain. It has been hypothesized that destruction of elastic fibers in the walls of bronchi and bronchioles plays an important role in this process.

Treatment approaches targeting the molecular basis of this disease are currently under investigation and include AAT replacement, gene therapy, and stem cell therapy.

REFERENCES

Stockley RA. Alpha1-antitrypsin review. *Clin Chest Med*. 2014 Mar;35(1):39–50.
Thoracic Radiology: The Requisites, 3rd ed., pp. 391–404.

CASE 136

Thymic Cyst

1. **A, B, C, and D**. On the CT scan, the anterior mediastinal mass has intermediate attenuation (40 HU) and is homogeneous. There is no mass effect on the adjacent lung. A protein-rich thymic cyst could have this appearance. Thymoma and lymphoma usually have some mass effect on adjacent structures but still should be considered because lymphoma is often homogeneous and cystic thymomas can also be homogenous on CT. Normal thymus (hyperplasia) could also have this appearance.
2. **D**. Pericardial cysts are homogenous and lack solid components. Cystic foci may be present in thymoma, germ cell neoplasm, and Hodgkin lymphoma.
3. **D**. Thymoma is the most common cause of a thymic mass. Thymic cysts and thymic carcinoids are less common. Thymolipoma is rare.
4. **B**. The presence of methemoglobin would result in high T1 signal intensity. Methemoglobin does not cause absent, low, or intermediate T1 signal intensity on MRI.

Comment

Differential Diagnosis

CT (Fig. 136.1) shows a homogeneous anterior mediastinal mass, which does not exert mass effect on adjacent structures. Attenuation is similar to chest wall musculature. MRI can be used for indeterminate lesions such as this. An axial T2-weighted image (Fig. 136.2) shows homogeneous high signal intensity. Pre- and postcontrast (Figs. 136.3 and 136.4, respectively) axial T1 weighted images show intermediate signal intensity and no enhancement.

Discussion

Thymic cysts are an uncommon cause of an anterior mediastinal mass. They may be congenital or acquired. Congenital cysts are probably derived from remnants of the fetal thymopharyngeal duct. Acquired cysts can develop following radiation therapy for Hodgkin lymphoma. Less commonly, they can occur following

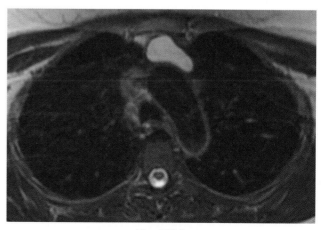

Fig. 136.2

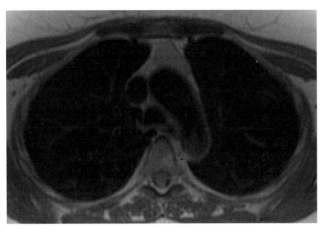

Fig. 136.3

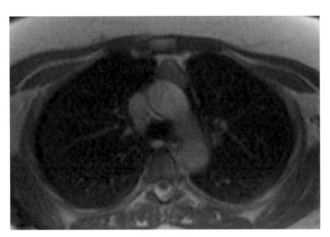

Fig. 136.4

thoracotomy or after chemotherapy for a malignant neoplasm. An association with human immunodeficiency virus (HIV) infection has also been reported.

On imaging studies, a thymic cyst typically appears as a well-defined, cystic mass with an imperceptible wall. In a minority of patients, curvilinear calcifications are present in the wall. On CT, thymic cysts typically have fluid attenuation but occasionally the attenuation value can be higher. Mass effect on adjacent structures (especially the lungs) is usually absent. MRI can be used to assess indeterminate thymic lesions. Thymic cysts usually demonstrate low signal intensity on T1-weighted images and increased signal intensity on T2-weighted images. However, the appearance can vary if the cyst has been complicated by hemorrhage or infection. The imaging features in this case are typical of an uncomplicated thymic cyst. Cysts will not enhance after the administration of contrast.

The presence of an anterior mediastinal mass with solid and cystic components may represent a solid anterior mediastinal mass that has undergone cystic necrosis. For example, thymoma and Hodgkin lymphoma can contain cystic areas, occasionally associated with a relatively small amount of neoplastic tissue. Germ cell neoplasms such as mature teratomas often contain cystic components intermixed with solid elements.

The identification of cystic elements in conjunction with fat, calcium, or both should suggest this diagnosis. No treatment is required for thymic cysts.

REFERENCES

McInnis MC, Flores EJ, Shepard JA, Ackman JB. Pitfalls in the imaging and interpretation of benign thymic lesions: how thymic MRI can help. *AJR Am J Roentgenol.* 2016 Jan;206(1):W1–8.

Thoracic Radiology: The Requisites, 3rd ed., pp. 61–87, 97–136.

CASE 137
Tracheal Bronchus

1. **B**. A supernumerary or replaced bronchus arising directly from the trachea is called a *tracheal bronchus*. A pulmonary sling is a condition in which the left pulmonary artery arises from the right pulmonary artery and crosses from right to left between the trachea and esophagus. Other airway anomalies may also be present. A cardiac bronchus arises from the inferomedial wall of the bronchus intermedius. The image does not show evidence of complete tracheal rings.
2. **A**. A tracheal bronchus almost always supplies the entire or a portion of the right upper lobe, most commonly the apical segment. A tracheal bronchus does not supply the right middle or left lower lobe. A left tracheal bronchus is exceedingly rare.
3. **D**. Most patients with a tracheal bronchus are asymptomatic, and the anomalous airway is detected incidentally on computed tomography (CT). Recurrent infection and hemoptysis are rare complications, usually related to bronchiectasis. A tracheal bronchus does not cause stridor.
4. **B**. When the tracheal bronchus supplies the entire right upper lobe, it is also referred to as a *pig bronchus* or *bronchus suis* because it represents the normal swine bronchial anatomy. Cows, sheep, and horses do not normally have tracheal bronchi.

Comment
Differential Diagnosis

Axial (Fig. 137.1) and coronal reformatted (Fig. 137.2) CT images show an anomalous bronchus arising from the right lateral wall of the trachea, proximal to the origin of the right main bronchus. The proper right upper lobe bronchus arises at its normal origin. CT is diagnostic, and there is no differential diagnosis.

Discussion

The term *tracheal bronchus* has been used to describe this congenital bronchial anomaly, which can supply a portion of the right upper lobe (usually the apical segment) or the entire right upper lobe. The latter configuration is also referred to as a pig bronchus or bronchus suis. Affected patients are usually asymptomatic. In a minority of patients, the bronchial orifice is narrow, which can lead to recurrent infection and bronchiectasis. Following intubation, the aberrant bronchus can become occluded by the endotracheal tube balloon cuff, resulting in atelectasis within the corresponding segment or lobe that is supplied by the aberrant bronchus. Treatment is generally not required.

REFERENCES

Ghaye B, Szapiro D, Fanchamps JM, Dondelinger RF. Congenital bronchial abnormalities revisited. *Radiographics.* 2001;21:105–119.

Chassagnon G, Morel B, Carpentier E, Ducou Le Pointe H, Sirinelli D. Tracheobronchial branching abnormalities: lobe-based classification scheme. *Radiographics*. 2016 Mar–Apr;36(2):358–373.
Thoracic Radiology: The Requisites, 3rd ed., pp. 193–209.

CASE 138

Amiodarone Toxicity

1. **A and C**. Amiodarone and talc deposition in the lungs can result in foci or nodules of consolidation with high attenuation. Renal cell carcinoma metastases are often hypervascular; however, high attenuation is not typical on unenhanced computed tomography (CT) scans. Bleomycin toxicity usually results in organizing pneumonia or fibrosis. High attenuation consolidation is not a feature.
2. **A**. Amiodarone deposition in the lungs can result in foci or nodules of consolidation with high attenuation. Amiodarone deposition also occurs in the liver and generally occurs before lung deposition. Renal cell carcinoma metastases are often hypervascular; however, high attenuation is not typical on unenhanced CT scans. Increased attenuation of the liver is not a feature of renal cell carcinoma. Talc deposition in the lungs cause high attenuation consolidation. However, high attenuation of the liver is not a feature of talcosis. Bleomycin toxicity usually results in organizing pneumonia or fibrosis. High attenuation lung consolidation and liver parenchyma are not features.
3. **B**. Amiodarone is used to treat some cardiac dysrhythmias. Amiodarone is not used to treat acute respiratory distress syndrome, myocarditis, and congestive heart failure.
4. **A**. 5% to 20% of patients treated with amiodarone develop lung toxicity or deposition.

Comment

Differential Diagnosis

Unenhanced CT images through the lungs (Figs. 138.1 and 138.2) show areas of high attenuation consolidation. These contrast to the lower attenuation atelectatic lung. Pleural and pericardial effusions are also present. Unenhanced CT image through the upper abdomen (Fig. 138.3) shows diffusely increased attenuation of the liver. Causes of increased attenuation of lung disease include amiodarone deposition, talcosis, and various forms of calcification.

Comment

Amiodarone is a tri-iodinated compound used to treat cardiac arrhythmias and has a long biologic half life. Lung toxicity occurs in 5% to 20% of patients treated with amiodarone and is dose related.

There are three distinct clinical presentations of amiodarone toxicity. The most common presentation is a subacute onset of dyspnea, nonproductive cough, and weight loss. Radiographs typically show a diffuse linear pattern that may be difficult to distinguish from congestive heart failure. This usually correlates pathologically with a nonspecific interstitial pneumonia (NSIP) pattern. A less-common presentation (observed in approximately one third of patients) is characterized by an acute onset of symptoms that mimic an infection. Radiographs of these patients typically show patchy opacities with a peripheral distribution that correlate pathologically with organizing pneumonia. Unenhanced CT scans of these patients typically show high-attenuation foci of parenchymal opacity, with attenuation values ranging from approximately 80 to 175 Hounsfield units. This appearance reflects the high concentration of amiodarone within these regions of lung parenchyma. A third rare but potentially fatal form of pulmonary toxicity is acute respiratory distress syndrome (ARDS).

High attenuation of the liver (Fig. 138.3) is a common finding in patients treated with amiodarone toxicity. Thus, the combination of high-attenuation focal parenchymal opacities and a high-attenuation liver is highly suggestive of amiodarone pulmonary toxicity. Prompt recognition is important because amiodarone pulmonary toxicity is frequently reversible after withdrawal of the drug. Although clinical symptoms usually resolve within 2 to 4 weeks of drug withdrawal, chest radiographic abnormalities typically clear more slowly, in approximately 3 months.

REFERENCES
Rossi SE, Erasmus JJ, McAdams HP, et al. Pulmonary drug toxicity: radiologic and pathologic manifestations. *Radiographics*. 2000;20:1245–1259.
Thoracic Radiology: The Requisites, 3rd ed., pp. 355–376.

CASE 139

Saphenous Vein Graft Aneurysm Following CABG Surgery

1. **B, C**. The anterior mediastinal mass contains small foci of contrast enhancement, indicating that it is vascular in nature, either an aneurysm or pseudoaneurysm. The remainder of the mass consists of thrombus. Furthermore, it lies in continuity with a venous bypass graft. The collections of contrast within the mass and association with the venous bypass graft argue against lymphoma or thymoma.
2. **A**. Rupture of a (pseudo)aneurysm can lead to life-threatening hemorrhage. Patients can present with symptoms of myocardial ischemia without acute infarct, either from decreased coronary flow or rupture into a vein or cardiac chamber causing a fistula. This myocardial ischemia may not be acutely life threatening. Although potentially serious, gradual SVC compression is not acutely life threatening in most cases.
3. **D**. Approximately 50% of venous bypass graft aneurysms contain thrombus.
4. **C**. The best next step in the management of this patient is surgical repair. The size of the aneurysm warrants repair and follow-up imaging will have little to no impact on management. Because the computed tomography (CT) scan is diagnostic, cardiac MRI will not offer additional information. However, cardiac MRI could be useful if there were concerns for myocardial ischemia. Coil embolization is usually reserved for patients who are not candidates for surgery.

Comment

Differential Diagnosis

Contrast-enhanced CT (Fig. 139.1) shows a large low-attenuation mass containing small foci of contrast (*arrowheads*), which is associated with an aortocoronary venous bypass graft (*arrow*), representing a partially thrombosed aneurysm or pseudoaneurysm.

Discussion

Aneurysms of saphenous vein grafts are a rare but serious complication of CABG and are typically detected 10 to 20 years after the surgery. False aneurysms (pseudoaneurysms), which are characterized by a disrupted vessel wall, are more common than true aneurysms, which are characterized by an intact vessel wall. False aneurysms are most commonly located at the anastomotic sites. Such aneurysms have been described in association with wound infection, intrinsic weakness of the graft wall, and iatrogenic trauma to the vein during harvesting. In contrast, true aneurysms occur most commonly within the body of the graft. True aneurysms are thought to arise because of progressive atherosclerosis related to exposure of saphenous vein grafts to systemic blood pressure.

Patients with venous graft aneurysms are often asymptomatic, and these aneurysms are discovered incidentally on chest radiographs or CT obtained for other reasons. Symptomatic patients generally present with symptoms of myocardial ischemia. Complications of venous graft aneurysms include myocardial infarction, distal embolization, fistula formation to the right atrium or right ventricle, and rupture with secondary hemorrhage. Treatment includes resection of the aneurysm and myocardial revascularization. Catheter-based coil embolization may be considered in high-risk surgical patients.

REFERENCES

Nishimura K, Nakamura Y, Harada S, et al. Saphenous vein graft aneurysm after coronary artery bypass grafting. *Ann Thorac Cardiovasc Surg.* 2009;15:61–63.

Thoracic Radiology: The Requisites, 3rd ed., pp. 259–278.

CASE 140
Infectious Bronchiolitis

1. **A and C.** *Mycoplasma* and respiratory syncytial virus are common causes of infectious bronchiolitis. *Staphylococcus* and *Streptococcus* typically do not cause a pure bronchiolitis, but small airway inflammation usually accompanies a pneumonia. However, in most cases, imaging is not specific enough to include or exclude any causative organism or group of organisms.
2. **B.** Tree-in-bud opacities are nodular and linear branching centrilobular opacities that nearly always indicate bronchiolitis. An acinar nodule does not describe a nodular and linear branching centrilobular opacity but is sometimes used to describe a nodule that occupies most of a lobule, sparing the periphery. The term is seldom used. The nodules are often ill defined. Ring shadow is an older term that that is used in chest radiography to describe a bronchus which is dilated with a thickened wall seen in cross section e.g., in bronchiectasis. Mosaic attenuation describes heterogeneity of the lungs. Small airway disease is a cause of mosaic attenuation due to air trapping, but infiltrative lung diseases and pulmonary vascular disease can also cause mosaic attenuation.
3. **C.** Respiratory bronchioles communicate directly with alveoli. Unlike bronchi, bronchioles lack cartilage and are below the resolution of CT. Terminal bronchioles do not participate in gas exchange but are conduits between the smallest bronchi and the respiratory bronchioles.
4. **A.** Bronchioles are adjacent to the pulmonary artery within the center of the pulmonary lobule. Bronchioles are not located in the interlobular septa, the subpleural interstitium, or adjacent to the pulmonary vein.

Comment
Differential Diagnosis

Axial (Fig. 140.1) and coronal (Fig. 140.2) CT images show diffuse centrilobular tree-in-bud opacities and mild bronchial wall thickening. Tree-in-bud opacities nearly always represent a cellular bronchiolitis, usually the result of infection or aspiration. In the correct clinical setting, tree-in-bud opacities can be a manifestation of infection including tuberculosis. Rare causes of tree-in-bud opacities include follicular bronchiolitis and

vascular causes such as small vessel occlusion due to IV drug use (excipient lung disease due to the injection of crushed tablets) and arteriolar metastases.

Discussion

The CT appearance is characteristic of a cellular bronchiolitis, a pattern that is often described as *tree-in-bud* because of its resemblance to a tree budding in springtime. Although the tree-in-bud pattern was originally described in conjunction with tuberculosis, it is by no means pathognomonic for this process. Rather, it may be associated with a wide variety of bronchiolar diseases.

Infection is the most common cause of a tree-in-bud pattern. Acute infectious bronchiolitis is most commonly associated with respiratory syncytial virus, adenovirus, and *Mycoplasma* pneumonia. Other important infections include mycobacterial and fungal disease. However, nearly any organism can cause a bronchiolitis pattern. Other causes of cellular bronchiolitis include aspiration and diffuse panbronchiolitis. Panbronchiolitis is a chronic disease of unclear etiology that occurs almost exclusively in Asian males. It is associated with large airway infection causing bronchiectasis.

Chest radiographs of patients with minimal small airways disease may be normal. In patients with more-extensive disease, a fine nodular pattern may be apparent, often accompanied by reticular opacities. CT is helpful in distinguishing small airways disease from a true miliary pattern. The latter is characterized by a random distribution of small nodules; in contrast, small airways disease is associated with a centrilobular distribution of small nodular and branching (tree-in-bud) opacities.

Treatment of bacterial bronchiolitis includes appropriate antibiotics. Viral infections generally resolve without treatment. Bronchodilators may be required for supportive treatment.

REFERENCES

Gosset N, Bankier AA, Eisenberg RL. Tree-in-bud pattern. *AJR Am J Roentgenol.* 2009 Dec;193(6):W472–477.

Winningham PJ, Martínez-Jiménez S, Rosado-de-Christenson ML, Betancourt SL, Restrepo CS, Eraso A. Bronchiolitis: a practical approach for the general radiologist. *Radiographics.* 2017 May–Jun;37(3):777–794. https://doi.org/10.1148/rg.2017160131.

Thoracic Radiology: The Requisites, 3rd ed., pp. 137–158.

CASE 141
Cytomegalovirus Pneumonia in a Lung Transplant Recipient

1. **B and C.** Viral pneumonias, and drug toxicity can manifest as patchy ground-glass opacity, sometime with superimposed intralobular lines (crazy-paving). Tuberculosis usually manifests as diffuse tiny (miliary) nodules in immunosuppressed patients. Post-transplant lymphoproliferative disorder can manifest as consolidation, a nodule or nodules, or lymphadenopathy.
2. **B.** *Pneumocystis jirovecii* pneumonia is very uncommon because of widespread prophylaxis and occurs primarily in those who are noncompliant with prophylaxis regimens. It is most commonly seen in patients on high steroid therapy.
3. **B.** CMV is the most common viral cause of pneumonia in solid organ transplant recipients. EBV, RSV, and adenovirus can occur but do so less frequently. EBV is associated with PTLD.
4. **D.** Because organ transplant recipients remain on immunosuppressive therapy, fungal infection continues to be a source of infection in renal transplant recipients. Opportunistic infections are uncommon during the first month after

transplant because the immunosuppressive therapy has not had its full effect on the patient's immune system. Community-acquired pathogens such as *S. pneumoniae* are common causes of pneumonia after the sixth month following transplant. T-cell mediated immunity is most severely depressed during this time because of intense immunosuppressive therapy.

Comment

Differential Diagnosis

Axial (Fig. 141.1) and coronal (Fig. 141.2) CT images show a region of ground-glass opacity with superimposed intralobular lines (crazy-paving) in the upper lobe of the right lung allograft. Pneumomediastinum developed as a result of vigorous coughing. The native left lung is fibrotic. The CT findings are nonspecific and include infection, rejection, and drug reaction. However, drug reactions are uncommon in the early transplant period because of heavy immunosuppression. Usually, infection and rejection cannot be distinguished by imaging alone.

Comment

Following lung transplantation, patients are at risk for a variety of infections because of the effects of immunosuppressive therapy and loss of normal lymphatic clearance of the transplanted lung. Knowledge of the interval between transplantation and the development of pulmonary infections can help predict the types of organisms that are likely to cause pulmonary infections.

During the first month following transplantation, the immunosuppressive agents have not yet had a profound effect on the patient's immune system. Opportunistic infections are unusual during this period. Organisms that are typically encountered in patients with normal immunity after surgery, particularly gram-negative organisms, usually cause infections. These result from aspiration or wound-related or catheter-related infections.

Immunosuppression is usually most severe during the second to sixth months following lung transplantation. T-cell–mediated immunity is most severely depressed, placing patients at highest risk for viral and fungal infections. CMV is the most common viral agent to affect these patients, but prophylactic preventive strategies have markedly reduced the prevalence of CMV infection in the post-transplant setting. Radiographs can show a reticular or nodular pattern and, less commonly, consolidation and discrete lung nodules and masses. Treatment of CMV includes antiviral therapy and prophylaxis as required.

After several months, the immunosuppression regimen may gradually decrease. As the patient's immune system recovers, the organisms that most commonly produce pneumonia in this period are those responsible for most community-acquired pneumonias, such as *Streptococcus pneumoniae*. Because immunosuppressive agents are tapered but not discontinued, patients continue to remain at risk for opportunistic infections, particularly fungal organisms.

REFERENCES

Jokerst C, Sirajuddin A, Mohammed TL. Imaging the complications of lung transplantation. *Radiol Clin North Am*. 2016 Mar;54(2):355–373.

Kim SJ, Azour L, Hutchinson BD, Shirsat H, Zhou F, Narula N, Moreira AL, Angel L, Ko JP, Moore WH. Imaging course of lung transplantation: from patient selection to postoperative complications. *Radiographics*. 2021 Jul–Aug;41(4):1043–1063.

Thoracic Radiology: The Requisites, 3rd ed., pp. 259–278, 310–322.

CASE 142

Pulmonary Veno-Occlusive Disease

1. **C and D**. Although a rare cause of pulmonary hypertension, PVOD is characterized by smooth interlobular septal thickening on high-resolution CT. The most common cause of smooth interlobular septal thickening is pulmonary edema. No findings to suggest diffuse alveolar hemorrhage or usual interstitial pneumonia are present.
2. **A**. The triad of pulmonary hypertension, pulmonary edema, and normal pulmonary venous wedge pressure is highly suggestive of PVOD. Chronic pulmonary thromboembolic disease can cause pulmonary hypertension but generally does not cause lung edema with normal left heart function. COPD can cause pulmonary hypertension but generally does not cause lung edema with normal left heart function. Pulmonary hypertension (primary) generally does not cause lung edema if left heart function is normal.
3. **C**. Intimal fibrosis in small pulmonary veins and venules leads to obstruction. The prognosis of PVOD is poor, and the disease is usually fatal. Most patients present with signs and symptoms such as dyspnea, orthopnea, fatigue, and syncope. The central pulmonary veins are normal caliber on CT because the obstruction is upstream in the smaller veins and venules.
4. **B**. The diagnosis of PVOD requires lung biopsy for confirmation. However, many patients are too ill at the time of presentation to undergo a biopsy. Cardiac MRI can provide functional cardiac information; however, it will not confirm the diagnosis of PVOD. BAL will not confirm nor exclude the diagnosis of PVOD, and FDG PET/CT currently has no role in evaluating patients with suspected PVOD.

Comment

Differential Diagnosis

CT images of the lungs (Figs. 142.1 and 142.2) show smooth septal thickening and mild peripheral ground glass opacity. The heart size is normal. Unenhanced CT image of the mediastinum (Fig. 142.3) shows mild lymphadenopathy. The most common cause of bilateral smooth septal thickening is cardiogenic edema. However, in the setting of pulmonary hypertension, PVOD and pulmonary capillary hemangiomatosis should also be considered. There is no evidence in this case of enlargement of the left atrium or left ventricle consistent with normal left heart function. Lymphangitic carcinomatosis can cause septal thickening, but the distribution of findings on CT is patchier. Furthermore, patients usually do not develop pulmonary hypertension.

Comment

Pulmonary veno-occlusive disease (PVOD) is a rare disorder characterized by obstruction of the pulmonary veins and venules by intimal fibrosis. Increased resistance to pulmonary venous drainage results in pulmonary hypertension. The classic triad associated with this condition includes severe pulmonary hypertension, radiographic evidence of pulmonary edema, and a normal wedge pressure. However, many affected patients do not have this triad. Affected patients usually present with orthopnea, progressive dyspnea, fatigue, and syncope.

The etiology of PVOD is unknown, but it has been described in association with viral infection, environmental toxins, chemotherapy, radiation injury, contraceptives, and intracardiac shunts. It has also been reported as a rare complication of sarcoidosis. A genetic predisposition has also been reported. There is no effective treatment for PVOD, and it is usually fatal within a few years of diagnosis. Currently, lung transplantation is the only therapy that appears to improve the prognosis of patients with this disorder.

The most commonly observed CT findings in PVOD are smoothly thickened septal lines, multifocal regions of ground-glass opacity, pleural effusions, enlarged central pulmonary arteries, pulmonary veins of normal caliber, and enlarged edematous mediastinal lymph nodes. Resten and colleagues compared CT findings in patients with PVOD with those with idiopathic pulmonary hypertension. They found that centrilobular ground-glass opacities, septal thickening, and mediastinal lymphadenopathy were significantly more common in patients with PVOD. Thus, the presence of these findings in a patient with pulmonary hypertension and no evidence of left sided heart disease (e.g., mitral stenosis) should suggest the diagnosis of PVOD. A definitive diagnosis requires lung biopsy, although many patients are too ill to undergo biopsy.

REFERENCES

Porres DV, Morenza OP, Pallisa E, Roque A, Andreu J, Martínez M. Learning from the pulmonary veins. *Radiographics*. 2013 Jul–Aug; 33(4):999–1022.

Resten A, Maitre S, Humbert M, Rabiller A, Sitbon O, Capron F, Simonneau G, Musset D. Pulmonary hypertension: CT of the chest in pulmonary venoocclusive disease. *AJR Am J Roentgenol.* 2004 Jul;183(1):65–70.

Thoracic Radiology: The Requisites, 3rd ed., pp. 238–258.

CASE 143

Tracheobronchial Papillomatosis

1. **A and D**. Tracheobronchial papillomatosis manifests as multiple endoluminal nodules and masses. Amyloidosis of the trachea can rarely present as multiple tracheal nodules and masses, although diffuse tracheobronchial thickening or a single tracheal nodule are more common. Amyloidosis in the lungs can rarely be associated with cystic lesions. Relapsing polychondritis presents as smooth thickening of the cartilaginous portion of the tracheal and bronchial walls. Bacterial tracheitis usually occurs as smooth or slightly nodular diffuse tracheal wall thickening.

2. **B**. Low signal intensity on T1- and T2-weighted images is the characteristic appearance of amyloid on MRI. The other choices are incorrect.

3. **B**. Human papilloma virus (HPV) is associated with respiratory papillomatosis. HIV does not directly cause respiratory papillomatosis, although patients with HIV may be at greater risk for HPV infection and papillomatosis. Epstein-Barr virus and cytomegalovirus are not associated with respiratory papillomatosis.

4. **C**. Malignant degeneration can occur within a papilloma. However, these tumors are squamous cell carcinomas and not adenocarcinomas. Large papillomas can result in severe airway obstruction, and papillomas can hemorrhage, resulting in hemoptysis. Obstruction of the airways can result in recurrent infection secondary to diminished mucociliary clearance.

Comment

Differential Diagnosis

Computed tomography (CT) images show small endoluminal nodules in the tracheal lumen (Fig. 143.1) and two cystic lesions in the posterior right upper lobe (Fig. 143.2). The differential

diagnosis for multiple tracheal endoluminal nodules includes tracheobronchial papillomatosis (sometimes referred to as respiratory papillomatosis), metastases, amyloidosis, and granulomatous disease (rare). The presence of cystic spaces, nodules, or both in the lungs in conjunction with tracheobronchial filling defects strongly favors tracheobronchial papillomatosis.

Discussion

Tracheobronchial papillomatosis is an uncommon condition characterized by the presence of multiple squamous papillomas within the larynx. This disorder is seen primarily in children but can also present in older adults. Extension of the disease into the trachea and bronchi occurs in roughly 5% of patients. Isolated tracheobronchial disease is seen more often in adults than in children. Rarely, there is dissemination into the lung parenchyma.

The radiographic and CT manifestations of papillomatosis include multiple wartlike and larger cauliflower-like growths projecting into the trachea and central airways. Larger lesions are less often observed but can cause significant airway obstruction. On MRI, the lesions demonstrate intermediate signal intensity, which contrasts with the characteristic low signal intensity associated with amyloidosis. When the lung parenchyma is involved, CT findings include centrilobular nodules, larger nodules, and cavitary nodules.

Presenting symptoms depend on the site of involvement. Laryngeal involvement often results in hoarseness. Tracheobronchial involvement is associated with stridor, wheezing, hemoptysis, and recurrent infections. In children with isolated laryngeal involvement, spontaneous remission is commonly observed. With airway involvement distal to the larynx, however, spontaneous remission is less common. Treatment for obstructing lesions includes cryotherapy and laser ablation. Local and distal recurrence is not uncommon. The most severe complication is development of squamous cell carcinoma within a papilloma.

REFERENCES

Lawrence DA, Branson B, Oliva I, Rubinowitz A. The wonderful world of the windpipe: a review of central airway anatomy and pathology. *Can Assoc Radiol J.* 2015 Feb;66(1):30–43.

Thoracic Radiology: The Requisites, 3rd ed., pp. 137–158.

CASE 144

Echinococcal Cyst

1. **C**. Echinococcosis may present with a mass within a cyst appearance. Aspergillosis, nocardiosis, and mucormycosis typically do not present with this appearance. These infections usually are associated with thick-walled cavities.

2. **A**. The crescent or meniscus sign describes the air collection within the cyst. The water lily sign describes a cyst membrane floating on the cyst fluid. The tip of the iceberg sign is used in ultrasonography to describe the appearance of an ovarian dermoid cyst. The collar sign describes the appearance of an abdominal viscus as it passes through a diaphragmatic defect, which is typically a result of trauma.

3. **B**. The crescent sign in the setting of an echinococcal cyst has been associated with impending rupture. The crescent sign in the setting of an echinococcal cyst does not indicate secondary infection, healing, or hemorrhage.

4. **C**. Approximately 70% of hydatid cysts in humans occur in the liver. The lung is the second most common site of hydatid cysts in humans. Brain and spleen involvement are not common in humans.

Comment

Differential Diagnosis

The initial computed tomography (CT) image (Fig. 144.1) shows both air and mass like fluid (there is no air fluid level) within a cyst in the left lower lobe. Note the crescent of air between the inner cyst and outer cyst wall. CT image obtained two weeks later (Fig. 144.2) shows the enfolded cysts membrane *layering* dependently in the cyst which is now air filled.

Comment

Echinococcus granulosus is the cause of most human forms of hydatid disease. It occurs in two forms: pastoral and sylvatic. The pastoral form is more common. In this form, sheep, cows, or pigs are the intermediate hosts, and dogs are the definitive host. This form of infection is particularly common in the sheep-raising regions of southeastern Europe, the Middle East, Northern Africa, South America, Australia, and New Zealand.

The hydatid cyst contains three layers: the pericyst, an acellular laminated membrane, and an inner germinal layer that generates daughter cysts. The liver is the most common site for echinococcal cysts, accounting for about 70% of cysts. The lung is the second most common site.

On chest radiographs and CT scans of patients with echinococcal cysts, single or multiple well-circumscribed spherical or oval masses may be present. If a cyst communicates with the bronchial tree, air can enter the space between the pericyst and the laminated membrane, producing a thin crescent of air around the periphery of the cyst. In this case, the first image (see (Fig. 144.1) shows a meniscus sign, which has been reported to indicate impending cyst rupture. Note the presence of cyst rupture on the second image (see (Fig. 144.2), which was obtained two weeks after the first image.

When bronchial communication occurs directly into the endocyst, expulsion of the cyst contents can produce an air-fluid level. Once the cyst has ruptured, its membrane can float on the fluid. The term *water lily sign* has been used to describe this characteristic appearance. It is important to know that these characteristic radiographic signs are rarely observed in association with this entity.

When intact, most hydatid cysts result in no symptoms. On cyst rupture there is usually an abrupt onset of cough, expectoration, and fever. Other manifestations include pneumothorax, pleuritis, lung abscess, parasitic embolism, and anaphylaxis. Percutaneous aspiration of such cysts has generally not been considered safe owing to the possibility of inciting an anaphylactic reaction or spreading the infection. Treatment includes antihelminthic therapy without or with surgical resection.

REFERENCES

Santivanez S, Garcia HH. Pulmonary cystic echinococcosis. *Curr Opin Pulm Med*. 2010 May;16(3):257–261.

Thoracic Radiology: The Requisites, 3rd ed., pp. 289–309.

CASE 145

Congenital Pulmonary Airway Malformation (CPAM)

1. **C.** Congenital pulmonary airway malformation (previously known as *congenital cystic adenomatoid malformation*, i.e., CCAM) can have the appearance of a multiloculated air cyst in the lung. A lung abscess typically contains fluid and has a thick irregular wall. Lymphangioleiomyomatosis is characterized by diffuse thin-walled lung cysts. Intrapulmonary bronchogenic cysts are usually filled with fluid ranging from water to higher-attenuation fluid depending on protein content. Occasionally, an air-fluid level is present.

2. **C.** Pulmonary sequestrations are characterized by systemic arterial supply. Congenital pulmonary airway malformations themselves do not have systemic arterial supply, but hybrid lesions do occur (e.g. CPAM + sequestration), so the presence of systemic aterial supply should suggest a component of sequestration. Bronchogenic cysts and congenital lobar overinflation are not characterized by systemic arterial supply.

3. **D.** Most bronchogenic cysts occur in the middle mediastinum (visceral compartment) in the subcarinal space or in the paratracheal regions. Intrapulmonary bronchogenic cysts are uncommon, approximately 10% of all bronchogenic cysts. The anterior mediastinum (prevascular compartment) is an unsual location for a bronchogenic cyst. Most cysts in this location are related to the pericardium or thymus.

4. **C.** Patients with congenital pulmonary airway malformation may be at increased risk for developing lung adenocarcinoma. Lymphoma, pleuropulmonary blastoma, and small cell lung carcinoma have not been associated with this malformation.

Comment

Differential Diagnosis

Axial (Fig. 145.1) and coronal reformated (Fig. 145.2) computed tomography (CT) images show a discrete low attenuation lesion in the superior segment of the right cystic lower lobe. Within the lesion are multiple poorly defined cystic spaces. This appearance is characteristic of a CPAM. Depending on the degree of cystic change and soft tissue, the differential diagnosis may include emphysema, necrotic pneumonia, pulmonary abscess, primary lung cancer, congenital lobar overinflation, bronchogenic cyst, and pulmonary sequestration.

Discussion

CPAM is a rare hamartomatous lesion that represents anomalous development of lung bud elements that would have become terminal bronchioles and alveolar ducts; its cystic components communicate with the major bronchi. CPAM is usually detected in the first 2 years of life but may not be detected until adulthood (10% to 20%). Affected adult patients may be asymptomatic or can present with recurrent infection or hemoptysis.

The imaging manifestations correlate with the updated classification scheme that includes five types of CPAM. Type I (see (Fig. 145.1) manifests as unilateral single or multiple air-filled cysts; in some cases a single dominant cyst is surrounded by smaller cysts. Type II manifests as multiple small uniform cysts. Type III lesions typically manifest as a solid mass or area of consolidation comprised of adenomatoid tissue at histology (the only true CCAM). Types 0 and IV are less common, with Type 0 representing acinar dysplasia involving all lobes and is incompatible with life. Type IV CPAM manifests as a large unlined cyst like that of a Type I lesion. Although CPAM has been considered a unilateral disease, CT has been reported to show bilateral involvement in some patients. Older reports link CPAM with an increased risk of developing primary lung adenocarcinoma. However, this relationship is controversial, and direct causation is less clear. Two schools of thought exist regarding management of CPAM. For symptomatic patients, most authorities agree that surgical resection is most appropriate. For incidentally detected lesions, especially in adults, disagreement exists as to whether or not resection or observation is most appropriate.

REFERENCES

Biyyam DR, Chapman T, Ferguson MR, Deutsch G, Dighe MK. Congenital lung abnormalities: embryologic features, prenatal diagnosis, and postnatal radiologic-pathologic correlation. *Radiographics*. 2010 Oct;30(6):1721–1738.

Thoracic Radiology: The Requisites, 3rd ed., pp. 193–209.

CASE 146

Lymphoid Interstitial Pneumonia (LIP)

1. **D.** Scattered basal predominant perivascular cysts characterize LIP. Nodules and variable amounts of ground-glass opacity might also be present. Usual interstitial pneumonia is characterized by subpleural and basal-predominant reticulation and honeycombing with varying degrees of traction bronchiectasis. Scattered discrete non-honeycomb cysts are not a feature of UIP. Lymphangioleiomyomatosis is characterized by multiple diffuse bilateral cysts scattered throughout an otherwise normal pulmonary parenchyma. Ground glass and nodular opacities do not occur. Langerhans cell histiocytosis has an upper lobe distribution with bizarre, shaped cysts in addition to solid and cavitary lung nodules.

2. **B.** Lymphoid interstitial pneumonia is most commonly associated with Sjögren syndrome but can occur in patients with immunodeficiency and children with HIV. LIP is not commonly associated with systemic lupus erythematosus. Idiopathic pulmonary fibrosis (UIP) is not associated with LIP. Acute interstitial pneumonia is an idiopathic form of diffuse alveolar damage and is not associated with LIP.

3. **A.** Ground-glass opacity is the predominant CT finding of *P. jirovecii* pneumonia. Lung consolidation and cysts can occur with *P. jirovecii* pneumonia but are not the predominant features. Lymphadenopathy is not a typical feature of *P. jirovecii* pneumonia.

4. **C.** Cysts are not a feature of respiratory bronchiolitis–associated interstitial lung disease, which is characterized by upper lung predominant ground-glass opacity and poorly-defined centrilobular nodules. Lung cysts are typical features of lymphangioleiomyomatosis, pulmonary Langerhans cell histiocytosis, and Birt-Hogg-Dubé syndrome.

Comment

Differential Diagnosis

CT images (Figs. 146.1 and 146.2) show basal predominant thin-walled perivascular cysts and a few scattered nodules. The three most common causes of cystic lung disease are pulmonary Langerhans cell histiocytosis (PLCH), lymphangioleiomyomatosis (LAM), and LIP. PLCH occurs almost exclusively in patients who smoke and is characterized by upper lobe predominant nodules and irregular cysts. LAM occurs in patients with tuberous sclerosis complex or sporadically in women of childbearing age and has a diffuse distribution of relatively uniform cysts. LIP most often occurs in the setting of Sjögren syndrome and typically has fewer cysts than LAM, and the cysts are basal predominant with vessels coursing along their walls.

Discussion

LIP is still included as part of the spectrum of idiopathic interstitial pneumonias but is now also classified as a lymphoproliferative disorder within a spectrum that ranges from follicular bronchiolitis to low-grade lymphoma. The diffuse form of this spectrum is referred to as LIP; the focal form is referred to as pseudolymphoma which is often cutaneous in location. The non-neoplastic entity of LIP must be distinguished from lymphoma by immunologic stains.

Although the cause of LIP is unknown, it is commonly associated with Sjögren syndrome but can also occur in the setting of immunodeficiency such as hypogammaglobulinemia and, in children, HIV infection. Idiopathic LIP is extremely rare.

The best imaging clue is the presence of patchy ground-glass opacity and scattered thin-walled cysts. The cysts tend to be basal predominant and often have a perivascular distribution with vessels coursing along their walls. Other CT findings of LIP may be arrayed along the lymphatic pathways of the lung: centrilobular nodules and thickening of interlobular septa and bronchovascular bundles. Larger nodules, which frequently calcify, usually are a sign of amyloid deposition. Symptomatic patients may be treated with steroids and other immunosuppressive agents; some cases show spontaneous remission without treatment.

REFERENCES

Tian X, Yi ES, Ryu JH. Lymphocytic interstitial pneumonia and other benign lymphoid disorders. *Semin Respir Crit Care Med.* 2012 Oct;33(5):450–461.

Escalon JG, Richards JC, Koelsch T, Downey GP, Lynch DA. Isolated Cystic Lung Disease: An algorithmic approach to distinguishing Birt-Hogg-Dubé syndrome, lymphangioleiomyomatosis, and lymphocytic interstitial pneumonia. *AJR Am J Roentgenol.* 2019 Mar;19:1–5.

Thoracic Radiology: The Requisites, 3rd ed., pp. 355–376.

Index

Note: Page numbers followed by *f* refer to illustrations